Renal Disease in Pregnancy

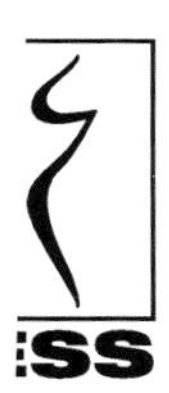

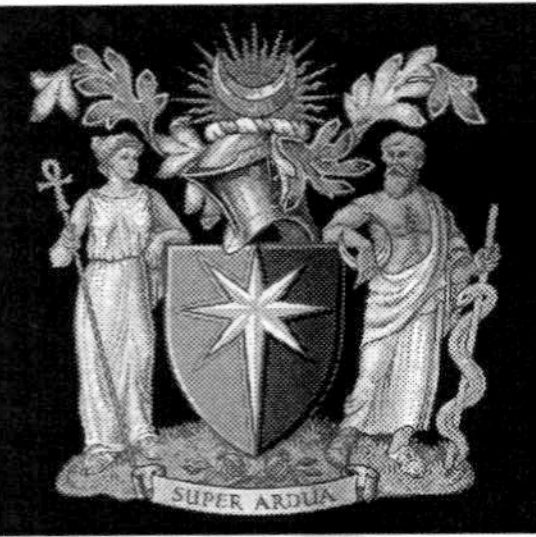

Since 1973 the Royal College of Obstetricians and Gynaecologists has regularly convened Study Groups to address important growth areas within obstetrics and gynaecology. An international group of eminent clinicians and scientists from various disciplines is invited to present the results of recent research and to take part in in-depth discussions. The resulting volume, containing enhanced versions of the papers presented, is published within a few months of the meeting and provides a summary of the subject that is both authoritative and up to date.

SOME PREVIOUS STUDY GROUP PUBLICATIONS AVAILABLE

Infertility
Edited by AA Templeton and JO Drife

Intrapartum Fetal Surveillance
Edited by JAD Spencer and RHT Ward

Early Fetal Growth and Development
Edited by RHT Ward, SK Smith and D Donnai

Ethics in Obstetrics and Gynaecology
Edited by S Bewley and RHT Ward

The Biology of Gynaecological Cancer
Edited by R Leake, M Gore and RHT Ward

Multiple Pregnancy
Edited by RHT Ward and M Whittle

The Prevention of Pelvic Infection
Edited by AA Templeton

Screening for Down Syndrome in the First Trimester
Edited by JG Grudzinskas and RHT Ward

Problems in Early Pregnancy: Advances in Diagnosis and Management
Edited by JG Grudzinskas and PMS O'Brien

Gene Identification, Manipulation and Treatment
Edited by SK Smith, EJ Thomas and PMS O'Brien

Evidence-based Fertility Treatment
Edited by AA Templeton, ID Cooke and PMS O'Brien

Fetal Programming: Influences on Development and Disease in Later Life
Edited by PMS O'Brien, T Wheeler and DJP Barker

Hormones and Cancer
Edited by PMS O'Brien and AB MacLean

The Placenta: Basic Science and Clinical Practice
Edited by JCP Kingdom, ERM Jauniaux and PMS O'Brien

Disorders of the Menstrual Cycle
Edited by PMS O'Brien, IT Cameron and AB MacLean

Infection and Pregnancy
Edited by AB MacLean, L Regan and D Carrington

Pain in Obstetrics and Gynaecology
Edited by A MacLean, R Stones and S Thornton

Incontinence in Women
Edited by AB MacLean and L Cardozo

Maternal Morbidity and Mortality
Edited by AB MacLean and J Neilson

Lower Genital Tract Neoplasia
Edited by Allan B MacLean, Albert Singer and Hilary Critchley

Pre-eclampsia
Edited by Hilary Critchley, Allan MacLean, Lucilla Poston and James Walker

Preterm Birth
Edited by Hilary Critchley, Phillip Bennett and Steven Thornton

Menopause and Hormone Replacement
Edited by Hilary Critchley, Ailsa Gebbie and Valerie Beral

Implantation and Early Development
Edited by Hilary Critchley, Iain Cameron and Stephen Smith

Contraception and Contraceptive Use
Edited by Anna Glasier, Kaye Wellings and Hilary Critchley

Multiple Pregnancy
Edited by Mark Kilby, Phil Baker, Hilary Critchley and David Field

Heart Disease and Pregnancy
Edited by Philip J Steer, Michael A Gatzoulis and Philip Baker

Teenage Pregnancy and Reproductive Health
Edited by Philip Baker, Kate Guthrie, Cindy Hutchinson, Roslyn Kane and Kaye Wellings

Obesity and Reproductive Health
Edited by Philip Baker, Adam Balen, Lucilla Poston and Naveed Sattar

Renal Disease in Pregnancy

Edited by

John M Davison, Catherine Nelson-Piercy,
Sean Kehoe and Philip Baker

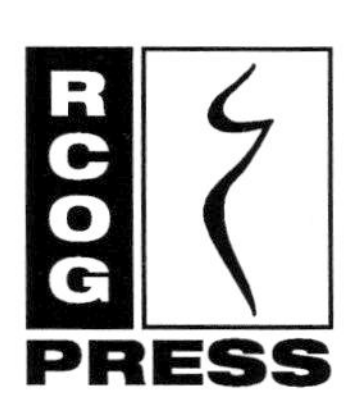

John M Davison MD FRCOG
Emeritus Professor of Obstetric Medicine, School of Surgical and Reproductive Sciences (Obstetrics and Gynaecology), 3rd Floor, William Leech Building, Medical School, Framlington Place, Newcastle upon Tyne NE2 4HH, and Part-time Consultant Obstetrician, Newcastle Hospitals NHS Foundation Trust

Catherine Nelson-Piercy MA FRCP FRCOG
Consultant Obstetric Physician, Guy's & St Thomas' NHS Foundation Trust, 10th Floor Directorate Office, North Wing, St Thomas' Hospital, Westminster Bridge Road, London SE1 7EH, and Queen Charlotte's & Chelsea Hospital, Imperial Healthcare NHS Trust.

Sean Kehoe MD FRCOG
Lead in Gynaecological Oncology, The Women's Centre, John Radcliffe Hospital, Headington, Oxford OX3 9DU

Philip Baker DM FRCOG
Professor of Maternal and Fetal Health, Maternal and Fetal Health Research Centre, St Mary's Hospital, Whitworth Park, Manchester M13 0JH

Published by the **RCOG Press** at the Royal College of Obstetricians and Gynaecologists, 27 Sussex Place, Regent's Park, London NW1 4RG

www.rcog.org.uk

Registered charity no. 213280

First published 2008

ISBN 978-1-904752-59-2

Cover image: False-colour gamma camera scan of the human kidneys, revealing an infection in the right kidney (right on this posterior incidence image). Gamma camera imaging using the radioisotope Technetium-99m (^{99m}Tc) linked to dimercaptosuccinic acid (DMSA), a compound absorbed by the kidneys, is used to obtain a comparison of their relative function. In this image, reduced function of the right kidney is indicated by decreased activity, represented in shades of purple, compared with the normal left kidney. © 2008 CNRI/Science Photo Library.

RCOG Editor: Andrew Welsh
Original design by Karl Harrington, FiSH Books, London
Typesetting by Andrew Welsh
Index by Jan Ross (Merrall-Ross (Wales) Ltd)
Printed by Henry Ling Ltd, The Dorset Press, Dorchester DT1 1HD

Contents

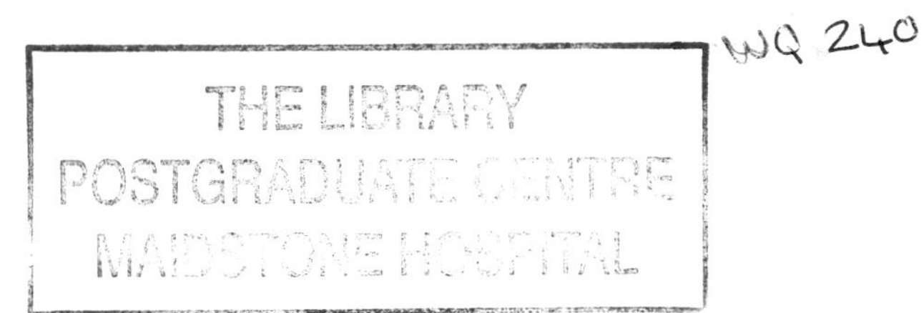

Participants vii

Preface xi

SECTION 1 RENAL PHYSIOLOGY IN PREGNANCY

1 **Recent advances in renal physiology in pregnancy**
Chris Baylis 3

SECTION 2 PATTERNS OF CARE

2 **Prepregnancy counselling and risk assessment: general overview**
Liz Lightstone 21

3 **Chronic kidney disease in pregnancy: patterns of care and general principles of management**
Mark A Brown 31

4 **Midwifery issues**
Kylie Watson 45

5 **Postpartum follow-up of antenatally identified renal problems**
Liz Lightstone 53

SECTION 3 CHRONIC KIDNEY DISEASE

6 **Pregnancy and dialysis**
Liam Plant 61

7 **Pregnancy and the renal transplant recipient**
Sue Carr 69

8 **Reflux nephropathy in pregnancy**
Nigel J Brunskill 89

9 **Lupus and connective tissue disease in pregnancy**
Mike Venning and Mumtaz Patel 95

10 **Diabetic nephropathy in pregnancy**
Andrew McCarthy 111

SECTION 4 DRUGS USED IN RENAL DISEASE IN PREGNANCY

11 Drugs in women with renal disease and transplant recipients in pregnancy
Graham W Lipkin, Mark Kilby and Asif Sarwar 129

12 Management of hypertension in renal disease in pregnancy
Mark Kilby and Graham W Lipkin 149

13 Assisted reproduction in women with renal disease
Jason Waugh 167

SECTION 5 ACUTE RENAL IMPAIRMENT

14 Acute renal failure in pregnancy: causes not due to pre-eclampsia
David Williams 179

15 Pre-eclampsia-related renal impairment
Louise Kenny 189

16 Renal biopsy in pregnancy
Nigel J Brunskill 201

SECTION 6 UROLOGY AND PREGNANCY

17 Urological problems in pregnancy
Jonathon Olsburgh 209

SECTION 7 SURGICAL AND MEDICAL ISSUES SPECIFIC TO RENAL TRANSPLANT PATIENTS

18 Surgical issues of renal and renal/pancreas transplantation in pregnancy
John Taylor 223

19 Comorbid conditions that can affect pregnancy outcome in the renal transplant patient
Sue Carr 229

SECTION 8 CONSENSUS VIEWS

20 Consensus views arising from the 54th Study Group: Renal Disease in Pregnancy 249

Index 253

Participants

Philip Baker
Convenor of RCOG Study Groups and Professor of Maternal and Fetal Health, Maternal and Fetal Health Research Centre, The University of Manchester, St Mary's Hospital, Hathersage Road, Manchester M13 0JH, UK.

Chris Baylis
Professor of Physiology and Medicine, Director of the Hypertension Center, 1600 SW Archer Road, Room M544, University of Florida, POB 100274, Gainesville, Fl 32667, USA.

Mark Brown
Professor of Medicine and Senior Staff Nephrologist, Department of Renal Medicine, St George Hospital, Kogarah, Sydney, NSW 2217, Australia.

Nigel J Brunskill
Professor of Renal Medicine, University Hospitals of Leicester NHS Trust, Leicester General Hospital, Gwendolen Road, Leicester LE5 4PW, UK.

Sue Carr
Consultant Nephrologist and Honorary Senior Lecturer, John Walls Renal Unit, University Hospitals of Leicester, Leicester General Hospital, Gwendolen Road, Leicester LE5 4PW, UK.

John M Davison
Emeritus Professor of Obstetric Medicine, School of Surgical and Reproductive Sciences (Obstetrics and Gynaecology), 3rd Floor, William Leech Building, Medical School, Framlington Place, Newcastle upon Tyne NE2 4HH, UK, and Part-time Consultant Obstetrician, Newcastle Hospitals NHS Foundation Trust, UK.

Sean Kehoe
Lead in Gynaecological Oncology, The Women's Centre, John Radcliffe Hospital, Headington, Oxford OX3 9DU, UK.

Louise Kenny
Senior Lecturer in Obstetrics and Gynaecology, Anu Research Centre, National University of Ireland, University College Cork, Cork University Maternity Hospital, Wilton, Cork, Ireland

Mark Kilby
Dame Hilda Lloyd Professor of Fetal Medicine, Department of Fetal Medicine, Division of Reproduction and Child Health, Birmingham Women's Hospital, Edgbaston, Birmingham B15 2TG, UK.

Liz Lightstone
Senior Lecturer and Honorary Consultant Physician, Renal Section, Division of Medicine, Faculty of Medicine, Imperial College London and West London Renal and Transplant Centre, Hammersmith Hospital, Du Cane Road, London W12 0NN, UK.

Graham Lipkin
Consultant Nephrologist and Honorary Senior Lecturer, Department of Nephrology, Queen Elizabeth Hospital, UHBNHSFT, Edgbaston, Birmingham B15 2TH, UK.

Andrew McCarthy
Consultant Obstetrician, Hammersmith and Queen Charlotte's Hospitals, Du Cane Road, London W12 0HS, UK.

Catherine Nelson-Piercy
Consultant Obstetric Physician, Guy's & St Thomas' NHS Foundation Trust, 10th Floor Directorate Office, North Wing, St Thomas' Hospital, Westminster Bridge Road, London SE1 7EH, UK, and Queen Charlotte's & Chelsea Hospital, Imperial Healthcare NHS Trust.

Jonathon Olsburgh
Consultant Transplant and Urological Surgeon, Renal Unit, Guy's Hospital, St Thomas Street, London SE1 9RT, UK.

Liam Plant
Consultant Renal Physician and Clinical Senior Lecturer in Nephrology, Department of Renal Medicine, Cork University Hospital, Wilton, Cork, Ireland.

John Taylor
Consultant Transplant Surgeon, Renal Unit, 6th Floor, New Guy's House, Guy's Hospital, London SE1 9RT, UK.

Mike Venning
Consultant Renal Physician, Renal Unit, Manchester Royal Infirmary, Manchester M13 9LT, UK.

Kylie Watson
Midwifery Practice Leader, Hospital Birth Centre, 7th Floor, North Wing, St Thomas' Hospital, Lambeth Palace Road, London SE1 7EH, UK.

Jason Waugh
Consultant in Obstetrics and Maternal Medicine, Royal Victoria Infirmary, Queen Victoria Road, Newcastle upon Tyne NE1 4LP, UK.

David Williams
Consultant Obstetric Physician, Institute for Women's Health, University College London Hospital, Huntley Street, London WC1E 6DH, UK.

Additional contributors

Mumtaz Patel
Consultant Nephrologist, Department of Renal Medicine, Manchester Royal Infirmary, Oxford Road, Manchester M13 9WL, UK.

Asif Sarwar
Lead Pharmacist for Renal Services, Pharmacy Department, Queen Elizabeth Hospital, UHBNHSFT, Edgbaston, Birmingham B15 2TH, UK.

DECLARATIONS OF PERSONAL INTEREST

All contributors to the Study Group were invited to make a specific Declaration of Interest in relation to the subject of the Study Group. This was undertaken and all contributors complied with this request. Philip Baker has declared that the Maternal and Fetal Health Research Centre in Manchester receives core support from Tommy's, the Baby Charity. Proportions of his salary are from Tommy's, the Baby Charity and from the National Institute of Health Research. He edits the undergraduate and postgraduate textbooks *Obstetrics by Ten Teachers* and *Obstetrics & Gynaecology: a Guide for MRCOG*, and is on the editorial board of *Obstetrics, Gynaecology and Reproductive Medicine*. Sean Kehoe has acted as an adviser for Sanofi Pasteur and received support to attend educational meetings. He is a member of the BGCS Council and the NCRI Ovarian Subgroup, and a spokesperson for WOW. Mark Kilby has acted as a consultant to the National Institute for Health and Clinical Excellence (NICE) and has done paid editorial work for *Maternal and Fetal Medicine Reviews*. Liz Lightstone has received honoraria for chapters in *Medicine 2003* and *Medicine 2005*. Catherine Nelson-Piercy is on the editorial boards of *Obstetrics, Gynaecology and Reproductive Medicine* and the *International Journal of Obstetric Anaesthesia* and is editor-in-chief of the journal *Obstetric Medicine*. She edits the postgraduate textbooks *Maternal Medicine* and *Obstetric Medicine: a Problem-based Approach* and has written the *Handbook of Obstetric Medicine*. She is a trustee for the charity Action on Pre-eclampsia and patron of the Lauren Page Trust. Jason Waugh is a clinical expert for Action on Pre-eclampsia.

P

Preface

Women with renal problems, including kidney transplant patients and those receiving dialysis, often consult clinicians on the advisability of becoming pregnant or continuing a pregnancy already in progress. Pre-existing renal disease is encountered with increasing frequency in pregnant women. When counselling and caring for such women it is crucial that the clinician understands the striking physiological alterations that occur during normal pregnancy (most marked in the renal and cardiovascular systems) as well as the need for expert multidisciplinary antenatal care with awareness of the technology for fetal surveillance and the role of neonatal intensive care. Renal problems may also arise *de novo* in pregnancy and again expert care is essential to ensure satisfactory short- and long-term outcomes for these women and their newborns.

This book stems from the 54th RCOG Study Group on 'Renal Disease in Pregnancy', which allowed specialists in many disciplines to sift the most up-to-date evidence on all aspects of diagnosis and management in women with renal problems before, during and after pregnancy. The chapters describe many of the issues likely to be faced in clinical practice, providing valuable information for all healthcare professionals working in this field.

General principles for optimal management are clearly defined and separate chapters are devoted to specific disease entities and/or clinical situations. Members of the Study Group were mindful of the need for the obstetric medicine literature to adopt the new internationally recommended five stage classification for chronic kidney disease. Also, they have not tried to avoid the many controversial areas – management of hypertension, diagnosis of pre-eclampsia, assisted conception, the rationalisation of the many medications used in nephrological practice, renal biopsy, surgical emergencies, patient input and responsibilities – all are carefully considered. Whatever the problem, the key to a successful service is multidisciplinary teamwork within appropriate facilities, requiring as a minimum an obstetrician, a renal/obstetric physician and a specialist midwife, all with the necessary expertise.

During the deliberations of the Study Group it became apparent that many of our conclusions and counselling advice are based on poorly controlled, retrospective evidence (although there have been improvements on this in the last 20 years), underscoring the need for prospectively acquired data as well as registries.

In summary, this book critically reviews current knowledge of renal physiology, chronic kidney disease and other renal problems in pregnancy and highlights areas of controversy. Much progress has been made in the last two decades but there still remains a paucity of investigative data behind many of the conflicting arguments. Nevertheless, the Study Group has concluded the book with a list of consensus views for the management of renal disease in pregnancy, which are not intended to be 'good practice guidelines' or 'evidence-based statements'. It is hoped that the book and the follow-up meeting will not only be a welcome and timely 'review of the art' but also a 'call to action' that will renew active interest in the field.

John M Davison
Catherine Nelson-Piercy
Sean Kehoe
Philip Baker

Section 1

Renal physiology in pregnancy

1

Chapter 1

Recent advances in renal physiology in pregnancy

Chris Baylis

Focus areas for this chapter

Mechanisms of increase in glomerular filtration rate

A robust and maintained renal vasodilation and increased glomerular filtration in pregnancy are good signs for both maternal and fetal outcome. In women with underlying chronic kidney disease (CKD), the level of prepregnancy renal function predicts outcome, with a serum creatinine (SCr) above approximately 120 μmol/l signalling increases in maternal and fetal risks. The presence of hypertension and/or heavy proteinuria increases the risk of accelerated loss of function. If the rise in glomerular filtration rate (GFR) occurs and persists during pregnancy in a woman with underlying CKD, the pregnancy outcome will probably be good and pregnancy is likely to have little long-term impact on maternal kidney function.[1–6] We still do not know the mechanisms that lead to the increased GFR or whether the requisite renal vasodilation is regulated separately from the systemic vasodilation that also occurs early in normal pregnancy.

What determines plasma volume expansion: primary vasodilation (underfill) or primary renal sodium retention and secondary vasodilation?

The systemic vasodilation is critical to accommodate the expanding plasma volume, another major haemodynamic event and prognostic of a successful outcome in both maternal and fetal terms.[7] Does the peripheral vasodilation occur first and drive renal sodium retention and volume expansion,[8] or does primary renal sodium retention begin the sequence of events?

Importance of vascular endothelial growth factor in glomerular health and disease, including pre-eclampsia

The remarkable studies by Karumanchi and colleagues have implicated derangements in vascular endothelial growth factor (VEGF) action in the pathogenesis of pre-eclampsia.[9–11] These observations have also focused attention on the fact that VEGF plays an important role in the maintenance of normal glomerular health in the nonpregnant adult.[12,13] There is a 'dose' effect of VEGF on glomerular structural and functional integrity and it seems that VEGF can either ameliorate or exacerbate glomerular injury in various models of CKD.[14] We need a better understanding of the role of the VEGF system in the control of normal glomerular function (during normal pregnancy and in the healthy nonpregnant individual) and in various types of renal disease, in order to unravel the role of derangements in VEGF signalling in pre-eclampsia.

Introduction

There are profound adaptations in renal function during pregnancy in normal women, including an early increase in GFR that is first detectable within 3–4 weeks of conception (Figure 1.1).[15] GFR continues to rise to a maximum of 40–50% above nonpregnant values by the end of the first trimester and this increase is maintained throughout most of the rest of the pregnancy, although a late fall in GFR occurs in the few weeks before delivery.[16] An optimal increase in GFR is a good prognosticator for a successful pregnancy outcome. For example, in a serial study of a small group of normal pregnant women, two women who failed to show the early rise in GFR subsequently suffered early miscarriage (Figure 1.1).[15] Also, in women with underlying CKD, those who show a gestational rise in GFR tend to have the best outcomes.[1] There are also marked systemic haemodynamic changes, including increases in plasma volume and cardiac output which, together with large reductions in total peripheral vascular resistance, lead to falls in blood pressure.[17–19]

How the renal and systemic changes are related is unclear. Does the renal vasodilation precede the systemic effects, perhaps driving them, or is there a coordinated, generalised vasodilatory response in early pregnancy that includes the kidney? Is the

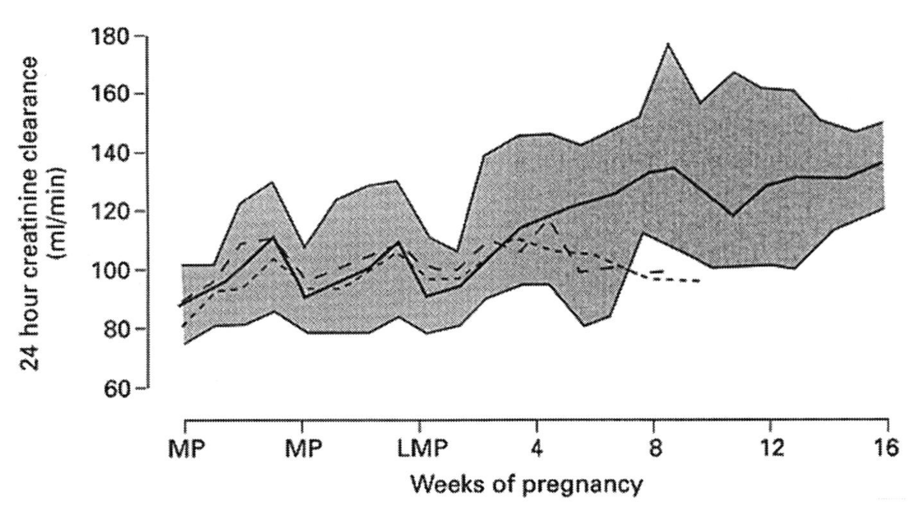

Figure 1.1. Changes in 24 hour creatinine clearance measured weekly before conception and throughout the first 16 weeks of normal pregnancy in nine women with successful obstetric outcome (the solid line represents the mean and the stippled area the range); the broken lines give the course in two women who progressed to miscarriage in the first trimester; MP = menstrual period; LMP = last menstrual period; reproduced with permission from Davison and Noble[15]

vasodilation the primary event that drives the renal sodium retention and plasma volume expansion, or is there a primary renal sodium retention that somehow triggers a vasodilatory vascular reply? One area for targeted research is for combined renal and systemic haemodynamic measurements, particularly during early pregnancy, to establish the relative relationship between systemic and renal vasodilation and the plasma volume expansion. The only study to attempt this, by Chapman *et al.*[20] in normal women, reported that by week 6 of pregnancy both the renal and systemic vasodilation was maximal, the renin–angiotensin system was activated and plasma volume expansion was underway. Unfortunately, there were no measurements earlier in pregnancy and thus the sequence of these events remains unknown.

Rats exhibit systemic and renal haemodynamic changes during normal pregnancy that are similar to those in humans, while the total gestation period is only 22 days. During pregnancy there is a progressive plasma volume expansion, a fall in blood pressure and a rise in GFR of approximately 30% (which falls toward nonpregnant values shortly before delivery).[21]

Mechanism of the gestational rise in GFR

Haemodynamics

Studies in the pregnant rat reveal that the increased GFR is accompanied by a parallel increase in renal plasma flow (RPF), due to renal vasodilation. Glomerular micropuncture studies have shown that both afferent and efferent arteriolar resistances (R_A and R_E, respectively) relax in parallel, which allows a selective increase in glomerular plasma flow to occur.[21] Importantly, parallel reductions in R_A and R_E allow the kidney to vasodilate and permit increases in RPF and GFR without an increase in glomerular blood pressure. Davison and colleagues[22] have used an indirect modelling approach to estimate the impact of normal pregnancy on glomerular haemodynamics. Much like in the rat, the majority of the increased GFR in pregnant women is due to increased RPF, although a small component may be due to falls in plasma protein concentration (reducing colloid osmotic pressure of blood entering the glomerulus). There is no evidence that the glomerular blood pressure increases during normal pregnancy, suggesting that parallel relaxation of R_A and R_E also occurs in normal pregnant women. This finding has important implications for the long-term effects of pregnancy on renal function, since states of chronic renal vasodilation where R_A is selectively relaxed lead to glomerular hypertension and development of injury.[23]

It is known that in the rat maternal factors initiate the gestational renal events since renal vasodilation and increases in GFR and RPF occur in pseudopregnant rats where fetoplacental tissue is absent.[24] In addition, both the peripheral vasodilation and plasma volume expansion are evident in pseudopregnant rats.[24,25] In pregnant women, renal and peripheral vasodilation is well established prior to complete placentation,[20] suggesting that the fetoplacental unit may not be necessary for initiation of the increase in GFR and/or the volume expansion of pregnancy.

Vasoactive factors

Studies in the rat have implicated nitric oxide (NO) as the renal vasodilatory agent of pregnancy. Both plasma and urinary levels of inorganic nitrite and nitrate (NO_x; oxidation products of NO) and cyclic guanosine monophosphate (cGMP; a major second messenger of NO) increase during pregnancy in rats,[26–28] suggesting an increase in total systemic NO production, which could include kidney. In women, 24 hour urinary excretions of cGMP and plasma cGMP increase in normal pregnancy[29,30] although the persistence of this increased cGMP excretion long after delivery[20] may reflect the prolonged postpartum rise in plasma atrial natriuretic peptide (ANP), since this agent also signals through cGMP.[31] The findings with plasma and urinary NO_x levels in women have been variable[32] and the only study conducted using a controlled low NO_x intake (a requirement for interpretation of NO_x values in the context of NO activity),[33] reported no elevation in plasma or 24 hour urinary NO_x excretion in late pregnancy compared with the nonpregnant state.[34] It should be noted that renal NO generation represents only a few percent of the total NO_x production[33] and thus a selective local increase in renal NO production would probably be undetected by NO_x measurement in body fluids.

Danielson and Conrad have reported that low-level, acute (nonselective) nitric oxide synthase (NOS) inhibition can reverse the pregnancy-induced rise in GFR without affecting the value of GFR in nonpregnant rats.[35] We reported that chronic nonselective NOS inhibition prevents the gestational rise in GFR and the renal vasodilation,[36] which has been confirmed by Schrier and colleagues.[37] Although *in vivo*, the specificity of 'isoform-specific' inhibitors is questionable, functional studies performed in rats have implicated both the neuronal and inducible NOS isoforms in mediating the renal vasodilation.[38,39] There are no endothelial NOS (eNOS)-specific inhibitors available but the *in vitro* data show midterm decreases in renal cortex total eNOS protein abundance,[40,41] activated phosphorylated (ser 1173) eNOS[41] and membrane fraction NOS activity (predominantly eNOS).[42] According to our *in vivo* and *in vitro* studies, the NOS isoform associated with the midterm renal vasodilation does exhibit functional characteristics of both the neuronal and inducible NOS.[42,43] We observed an increase in the NOS activity, *in vitro*, of renal cortex in the midterm pregnant rat, but only in the soluble fraction which houses predominantly the neuronal and inducible NOS (nNOS and iNOS, respectively). This agrees with a report by Alexander *et al.*[41] of increasing renal nNOS and iNOS protein during pregnancy in rat kidney although we have observed that the renal cortex nNOS protein abundance is unchanged at midterm.[41] However, our laboratories used different nNOS antibodies: one recognising the amino terminal (Baylis and colleagues) and one recognising the carboxy terminal (Alexander and colleagues) of the 160 kDa, nNOS-α protein. There are splice variants of the nNOS gene that encode for fully functional, amino-terminal truncated proteins and using a carboxy-terminal antibody we now report that one of these, the nNOS-β, is upregulated at both the mRNA and protein level in the renal cortex in pregnancy in phase with the renal vasodilation.[44] We are currently exploring the significance and mechanism of the nNOS-β activation in the kidney during pregnancy. It is important to point out that all these data were obtained in rats and that there is no evidence in pregnant women to confirm or exclude a role for NO in the renal response.

Signalling events leading to NO-dependent renal vasodilation

Functional and *in vitro* studies in rats suggest an important role for NO in the gestational renal vasodilation but what is the trigger? It is known that in the rat this is a maternal signal and estrogens have been implicated since they have a widespread stimulatory action on the NO system in nonpregnant women.[45] Estrogens, however, are unlikely to provide the primary stimulus to renal vasodilation since, in the rat, estrogen levels fall throughout pregnancy, increasing only just before term when the renal vasodilation is waning.[46] A novel and exciting possibility was raised by Conrad *et al.*,[47,48] who suggested that the ovarian hormone relaxin might provide the trigger. Exogenous relaxin has a powerful NO-dependent renal vasodilatory action in nonpregnant female rats, with and without ovaries, and in male rats. Chronic relaxin administration also dampens the renal vasoconstrictor response to angiotensin II and reduces the myogenic response in resistance-sized renal arteries,[47,49] changes also seen in the kidney during pregnancy.[50,51] The most direct evidence is that removal of relaxin from the pregnant rat, by neutralising antibody (Figure 1.2) or ovariectomy, eliminates the gestational renal vasodilation.[52]

There are limited clinical data, which so far are equivocal. Women who conceive by ovum donation have no circulating relaxin and have blunted increases in creatinine clearance.[53] Healthy women show an elevated GFR during the luteal phase of the menstrual cycle, when circulating relaxin levels are elevated.[20,54] Administration of human chorionic gonadotrophin (hCG), which stimulates further ovarian relaxin release in the late luteal phase, produced no further renal haemodynamic response

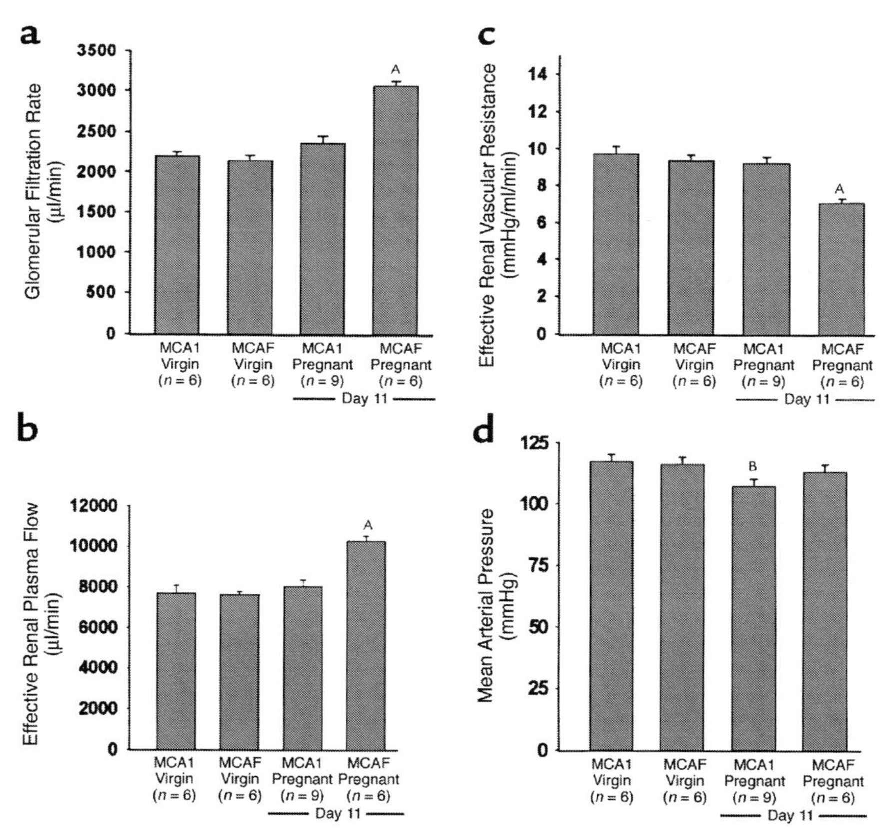

Figure 1.2. Renal function in virgin and 11 day pregnant, conscious rats treated with a relaxin-neutralising antibody (MCA1) or inactive antibody (MCAF); (a) glomerular filtration rate; (b) effective renal plasma flow; (c) effective renal vascular resistance; (d) mean arterial blood pressure; $^{A}P < 0.01$ versus other groups; $^{B}P < 0.05$ versus MCA1 and MCAF virgin; reproduced with permission from Novak *et al.*[52]

in cycling women, possibly because the elevation in relaxin achieved was below the pregnancy values.[54] Smith *et al.*[55] subsequently reported that acutely administered relaxin, to both nonpregnant women and to men, results in a marked increase in RPF, due to renal vasodilation. Unexpectedly, despite the large rise in RPF there was no accompanying increase in GFR, which must mean offsetting changes occurred in the other determinants of GFR.[56] Acutely administered relaxin, in humans, thus does not mimic all the renal haemodynamic responses of the rat, nor of normal pregnancy. Studies with chronic relaxin administration in humans are eagerly awaited.

The relaxin-mediated renal vasodilation in the rat requires NO since NOS inhibition/endothelium removal abrogates the response.[47,49,51] Endothelin also plays a role since the renal haemodynamic responses in normal pregnancy are prevented by blockade of the endothelin type B (ET_B) receptor.[57] ET_B blockade also prevents the relaxin-induced renal haemodynamic responses.[48,49] The link between relaxin and endothelin is probably mediated via relaxin-induced upregulation of the matrix metalloproteinase 2 (MMP2) which functions as an alternative endothelin-converting enzyme to stimulate endothelin production.[58,59] Most probably, endothelial ET_B-mediated NO release provides the vasodilatory stimulus to relaxin, although how this relates to the falls in eNOS abundance/activity reported in midterm pregnancy[40–42] and our recent finding of increased renal nNOS-β in midterm pregnancy are the subject of continuing investigations.

In summary, the animal literature suggests that NO plays an important role in mediating the gestational rise in GFR via a relaxin-mediated signalling cascade. While the studies in the rat are quite convincing, studies in women are needed that develop and test these hypotheses. Once the normal signals that evoke renal vasodilation in pregnant women have been established, it will be important to determine whether defects in this signalling system occur where pregnancy adversely impacts maternal renal function.

What determines the plasma volume expansion?

Volume perception in pregnancy

Net sodium accumulation in the extracellular fluid space must drive the maternal plasma volume expansion. Since plasma osmolality falls a little in normal pregnancy there must be excess net free water retention.[18] For a continual sodium retention to coexist in the presence of maintained plasma volume expansion, there must be drastic alterations in the volume sensing and regulatory systems of the body. Normal nonpregnancy physiology would prevent a prolonged rise in plasma volume expansion by activating natriuretic systems and suppressing antinatriuretic systems, to force plasma volume back to a set point considered 'normal'. In contrast, normal pregnancy is a state of continued plasma volume expansion coexisting with continued renal sodium retention. The activity of the primary antinatriuretic system, the renin–angiotensin–aldosterone system (RAAS), is markedly elevated. These findings have led Schrier and colleagues to suggest that normal pregnancy is in fact a chronically 'underfilled' state where the effective circulating volume is always seen as inadequate.[8] According to this hypothesis, there is a primary drive to peripheral vasodilation early in pregnancy that creates the underfill signal and precedes the plasma volume expansion. At present there are unfortunately no serial data early in pregnancy that can separate the cause and effect relationship between peripheral resistance and plasma volume expansion since, as reported by Chapman *et al.*,[20] all keys events are established as early as week 6 of pregnancy. Although difficult, serial studies in earlier pregnancy are required and should be conducted in women because the small size of rats and need for chronic instrumentation in this species will make detection of early haemodynamic changes in an unstressed preparation unlikely.

The underfill theory is persuasive when only the RAAS is considered but other volume regulatory systems do not conform. On the volume conservation side there are complex changes in the sympathetic nervous system in normal pregnancy but the acute sympathetic response to haemorrhage is reset in the pregnant rat so that the expanded blood volume is viewed as normal.[21,60–62] The arginine vasopressin (AVP) osmoregulatory system is markedly altered in normal pregnancy, with resetting of the osmotic threshold for AVP release to sense the lower plasma osmolality as normal.[63] The volume-dependent component of AVP release is also reset to recognise the continually expanding volume as normal,[63] as is the tubuloglomerular feedback system.[64] Thus, the volume conservation systems other than the RAAS apparently adapt throughout pregnancy to sense the expanding volume as 'normal fill'. Of the natriuretic systems that are activated by 'overfill', ANP shows a delayed small rise in pregnant women[20] and little increase until delivery in the rat,[65] more consistent with mild 'overfill' or 'normal fill' than an 'underfill' signal. The increased renal NO production (discussed above) is consistent with an 'overfill' signal, given the significant natriuretic as well as vasodilatory actions of renal NO.[65]

So, different volume perception pathways view the circulating volume in pregnancy quite differently and, while the 'underfill' theory of plasma volume expansion in pregnancy is very attractive, it requires some very sophisticated resetting of the majority of the individual control systems.

Signals influencing renal sodium excretion in pregnancy

There are many conflicting signals that influence renal sodium excretion in normal pregnancy. There is clearly net renal sodium retention throughout most of pregnancy leading to the plasma volume expansion, which suggests a dominant role for the activated RAAS. However, there are also significant natriuretic signals, including the rise in GFR, maintained or mild increases in ANP and marked increases in NO production (at least in the rat).

Pregnancy is an interesting haemodynamic state, where the renal tubular actions of the antinatriuretic, vasoconstrictor arm of the volume regulatory control predominate (to allow plasma volume expansion), whereas the vascular actions of the natriuretic, vasodilatory systems must predominate to allow peripheral vasodilation (to accommodate the expanded plasma volume). It is well known that vasoconstrictor responsiveness decreases in a normal pregnancy; the pressor response to angiotensin II is profoundly blunted early in normal pregnancy[66] while the antinatriuretic actions persist. Is it also possible that while the vasodilatory actions of the vasodilators persist, a refractoriness develops to their tubular natriuretic actions?

Some studies in the rat have suggested loss of natriuretic responsiveness to administered ANP during normal pregnancy.[67,68] The acute natriuretic response to volume expansion is dependent on endogenous ANP release and this is also blunted in the pregnant rat.[69] The pressure natriuresis (an NO-dependent event) is also blunted in the pregnant rat.[70,71] Since both ANP and NO signal through cGMP, this suggests that the tubular response to cGMP may become blunted and, indeed, we have reported increased cGMP breakdown in the inner medullary collecting duct of the pregnant rat kidney, a major site of natriuretic action of ANP and NP.[69] This effect is due to a selective, local increase in abundance/activity of phosphodiesterase 5 (PDE5).[69] We recently reported that the natriuretic response to administered ANP in pregnancy could be restored by local intrarenal PDE5 inhibition (Figure 1.3).[72] This natriuretic refractoriness in pregnancy does seem to be cGMP specific since dopamine-induced natriuresis (which signals via increased cyclic adenosine-3′,5′-monophosphate (cAMP)) is unblunted in the pregnant rat.[73]

The hypothesis of local renal tubular loss of cGMP responsiveness but with maintained systemic vascular responsiveness to cGMP is appealing, but whether this has any relevance to human pregnancy is unclear. The only study to directly address the question, by Irons *et al.*,[74] reported that a low dose of infused ANP produced a minimal natriuresis in normal women in late pregnancy and had no impact on sodium excretion in the same women when studied 4 months postpartum. This study was different in design to the animal studies in that a prolonged 60 minute equilibration time was allowed prior to measurement of sodium excretion. The tubular actions of ANP are very rapid and it is possible that a more robust and earlier natriuretic response was missed in the women when studied postpartum. This is an important area to target for further clinical study.

In summary, the volume expansion of normal pregnancy is critical for an optimal outcome for both mother and baby. An understanding of the basic physiological mechanisms is essential so that situations in which the volume expansion is suboptimal can, perhaps, be corrected.

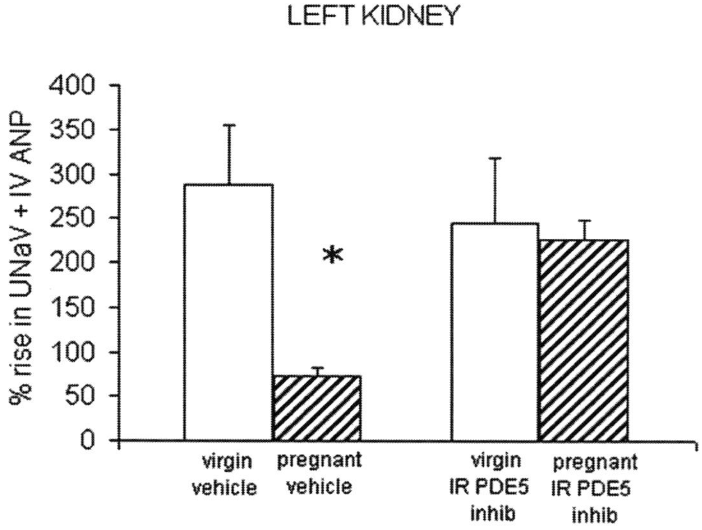

Figure 1.3. The blunted natriuretic response to systemic atrial natriuretic peptide (ANP; 11.6 ng/100 g body weight/minute) is shown in pregnant (versus virgin) rats that received vehicle infusion (2 µl/100 g body weight/minute isotonic NaCl into the left kidney); when the phosphodiesterase 5 (PDE5) inhibitor sildenafil (0.2 µg/100 g body weight/minute) was infused into the left kidney, the natriuretic response to ANP was restored in the pregnant rats; * denotes a significant difference ($P < 0.05$) between virgin and pregnant; IV = intravenous; IR = intrarenal; UNaV = urinary sodium excretion; data derived from Knight *et al.*[72]

VEGF and the glomerulus

Physiological actions of VEGF on the glomerulus

VEGF is essential for endothelial cell differentiation and angiogenesis, and it plays a key role in fetal and neonatal development. For example, it is particularly important in glomerular development in the neonate. Total deletion of VEGF-A is lethal at embryonic day 9–10 because of widespread failure of angiogenesis, while podocyte-specific total deletion leads to perinatal renal failure and death. A gene dosing effect is seen, with mice with a single VEGF-A allele developing nephrotic range proteinuria and death from renal failure by approximately 10 weeks of life. The normal complement of two alleles results in normal glomerular formation and, interestingly, too much VEGF-A produced by podocyte-specific overexpression in rats, and kidney and liver overexpression in rabbits, also leads to nephrotic range proteinuria and early death due to CKD.[13,75]

VEGF is also required for maintenance of vascular endothelial cell health and permeability in the adult.[13,76] The glomerular podocyte of the adult animal makes a large quantity of VEGF and the VEGF receptors Flt1 and KDR are expressed on endothelial cells – Flt1 is particularly abundant on glomerular endothelium.[13,76] There is considerable *in vivo* and *in vitro* evidence that VEGF is required to maintain the glomerular endothelial fenestrations. For example, as shown in Figure 1.4, administration of VEGF to glomerular endothelial cells in culture stimulates fenestra formation.[12] VEGF antagonism *in vivo* leads to loss of glomerular fenestrae and severe proteinuria, while administered VEGF reverses the injury.[9,11,76–78] The glomerular fenestrae are critical for the high water permeability at the glomerular wall that allows high rates of filtration[76] and the presence of VEGF increases the glomerular ultrafiltration coefficient in the isolated glomerulus.[79] In addition to allowing easy transglomerular passage to water, a glycocalyx layer covering the endothelial fenestrae is suggested to provide the primary filter for restriction of plasma protein, possibly restricting more than 95% of the delivered plasma protein.[76] This makes perfect sense from an engineering point of view, since the primary filter should be on the proximal, blood side to allow easy 'cleaning' of the filter and thus maintained patency. If the primary site of protein restriction lies at the epithelial slit pore, deep within the glomerular basement membrane (GBM), as often suggested, then the filter would rapidly 'clog' up with proteins. Studies by Quaggin and colleagues suggest that mesangial cell health is also dependent on podocyte-derived VEGF.[80] Furthermore, VEGF induces proximal tubular cell growth[81] and podocyte health is also controlled by an autocrine action of VEGF.[82]

Both major VEGF receptors are expressed on endothelium and the Flt1 (VEGFR1) triggers NO release while the KDR (VEGFR2 or Flk1) triggers endothelial proliferation and migration.[13,83] Flt1 is also expressed on vascular smooth muscle (VSM) where activation by VEGF stimulates proliferation and migration of VSM as well as migration of macrophages. VEGF can thus activate proliferative pathways by stimulation of KDR on endothelium and Flt1 on VSM and is antiproliferative via endothelial Flt1 stimulation of NO release (Figure 1.4).[13,83]

VEGF and renal disease

VEGF administration is protective in several animal models of CKD, including the renal mass reduction model, acute ciclosporin-induced renal injury, both anti-Thy1 and anti-GBM glomerulonephritis and the renal lesion of pre-eclampsia.[83] On the

A NO-dependent pathway (Coupling of VEGF with endothelial NO)

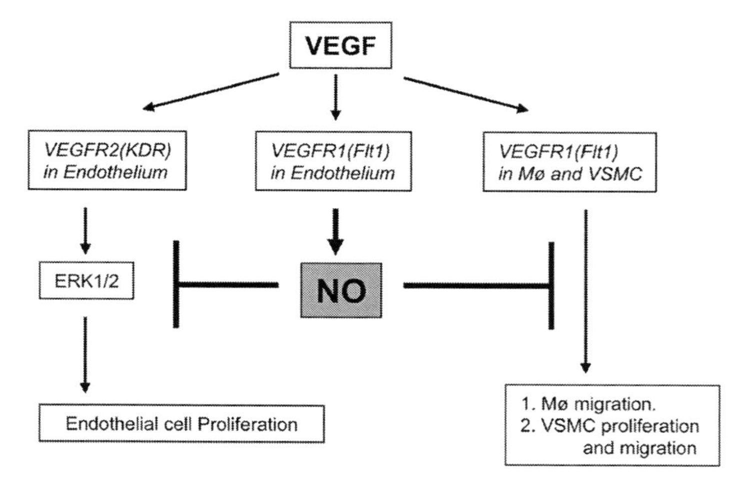

B NO-independent pathway (Uncoupling of VEGF with endothelial NO)

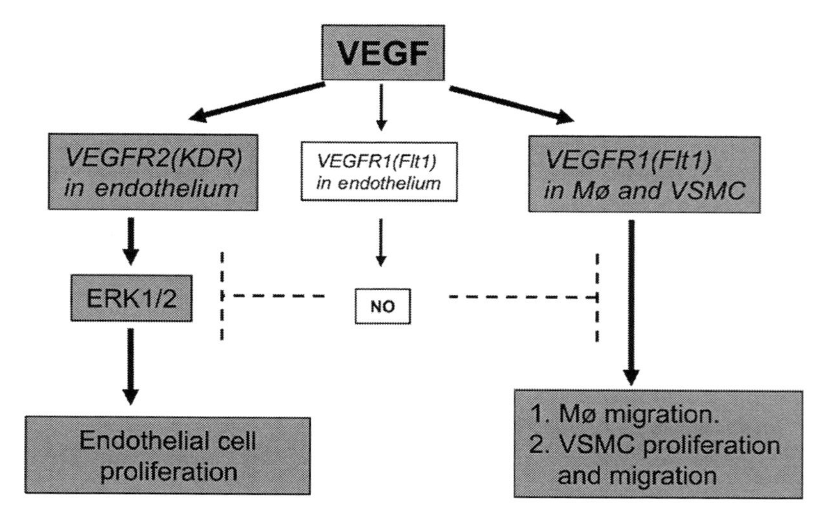

Figure 1.4. (A) The various vascular actions of vascular endothelial growth factor (VEGF) on its receptors VEGFR1 (Flt1) and VEGFR2 (KDR) in the presence of an intact endothelial nitric oxide (NO) system; Flt1 stimulates endothelial NO production, which inhibits the proliferative action of Flt1 stimulation on vascular smooth muscle and of KDR on endothelium; (B) the suggested effects of the VEGF pathway when endothelial NO becomes dysfunctional; this leads to loss of the antiproliferative effects of VEGF and allows endothelial cell, vascular smooth muscle and macrophage proliferation leading to vascular damage; ERK = extracellular signal-regulated kinase; Mø = macrophage; VSMC = vascular smooth muscle cell; reproduced with permission from Nakagawa[14]

other hand, VEGF antagonism is protective in diabetic nephropathy, high-dose angiotensin II infusion and chronic ciclosporin-induced renal injury and during chronic NOS inhibition.[83] Thus in some settings VEGF is protective of kidney function and structure, while in others it actually exacerbates the injury. These disparities may reflect which of the VEGF signalling systems predominates in a particular disease. Nakagawa has developed an interesting hypothesis suggesting that the state of the vascular endothelial NO-generating capacity is the critical determinant of whether VEGF is helpful or harmful. In models where VEGF is protective, such as renal mass reduction, there is loss of both glomerular and peritubular capillaries and administration of VEGF provokes new vessel growth and reduces or reverses fibrosis. Successful angiogenesis requires an intact eNOS system[84] and Nakagawa suggests that when the glomerular eNOS is dysfunctional (as in hyperglycaemia, oxidative stress and experimental NOS inhibition), normal angiogenesis is prevented and the NO-independent, proliferative and injurious VEGF-stimulated pathways predominate.[83]

A cautionary note on the relevance of animal studies in models of CKD was raised by Lindenmeyer *et al.*,[85] who reported that, in contrast to rodent models of diabetic nephropathy, there was a decrease in VEGF mRNA in the region of peritubular capillaries in biopsy samples from human established diabetic nephropathy. Furthermore, low VEGF expression was associated with greater proteinuria, suggesting that in humans diabetic nephropathy may be associated with decreased rather than increased VEGF actions.

VEGF deficiency in pre-eclampsia

Alternative splicing of Flt1 mRNA produces a soluble form of Flt1 that binds with and antagonises VEGF and also placental growth factor. Karumanchi and colleagues have published a series of studies showing that sFlt1 rises in pre-eclamptic pregnancy prior to the appearance of clinical signs of pre-eclampsia, proteinuria and hypertension.[9–11] Placental sFlt1 also correlates with the appearance and severity of pre-eclampsia. This group has also described a rat model of hypertension, proteinuria and glomerular endotheliosis (a hallmark of the pre-eclamptic kidney) produced by high sFlt1 levels (produced by sFlt1-expressing adenovirus) administered to pregnant rats.[9] It is notable that sFlt also produced similar symptoms in nonpregnant rats, and administered excess VEGF121 rescues the sFlt1-infused rat.[9,11] Furthermore, transient overexpression of VEGF at the mouse maternal–fetal interface in normal mid-pregnancy led to transient lowering of maternal blood pressure,[86] reinforcing the importance of placental-derived VEGF in control of maternal endothelial function.

Administered sFlt1 does not recapitulate the most severe versions of pre-eclampsia such as HELLP syndrome and this prompted a search for additional causal factors. Microarray analysis revealed an early increase in endoglin production, a soluble form of the transforming growth factor β (TGFβ) co-receptor[10] and in subsequent animal studies the combination of sFlt1 and endoglin produced severe symptoms of pre-eclampsia that included liver, central nervous system and coagulation disorders.[87] It is important to note that both sFlt1 and endoglin are splice variants of the normal genes that encode the respective functional receptors. In pre-eclamptic placentas there is a huge increase in the transcript for both the intact and truncated forms of the receptors[9–11] and the stimulus is presumed to be hypoxia at the maternal–fetal interface. Recent observations by Makris, Hennessey and colleagues in the pregnant baboon have provided the first direct *in vivo* evidence that uteroplacental ischaemia results in increased circulating Flt1.[88]

In summary, the adult glomerulus is exquisitely dependent on the presence of VEGF to maintain a normal phenotype and function. In some types of renal disease, VEGF deficiency is pathogenic whereas, in others, VEGF excess seems to be the culprit. There is thus an exact dose requirement for optimal glomerular function and structure that may also require optimal glomerular NO generation. In pre-eclampsia, functional VEGF deficiency is caused by excess circulating sFlt1 that originates from the hypoxic placenta and neutralises circulating VEGF. Similar antagonism of the TGFβ co-receptor by endoglin also contributes to the severity of the disease.

Acknowledgements

I thank past and present graduate students, postdoctoral students and collaborators who have contributed to this work in the past 28 years. In addition, I thank both John Davison and Marshall Lindheimer for their helpful discussions and friendship. Funding for these studies has been provided by the NIH (HL31933 and HD041571), The American Heart Association and the March of Dimes and also by a Wellcome Trust Senior Biomedical Research Fellowship (from 1977 to 1981).

References

1. Jones DC, Hayslett JP. Outcome of pregnancy in women with moderate or severe renal insufficiency. *New Engl J Med* 1996;335:226–32.
2. Katz AI, Davison JM, Hayslett JP, Singson E, Lindheimer MD. Pregnancy in women with kidney disease. *Kidney Int* 1980;18:192–206.
3. Cunningham FG, Cox SM, Harstad TW, Mason RA, Pritchard JA. Chronic renal disease and pregnancy outcome. *Am J Obstet Gynecol* 1990;163:453–9.
4. Reece EA, Coustan DR, Hayslett JP. Diabetic nephropathy. Pregnancy performance and fetal maternal outcome. *Am J Obstet Gynecol* 1998;159:56–66.
5. Purdy LP, Hantsch CE, Molitch ME, Metzger BE, Phelps RL, Dooley SL, *et al.* Effect of pregnancy on renal function in patients with moderate to severe diabetic renal insufficiency. *Diabetes Care* 1996;19:1067–74.
6. Jungers P, Houillier P, Forget D, Labrunie M, Skhiri H, Giatras I, *et al.* Influence of pregnancy on the course of primary chronic glomerulonephritis. *Lancet* 1995;346:1122–4.
7. Chesley LC, Lindheimer MD. Renal hemodynamics and intravascular volume in normal and hypertensive pregnancy. In: Rubin PC, editor. *Handbook of Hypertension*. Amsterdam: Elsevier; 1988. p. 38–52.
8. Schrier RW, Dürr JA. Pregnancy: an overfill or underfill state. *Am J Kidney Dis* 1987;9:284–9.
9. Maynard SE, Min JY, Merchan J, Lim KH, Li J, Mondal S, *et al.* Excess placental soluble fms-like tyrosine kinase 1 (sFlt1) may contribute to endothelial dysfunction, hypertension, and proteinuria in preeclampsia. *J Clin Invest* 2003;111:649–58.
10. Levine RJ, Lam C, Qian C, Yu KF, Maynard SE, Sachs BP, *et al.* Soluble endoglin and other circulating antiangiogenic factors in preeclampsia. *New Engl J Med* 2006;355:992–1005.
11. Baumwell S, Karumanchi SA. Pre-eclampsia: clinical manifestations and molecular mechanisms. *Nephron Clin Pract* 2007;106:72–81.
12. Satchell SC, Tasman CH, Singh A, Ni L, Geelen J, von Ruhland CJ, *et al.* Conditionally immortalized human glomerular endothelial cells expressing fenestrations in response to VEGF. *Kidney Int* 2006;69:1633–40.
13. Eremina V, Baelde HJ, Quaggin SE. Role of the VEGF – a signaling pathway in the glomerulus: evidence for crosstalk between components of the glomerular filtration barrier. *Nephron Physiol* 2007;106:32–7.
14. Nakagawa T. Uncoupling of the VEGF-endothelial nitric oxide axis in diabetic nephropathy: An explanation for the paradoxical effects of VEGF in renal disease. *Am J Physiol Renal Physiol* 2007;292:F1665–72.

15. Davison JM, Noble MCB. Serial changes in 24-hour creatinine clearance during normal menstrual cycles and the first trimester of pregnancy. *Br J Obstet Gynaecol* 1981;88:10–17.
16. Davison JM, Hytten FE. Glomerular filtration during and after pregnancy. *J Obstet Gynaecol Br Commonw* 1974;81:588–95.
17. De Swiet M. The physiology of normal pregnancy. In: Rubin PC, editor. *Handbook of Hypertension: Hypertension in Pregnancy.* Vol. 10. Amsterdam: Elsevier; 1988. p. 1–9.
18. Lindheimer MD, Katz AI. Normal and abnormal pregnancy. In: Arieff AI, DeFronzo R, editors. *Fluid, Electrolyte and Acid–Base Disorders.* New York: Churchill Livingstone; 1985. p. 1041–80.
19. Chesley LC. Blood pressure and circulation. In: Chesley LC, editor. *Hypertensive Disorders in Pregnancy.* New York: Appleton-Century-Crofts; 1978. p.119–54.
20. Chapman AB, Abraham WT, Zamudio S, Coffin C, Merouani A, Young D, *et al.* Temporal relationships between hormonal and hemodynamic changes in early human pregnancy. *Kidney Int* 1998;4:2056–63.
21. Baylis C. Glomerular filtration and volume regulation in gravid animal models. In: Lindheimer MD, Davison JM, editors. *Baillieres Clinical Obstetrics and Gynecology.* 2nd ed., vol. 8. London: Bailliere Tindall; 1994. p. 235–64.
22. Roberts M, Lindheimer MD, Davison JM. Altered glomerular permselectivity to neutral dextran and heteroporous membrane modeling in human pregnancy. *Am J Physiol* 1996;270:F338–43.
23. Brenner BM. Nephron adaptation to renal injury or ablation. *Am J Physiol* 1985;249:F324–37.
24. Baylis C. Glomerular ultrafiltration in the pseudopregnant rat. *Am J Physiol* 1982;243:F300–5.
25. Slangen BF, Out IC, Verkeste CM, Smits JF, Peeters LL. Hemodynamic changes in pseudopregnancy in chronically instrumented conscious rats. *Am J Physiol* 1997;272:H695–700.
26. Conrad KP, Vernier KA. Plasma levels, urinary excretion and metabolic production of cGMP during gestation in rats. *Am J Physiol* 1989;257:R847–53.
27. Conrad KP, Joffe GM, Kruszyna H, Kruszyna R, Rochelle LG, Smith RP, *et al.* Identification of increased nitric oxide biosynthesis during pregnancy in rats. *FASEB J* 1993;7:566–71.
28. Deng A, Engels K, Baylis C. Increased nitric oxide production plays a critical role in the maternal blood pressure and glomerular hemodynamic adaptations to pregnancy in the rat. *Kidney Int* 1996;50:1132–8.
29. Kopp L, Paradiz G, Tucci JR. Urinary excretion of cyclic 3′,5′-adenosine monophosphate and cyclic 3′,5′-guanosine monophosphate during and after pregnancy. *J Clin Endocrinol Metab* 1977;44:590–4.
30. López-Jaramillo P, Narváez M, Calle A, Rivera J, Jácome P, Ruano C, *et al.* Cyclic guanosine 3′,5′ monophosphate concentrations in pre-eclampsia: effects of hydralazine. *Br J Obstet Gynaecol* 1996;103:33–8.
31. Gregoire I, el Esper N, Gondry J, Boitte F, Fievet P, Makdassi R, *et al.* Plasma atrial natriuretic factor and urinary excretion of a ouabain displacing factor and dopamine in normotensive pregnant women before and after delivery. *Am J Obstet Gynecol* 1990;162:71–6.
32. Baylis C, Beinder E, Suto T, August P. Recent insights into the roles of nitric oxide and renin-angiotensin in the pathophysiology of preeclampsia pregnancy. *Semin Nephrol* 1998;18:208–30.
33. Baylis C, Vallance P. Measurement of nitrite and nitrate levels in plasma and urine – what does this measure tell us about the activity of the endogenous nitric oxide system? *Curr Opin Nephrol Hypertens* 1998;7:59–62.
34. Conrad KP, Kerchner LJ, Mosher MD. Plasma and 24-h NOx and cGMP during normal pregnancy and preeclampsia in women on a reduced NOx diet. *Am J Physiol Renal Physiol* 1999;277 F48–57.
35. Danielson LA, Conrad KP. Acute blockade of nitric oxide synthase inhibits renal vasodilation and hyperfiltration during pregnancy in chronically instrumented conscious rats. *J Clin Invest* 1995;96:482–90.
36. Baylis C, Engels K. Adverse interactions between pregnancy and a new model of systemic hypertension produced by chronic blockade of endothelial derived relaxing factor (EDRF) in the rat. *Clin Exp Hypertens* 1992;B11:117–29.
37. Cadnapaphornchai MA, Ohara M, Morris KG, Knotek M, Rogachev B, Ladtkow T, *et al.* Chronic NOS inhibition reverses systemic vasodilation and glomerular hyperfiltration in pregnancy. *Am J Physiol Renal Physiol* 2001;280:F592–8.

38. Abram SR, Alexander BT, Bennett WA, Granger JP. Role of neuronal nitric oxide synthase in mediating renal hemodynamic changes during pregnancy. *Am J Physiol Regul Integr Comp Physiol* 2001;281:R1390–3.
39. Alexander BT, Cockrell K, Cline FD, Granger JP. Inducible nitric oxide synthase inhibition attenuates renal hemodynamics during pregnancy. *Hypertension* 2002;39:586–90.
40. Santmyire BR, Baylis C. Isoform specific changes in kidney NOS activity during rat pregnancy. *J Am Soc Nephrol* 1998;9:346.
41. Alexander BT, Miller T, Kassab S, Novak J, Reckelhoff JF, Kruckeberg WC, *et al.* Differential expression of renal nitric oxide synthase isoforms during pregnancy in rats. *Hypertension* 1999;33:435–9.
42. Narayanasamy V, Erdely A, Baylis C. Comparison of expression of Endothelial nitric oxide synthase (eNOS), phosphorylated eNOS (p-eNOS) and neuronal NOS (nNOS) in renal cortex (C) and medulla (M) in virgin (V), mid pregnant (MP) and late pregnant (LP) rats. *FASEB J* 2002;16:A1173.
43. Santmyire BR, Baylis C. The inducible nitric oxide synthase inhibitor aminoguanidine inhibits the pregnancy induced renal vasodilation and increase in kidney NOS activity in the rat. *J Am Soc Nephrol* 1999;10:386.
44. Smith C, Baylis C. Neuronal nitric oxide synthase (nNOS) in rat kidney during pregnancy. *J Am Soc Nephrol* 2006;17:302A.
45. Neugarten J, Ding Q, Friedman A, Lei J, Silbiger S. Sex hormones and renal nitric oxide synthases. *J Am Soc Nephrol* 1997;8:1240–6.
46. Garland HO, Atherton JC, Baylis C, Morgan MRA, Milne CM. Hormone profiles for progesterone, ostradiol, prolactin, plasma renin activity, aldosterone and corticosterone during pregnancy and pseudopregnancy in two strains of rats: Correlation with renal studies. *J Endocrinol* 1987;113:435–44.
47. Danielson LA, Sherwood OD, Conrad KP. Relaxin is a potent renal vasodilator in conscious rats. *J Clin Invest* 1999;103:525–33.
48. Danielson LA, Kerchner LJ, Conrad KP. Impact of gender and endothelin on renal vasodilation and hyperfiltration induced by relaxin in conscious rats. *Am J Physiol* 2000;279:R1298–304.
49. Novak J, Ramirez RJ, Gandley RE, Sherwood OD, Conrad KP. Myogenic reactivity is reduced in small renal arteries isolated from relaxin-treated rats. *Am J Physiol* 2002;283:R349–55.
50. Novak J, Reckelhoff J, Bumgarner L, Cockrell K, Kassab S, Granger JP. Reduced sensitivity of the renal circulation to angiotensin II in pregnant rats. *Hypertension* 1997;30:580–4.
51. Gandley RE, Conrad KP, McLaughlin MK. Endothelin and nitric oxide mediate reduced myogenic reactivity of small renal arteries from pregnant rats. *Am J Physiol* 2001;280:R1–7.
52. Novak J, Danielson LA, Kerchner LJ, Sherwood OD, Ramirez RJ, Moalli PA, *et al.* Relaxin is essential for renal vasodilation during pregnancy in conscious rats. *J Clin Invest* 2001;107:1469–75.
53. Smith MC, Murdoch AP, Danielson LA, Conrad KP, Davison JM. Relaxin has a role in establishing a renal response in pregnancy. *Fertil Steril* 2006;86:253–5.
54. Smith M, Davison J, Conrad K, Danielson L. Renal hemodynamic effects of relaxin in humans. *Ann N Y Acad Sci* 2005;1041:163–72.
55. Smith MC, Danielson LA, Conrad KP, Davison JM. Influence of recombinant human relaxin on renal hemodynamics in healthy volunteers. *J Am Soc Nephrol* 2006;17:3192–7.
56. Sasser JM, Lindheimer MD, Baylis C. Invited Editorial: An emerging role for relaxin as a renal vasodilator. *J Am Soc Nephrol* 2006;17:2960–1.
57. Danielson LA, Kercher LJ, Conrad KP. Impact of gender and endothelin on renal vasodilation and hyperfiltration induced by relaxin in conscious rats. *Am J Physiol Regul Integr Comp Physiol* 2000;279:R1298–304.
58. Fernandez-Patron C, Radomski MW, Davidge ST. Vascular matrix metalloproteinase-2 cleaves big endothelin-1 yielding a novel vasoconstrictor. *Circ Res* 1999;85:906–11.
59. Jeyabalan A, Novak J, Danielson LA, Kerchner LJ, Opett SL, Conrad KP. Essential role for vascular gelatinase activity in relaxin-induced renal vasodilation, hyperfiltration and reduced myogenic reactivity of small arteries. *Circ Res* 2003;93:1249–57.
60. Hines T. Baroreceptor afferent discharge in the pregnant rat. *Am J Physiol Regul Integr Comp Physiol* 2000;278:R1433–40.

61. Masilamani S, Heesch CM. Effects of pregnancy and progesterone metabolites on arterial baroreflex in conscious rats. *Am J Physiol* 1997;272:R924–34.
62. Baylis C, Brango C, Engels K. Renal effects of moderate hemorrhage in the pregnant rat. *Am J Physiol* 1990;259:F945–9.
63. Barron WM, Dürr JA, Schrier RW, Lindheimer MD. Role of hemodynamic factors in osmoregulatory alterations of rat pregnancy. *Am J Physiol* 1989;257:R909–16.
64. Baylis C, Blantz RC. Tubuloglomerular feedback activity in virgin and 12 day pregnant rats. *Am J Physiol* 1985;249:F169–73.
65. Kone BC, Baylis C. Biosynthesis and homeostatic roles of nitric oxide in the kidney. Editorial review. *Am J Physiol* 1997;272:F561–78.
66. Gant NF, Whalley PJ, Everett RB, Worley RJ, MacDonald PC. Control of vascular reactivity in pregnancy. *Am J Kidney Dis* 1987;9:303–7.
67. Masilamani S, Castro L, Baylis C. Pregnant rats are refractory to the natriuretic actions of atrial natriuretic peptide. *Am J Physiol* 1994;267:R1611–16.
68. Omer S, Mulay S, Cernacek P, Varma DR. Attenuation of renal effects of atrial natriuretic factor during rat pregnancy. *Am J Physiol.* 1995;268:F416–22.
69. Ni XN, Safai M, Rishi R, Baylis C, Humphreys MH. Increased activity of cGMP-specific phosphodiesterase (PDE5) contributes to resistance to atrial natriuretic peptide natriuresis in the pregnant rat. *J Am Soc Nephrol* 2004;15:1254–60.
70. Masilamani S, Hobbs GR, Baylis C. The acute pressure natriuresis response blunted and the blood pressure response reset in the normal pregnant rat. *Am J Obstet Gynecol* 1998;179:486–91.
71. Khraibi A. Renal interstitial hydrostatic pressure and pressure natriuresis in pregnant rats. *Am J Physiol* 2000;279:F353–7.
72. Knight S, Snellen H, Humphreys M, Baylis C. Increased renal phosphodiesterase (PDE)-5 activity mediates the blunted natriuretic response to ANP in the pregnant rat. *Am J Physiol Renal Physiol* 2007;292:F655–9.
73. Sasser JM, Snellen H, Baylis C. The natriuretic and diuretic response to dopamine is maintained during rat pregnancy. *J Am Soc Nephrol* 2007;18:595A.
74. Irons DW, Baylis PH, Davison JM. Effect of atrial natriuretic peptide on renal hemodynamics and sodium excretion during human pregnancy. *Am J Physiol Renal Physiol* 1996;271:F239–42.
75. Liu E, Morimoto M, Kitajima S, Koike T, Yu Y, Shiiki H, *et al.* Increased expression of vascular endothelial growth factor in kidney leads to progressive impairment of glomerular functions. *J Am Soc Nephrol.* 2007;18:2094–104.
76. Ballermann BJ. Contribution of the endothelium to the glomerular permselectivity barrier in health and disease. *Nephron Physiol* 2007;106:19–25.
77. Sugimoto H, Hamano Y, Charytan D, Cosgrove D, Kieran M, Sudhakar A, Kalluri R. Neutralization of circulating vascular endothelial growth factor (VEGF) by anti-VEGF antibodies and soluble VEGF receptor 1 (sFlt-1) induces proteinuria. *J Biol Chem* 2003;278:12605–8.
78. Yang JC, Haworth L, Sherry RM, Hwu P, Schwartzentruber DJ, Topalian SL, *et al.* A randomized trial of bevacizumab, an anti-vascular endothelial growth factor antibody, for metastatic renal cancer. *N Engl J Med* 2003;349:427–34.
79. Salmon AH, Neal CR, Bates DO, Harper SJ. Vascular endothelial growth factor increases the ultrafiltration coefficient in isolated intact Wistar rat glomeruli. *J Physiol* 2006;570:141–56.
80. Eremina V, Cui S, Gerber H, Ferrara N, Haigh J, Nagy A, *et al.* Vascular endothelial growth factor a signaling in the podocyte-endothelial compartment is required for mesangial cell migration and survival. *J Am Soc Nephrol* 2006;17:724–35.
81. Karihaloo A, Karumanchi SA, Cantley WL, Venkatesha S, Cantley LG, Kale S. Vascular endothelial growth factor induces branching morphogenesis/tubulogenesis in renal epithelial cells in a neuropilin-dependent fashion. *Mol Cell Biol* 2005;25:7441–8.
82. Guan F, Villegas G, Teichman J, Mundel P, Tufro A. Autocrine VEGF-A system in podocytes regulates podocin and its interaction with CD2AP. *Am J Physiol Renal Physiol* 2006;291:F422–8.
83. Nakagawa T. Uncoupling of the VEGF-endothelial nitric oxide axis in diabetic nephropathy: an explanation for the paradoxical effects of VEGF in renal disease. *Am J Physiol Renal Physiol* 2007;292:F1665–72.

84. Noiri E, Lee E, Testa J, Quigley J, Colflesh D, Keese CR, *et al.* Podokinesis in endothelial cell migration: role of nitric oxide. *Am J Physiol* 1998;274:C236–44.
85. Lindenmeyer MT, Kretzler M, Boucherot A, Berra S, Yasuda Y, Henger A, *et al.* Interstitial vascular rarefaction and reduced VEGF-A expression in human diabetic nephropathy. *J Am Soc Nephrol* 2007;18:1765–76.
86. Koyama S, Kimura T, Ogita K, Nakamura H, Khan MA, Yoshida S, *et al.* Transient local overexpression of human vascular endothelial growth factor (VEGF) in mouse feto-maternal interface during mid-term pregnancy lowers systemic maternal blood pressure. *Horm Metab Res* 2006;38:619–24.
87. Venkatesha S, Toporsian M, Lam C, Hanai J, Mammoto T, Kim YM, *et al.* Soluble endoglin contributes to the pathogenesis of preeclampsia. *Nat Med* 2006;12:642–9.
88. Makris A, Thornton C, Thompson J, Thomson S, Martin R, Ogle R, *et al.* Uteroplacental ischemia results in proteinuric hypertension and elevated sFLT-1. *Kidney Int* 2007;71:977–84.

Section 2

Patterns of care

2

Chapter 2

Prepregnancy counselling and risk assessment: general overview

Liz Lightstone

Introduction

Women with kidney disease have an increased risk of adverse maternal and fetal outcomes and it is now recognised that kidney disease is much more common than previously appreciated. By using an estimation of glomerular filtration rate (eGFR) rather than serum creatinine to assess renal function, between 3% and 10% of women of childbearing age might be defined as having chronic kidney disease (CKD).[1] Physicians in both primary and secondary care need to be alert to advising women with renal disease that they might be at risk, but they need guidelines as to who to alert and how to advise on the degree of risk. This chapter will address these issues in more detail. The aim is to advise all women who are at increased risk of that risk prior to conception – not only so that appropriate investigations and medication changes can be implemented safely well in advance but to avoid the emotional trauma of only discovering, once pregnant, that pregnancy might be associated with long-term complications. Importantly, many women with kidney disease may be entirely unaware that their condition could affect a pregnancy.

Who should have prepregnancy counselling?

The role of prepregnancy advice is to make a woman and her partner aware of the risks a pregnancy may pose to her health and that of the fetus, to give guidance as to the best time to contemplate pregnancy (i.e. sooner, if she has progressive renal disease, or later, if she has a relapsing condition that has recently flared), and to provide the opportunity to optimise treatment to ensure she is not on teratogenic medications at the time of conception and to focus her on the need for optimal control of risk factors such as hypertension and hyperglycaemia. All physicians should contemplate whether a woman of childbearing age has a condition that either itself, or the treatment of which, might influence the ability to become pregnant and the likelihood of complications both for mother and baby. This is particularly so with renal disease where the treatment of even those with mild disease could have a major impact on the fetus. In women with only minor disease, prepregnancy counselling can offer reassurance regarding a likely successful pregnancy outcome.

There has recently been a small revolution in the way CKD is considered – the introduction of the Modification of Diet in Renal Disease (MDRD) equation for eGFR rather than relying on serum creatinine alone.[2] This followed recognition that the serum creatinine does not rise until about 70% of function has been lost and it is unduly influenced by age, gender, ethnicity, diet and muscle mass, as well as other variables. Furthermore, even mild reductions in eGFR are associated with increased cardiovascular risk.[3] It is hoped that use of the MDRD equation to define renal function will lead to earlier identification of renal impairment and thus allow interventions to halt or delay progression of CKD and reduce cardiovascular risk. Approximately 10–15% of the general population have CKD as defined by an eGFR below 60 ml/minute/1.73 m^2 body surface area (stage 3–5 CKD) or structural abnormalities or proteinuria associated with either normal or slightly impaired GFR (stage 1–2 CKD) (Table 2.1).[2] The prevalence of CKD in women of childbearing age is approximately 3–10% and likely to rise in the light of the rising prevalence of type 2 diabetes in younger people.[4] The prevalence is much higher than previously thought based on serum creatinine alone. In the UK, all NHS laboratories now report eGFR and GPs are required to record all those with CKD 3 or worse. There is thus a much greater awareness of individuals having mild renal impairment. It is important to note that the MDRD equation does not work well during pregnancy.[5]

This then raises questions as to who requires prepregnancy counselling (Box 2.1) and whether all women with CKD should be referred for formal advice. It is unlikely that this would be practical or reasonable as, in many women with very mild disease, the risks are fairly low. However, even mild renal impairment is associated with a doubling of the risk of pre-eclampsia and, since virtually all women with CKD and any degree of proteinuria and/or hypertension are likely to be on an angiotensin-converting enzyme (ACE) inhibitor or angiotensin II receptor blocker, primary and secondary

Table 2.1. Stages of chronic kidney disease (CKD) using the Modification of Diet in Renal Disease (MDRD) formula to calculate the estimated glomerular filtration rate (eGFR)

CKD stage	eGFR (ml/minute/1.73 m^2)	Description	Approximate creatinine in nonpregnant woman (μmol/l)
1	>90	Kidney damage[a] with normal or raised GFR	<70
2	60–90	Kidney damage[a] with mild or reduced GFR	70–100
3	30–59	Moderately reduced GFR	100–180
4	15–29	Severely reduced GFR	180–350
5	<15	Kidney failure	>350

[a] Kidney damage with evidence of structural damage or proteinuria; cannot classify as CKD 1 or 2 on the basis of eGFR alone

Box 2.1. Women with renal disease who should be referred for prepregnancy counselling

- Women with CKD stage 4 or 5.
- Women with CKD stage 3 and adverse risk factors, e.g. significant proteinuria, hypertension or previous adverse obstetric history.
- Women with kidney transplants.
- Women on dialysis who are contemplating pregnancy.
- Women with CKD stage 1 or 2 and adverse risk factors, e.g. systemic disease such as lupus or vasculitis, significant proteinuria, hypertension or previous adverse obstetric history.
- Women with a family history of heritable renal disease.

care physicians need to be ready to advise about the risks and about prepregnancy discontinuation of such drugs. All high-risk women should be referred, i.e. those with CKD stage 4 or 5, those with renal transplants, probably all those with significant proteinuria (even if function preserved), and all women with inherited renal disease. All women with systemic disease, such as systemic lupus erythematosus (SLE) or vasculitis, that has involved the kidney should be referred regardless of renal function, not least because they will often be on medication that poses problems during pregnancy. Sadly, the women who are probably least likely to be referred are those with the worst prognosis, namely those on dialysis. Conception on dialysis is rare but more frequent than realised and the pregnancies have poor outcomes; however, it is often overlooked that such women may be fertile or contemplating pregnancy and hence they often present late in pregnancy with no idea of how risky the pregnancy is and/or the likelihood of severe prematurity or fetal loss (see Chapter 6).

It is probably unnecessary to refer women with isolated microscopic haematuria who have normal function and normal blood pressure. Women with recurrent urinary tract infections (UTIs) may have underlying vesicoureteric reflux and scarred kidneys, often picked up in pregnancy by ultrasound scans undertaken to identify a cause for frequent UTIs. These women are, however, rarely referred before their first pregnancy. Women known to have structural abnormalities of the kidney may require referral, especially if associated with hypertension, proteinuria, impaired function and/or recurrent UTIs.

Prepregnancy evaluation of women with kidney disease

The key aspects of assessment, as these are the main determinants of prognosis, are evaluation of the degree and progression of kidney injury as well as identification of medications and comorbidities that impact on pregnancy prognosis. The minimum data set (Box 2.2) would thus include eGFR and its rate of change over the previous 1–2 years, quantification of proteinuria/albuminuria (assessed by urine protein/creatinine ratio (PCR) or albumin/creatinine ratio (ACR), or a timed urine collection),[6] as well as imaging and, where indicated, a renal biopsy to make a formal diagnosis or to stage the degree of damage. An important consideration is to assess which tests

Box 2.2. Minimum data set required for prepregnancy counselling; ACR = albumin/creatinine ratio; CKD = chronic kidney disease; eGFR = estimated glomerular filtration rate; PCR = protein/creatinine ratio

- Degree of kidney injury and control of kidney disease:
  – eGFR
  – rate of change of eGFR over previous 12–24 months
  – spot urine ACR (if proteinuria 1+ or < on dipstick) or PCR (if proteinuria > 1+ on dipstick)
  – degree of anaemia and whether attributable to CKD
  – imaging and, where appropriate, diagnostic or staging biopsy
  – blood pressure control (and drugs used, i.e. number and class)
  – disease activity, e.g. in lupus/vasculitis.
- Medications: identifying those that require changing and those that are safe.
- Associated comorbidities, e.g. diabetic control.
- Assessment of factors that increase risk, e.g. anticardiolipin antibodies (ACA) or lupus anticoagulant.
- Assessment of fertility: risk posed by condition/prior treatment.

would provide useful baseline prepregnancy information and which should be avoided during pregnancy. Examples would include divided function tests in women with asymmetric or scarred kidneys, or renal biopsy in those with significant proteinuria in whom it would be ideal to have a firm renal diagnosis before pregnancy.

Women need to be advised on the timing of pregnancy – if they are known to have progressive renal decline as judged by steadily falling GFR or a condition with a predictable course such as adult polycystic kidney disease (APKD), then the sooner they become pregnant the better, as worse renal function is an important determinant of outcome. However, for those with relapsing–remitting diseases, they need to be in a stable remission and no longer taking toxic medications, and they may be advised to wait a few months or longer before contemplating conception. Where delay is obviously needed, women must be advised about appropriate contraception. It is important to consider whether the kidney condition or its treatment will have impaired a woman's fertility and to have a low threshold for referring for assessment – advising a woman with impaired and declining renal function to wait a year or two before having fertility treatment might mean she only has the chance to get pregnant once her renal function has declined to unsafe levels.

Perhaps the most important aspect of prepregnancy counselling is to review medications, not only to identify those which require changing or to provide advice about the risks of continuing, but also to identify those which the woman herself might be tempted to stop but which, in fact, are safe for the fetus and dangerous for her to discontinue. The two most common areas of difficulty are antihypertensives and immunosuppressants. Some of these will be discussed in more detail elsewhere (see Chapters 11 and 12). However, it is important to note that advice changed in 2006 on the use of ACE inhibitors and angiotensin II receptor blockers. These drugs are very widely used in women with CKD as they not only control blood pressure but reduce proteinuria and are renoprotective. They are absolutely contraindicated beyond the first trimester as they are associated with an often-fatal fetopathy. Previous advice had been that, on balance, it was reasonable to stop them once pregnant. However, a publication[7] has demonstrated that even first-trimester exposure only is associated with a significant increased risk of congenital abnormalities, especially neurological and cardiological. The absolute risk remains low but is four times the background risk. Women with minimal proteinuria should be advised to stop these drugs before conception and to have their blood pressure controlled by agents known to be safe in pregnancy, such as labetalol (not unopposed beta blockade), methyldopa and nifedipine. For women with progressive proteinuric renal disease, however, and especially those with diabetic nephropathy, the risk of renal progression may outweigh the risk of congenital abnormality, in which case I counsel women on the risks but advise continuing the medication until they are pregnant and then stopping at no later than 7 weeks. However, it is critical not to lose the message that control of blood pressure remains of paramount importance, not simply to preserve renal function but to reduce the risk of a poor obstetric outcome. Since CKD is a major risk factor for cardiovascular disease, many women will be taking statins for lipid control and these should be stopped before conception.

Immunosuppressants are often necessary to prevent relapse of systemic diseases, to treat glomerulonephritis or to prevent rejection of transplants. Women need to know that they absolutely do not need to stop prednisolone, azathioprine, hydroxychloroquine or calcineurin inhibitors (ciclosporin and tacrolimus).[8,9] The current advice is that they should not be taking mycophenolate mofetil (MMF) or sirolimus when they conceive because of the risk of congenital abnormalities.[10]

However, some renal physicians believe the risk of stopping these drugs is much greater for the mother than the risk of congenital abnormalities. It is critical that such discussions are carefully documented and ideally repeated so that the woman goes into pregnancy fully cognisant of possible risks. Some drugs are predictably teratogenic if exposure occurs early in pregnancy and women need to be clearly advised against getting pregnant while taking them or for several months afterwards, e.g. cytotoxic agents such as cyclophosphamide or chlorambucil.

Quantifying risk in women with CKD

Overall, the risks to the mother and baby are proportional to three key factors prepregnancy: the degree of renal impairment, the level of baseline proteinuria and the degree of hypertension. There is a paucity of prospective outcome studies but the latest data suggest that maternal and fetal outcomes are significantly worse in women who have a baseline eGFR below 40 ml/minute/1.73 m^2 and proteinuria above 1 g/24 hour (equivalent to a PCR of approximately 100 or more).[1] However, even in women with mild primary renal disease, no proteinuria and no hypertension, the risk of pre-eclampsia is 2–3 times that of the general population (7–14% versus 5%).[11] It is therefore reasonable for even women with mild CKD to take low-dose aspirin through pregnancy. In women with eGFR below 40 ml/minute/1.73 m^2 and proteinuria above 1 g/24 hours at baseline, the percentage of women who develop pre-eclampsia rises to 30–54%. While distinguishing pre-eclampsia from worsening renal disease is difficult as both involve hypertension and proteinuria, and fetal growth restriction is often present in both conditions, in practice it matters little – severe hypertension, proteinuria and a small baby usually mandate delivery regardless of specific cause.

From the prospective mother's perspective, the key questions to be answered are: (i) will her kidney function worsen because of a pregnancy and (ii) will her baby be harmed by her kidney impairment. The literature suggests that those with mild renal impairment prepregnancy (traditionally serum creatinine below 120 μmol/l, although this almost certainly includes a number of women with significant reduction in eGFR), minimal proteinuria and well-controlled or no hypertension are very unlikely (below 3%) to suffer a permanent decline in renal function.[4] The risk increases with the degree of renal impairment, particularly if combined with significant proteinuria, presumably because of hyperfiltration-induced damage (Table 2.2). In those with advanced renal impairment, the risk of requiring dialysis during or soon after pregnancy is increased and women need to be prepared for what dialysis entails and, importantly, how it will impact on their lives, especially with a newborn who may be born preterm.[12]

With the increase in live donor transplantation, in some young women with advanced CKD (eGFR less than 20 ml/minute/1.73 m^2), it may be appropriate to advise pre-emptive transplantation and a year or two's wait (for stable renal function

Table 2.2. Risks associated with different levels of renal impairment in pregnant women; based on data from 1988 to 2005 in 676 women with 908 pregnancies, supplied by Prof. J Davison, University of Newcastle

Serum creatinine (μmol/l)	Problems during pregnancy	Successful obstetric outcome	Long-term renal problems
< 120	26%	96%	< 3%
120–250	47%	89%	30%
> 250	86%	46%	53%

and minimal immunosuppression) before contemplating pregnancy. However, where there is no prospect of a live donor or in older women, this may not be practical advice and they may decide to risk a pregnancy before starting dialysis, when the chances of a successful obstetric outcome plummet. Women with significant renal impairment need to be aware that they are likely to need erythropoietin (EPO) injections (with or without intravenous iron) to treat anaemia during pregnancy,[13] and an increase in their antihypertensive medications and possibly anticoagulation treatment if their proteinuria increases markedly.

Although fetal outcomes have undoubtedly improved owing to improved neonatal care it must not be forgotten that impaired function combined with significant proteinuria is associated with higher rates of preterm delivery, fetal growth restriction and neonatal death. In a prospective study of 49 white non-diabetic women with CKD stages 3–5, perinatal mortality was confined to those women with eGFR below 40 ml/minute/1.73 m^2 and proteinuria above 1 g/24 hour and was 4% which, although not a huge rate, is three times higher than in the general population.[1,14]

It is harder to advise those in the middle ground with moderate renal impairment and/or significant proteinuria. Retrospective data would suggest that a serum creatinine concentration over 120 μmol/l predicts a poorer outcome as does baseline nephrotic syndrome (Table 2.3). In a recent prospective study, however, it was only the combination of significant renal impairment and proteinuria that led to a statistically important increased risk to long-term renal function and to fetal outcome.[1] All women with significantly impaired kidney function should be advised that they are likely to be at increased risk of hypertension, pre-eclampsia, fetal growth restriction and preterm delivery as well as a possible long-term decline in renal function. While the latter is not entirely predictable, it is likely to be more of an issue for women with progressive renal dysfunction prepregnancy, such as those with diabetic nephropathy, than for those with stable moderate CKD, for example stage 3 CKD with minimal proteinuria but perhaps a serum creatinine concentration above 150 μmol/l. It is also worth noting that just as many women with poor renal risk factors will do well, and some apparently at low risk will do very badly with a marked decline in renal function. This is well illustrated by the study of a group of women with prepregnancy serum creatinine levels of above 180 μmol/l. While 50% did not lose renal function during pregnancy, 30% declined through pregnancy and continued to do so afterwards, 8% worsened during pregnancy but improved back to baseline by 6 months postpartum, and 10% were stable through pregnancy but declined significantly between 6 weeks and 6 months postpartum.[12] The counsel of perfection should thus be to warn of possible adverse outcomes while expecting generally good results.

While renal function and proteinuria are clearly important determinants of outcome, the influence of hypertension cannot be overstated. Women with quite

Table 2.3. Types of problem encountered with different levels of renal impairment in pregnant women; based on data from 1988 to 2005 in 676 women with 908 pregnancies, supplied by Prof. J Davison, University of Newcastle

Serum creatinine (μmol/l)	High blood pressure	Pre-eclampsia	Fetal growth restriction and/or preterm birth
< 120	Variable	10–20%	Increased
120–250	30–50%	40%	30–50%
$\geq$ 250	Most	80%	57–73%

significant kidney disease but who do not require antihypertensives tend to have excellent outcomes. In contrast, uncontrolled hypertension at baseline is associated with poor outcomes, although this can be improved if blood pressure is controlled during pregnancy.[15] Prepregnancy review should include not only adjustment of antihypertensive medications to those safe in pregnancy but to ensure the blood pressure is adequately controlled. The target for blood pressure control during pregnancy is discussed in Chapter 12.

Preterm delivery is common in women with kidney disease. This may partly reflect physician anxiety and a tendency to have a lower threshold to induce preterm, but data on birthweight and fetal growth restriction suggest that often it is for perceived fetal distress. While outcomes for neonates beyond 30 weeks of gestation are generally excellent, it must not be assumed that such prematurity is without risk to the offspring. Importantly, it is vital to note that, although neonatal outcomes have hugely improved in recent years, short gestation/very low birthweight can be associated with significant long-term handicap.[14] Women contemplating a high-risk pregnancy need to be very clear as to what the worst-case scenario might be even if the overall risk is relatively low.

The most difficult problem is when to advise someone not to get pregnant at all because of their kidney disease. It might be argued ethically that this is not the doctor's role – they are simply there to advise on risks and it is for the woman to decide whether she is prepared to take on the risks and that the doctor's role is to support her decision whatever it may be. However, many women seek an absolute answer and it is the doctor's role to judge whether the balance of risk weighs so heavily against the health of the mother with little chance of a 'take-home' baby that pregnancy really should not be contemplated. In reality this advice is rarely required and sometimes it is self-evident, for example for women with severe active lupus nephritis, pregnancy is very high risk and unlikely to be successful.

The much more subjective areas concern older women who perhaps need assisted conception and who have significantly impaired kidney function. They are likely to be menopausal before they get a transplant and yet pregnancy might well cause a rapid permanent decline leading to dialysis sooner than had they not become pregnant. If dialysis is required during pregnancy, then the risk of losing the fetus is high and the woman will have gained nothing and lost a lot. Anecdotally, there is a dichotomy of responses between women who have failing native kidney function and those with failing transplants. The latter group have often been on dialysis before and may well treasure their kidney function above their fertility; for those women who have never been dialysed and who perhaps do not fully appreciate the difficulties of life on dialysis, the desire to have a baby will often outweigh a theoretical risk of being on dialysis sooner rather than later. In most cases where the clinician believes pregnancy is not advisable, it is rarely because of just one issue but rather the sum of several medical problems which together suggest that pregnancy would simply be inadvisable. For example, consider a woman in her thirties who requires *in vitro* fertilisation (IVF), who has had her renal transplant for 14 years, who is on MMF and tacrolimus, who had a late episode of rejection resulting in poor graft function, and who has difficult hypertension that requires four agents to be controlled adequately, including an ACE inhibitor and angiotensin II receptor blocker. Each aspect on its own is not a contraindication but given the whole picture the risk–benefit analysis swings against going for a pregnancy. Clearly, the woman may choose to ignore the advice and the risks, and then all efforts have to be made to support her through any pregnancy that occurs and to ensure that appropriate multidisciplinary care in a high-risk obstetric setting is available.

It is important not to overlook those women who have had previous pregnancies. They may well assume that if a previous pregnancy went well then they have nothing to worry about. However, they may not have had kidney disease at that time, or it may have been much milder. Their risk may thus have changed significantly. Importantly, if they have a bad obstetric history, e.g. early pre-eclampsia, then, even if their renal disease is apparently mild, the risk to a subsequent pregnancy may be much greater. It is thus important to differentiate between nulliparous and parous women with kidney disease for prepregnancy advice and assessment.

Conclusion

Prepregnancy advice should be available to all women of childbearing age with significant kidney disease. Primary and secondary care physicians need to consider the medications such women are taking and advise them whether they need to stop prepregnancy or as soon as they are pregnant. All doctors who look after these women should remember to advise about contraception, cessation of smoking and taking folic acid if planning a pregnancy. All renal units should have at least one nephrologist who is able to undertake a proper risk assessment given the specifics of each case. Ideally, women would be advised in the setting of a joint renal–antenatal clinic where both the obstetric and medical aspects can be addressed by expert doctors in the same consultation. It is imperative that women with kidney disease are forewarned of the risks that a pregnancy may pose, the need to book early, the need for regular monitoring and the use of a centre where obstetric, nephrological and high-risk perinatal care are all available.

All of this requires education of primary and secondary care physicians as well as nephrologists on the risks of pregnancy associated with kidney disease. Women need to be told how their condition might impact on pregnancy and they should be given a fact sheet when they are diagnosed with kidney disease. While it may not be possible for all women with CKD to be seen in specialist prepregnancy clinics, it is advisable to refer all women with significant renal impairment *and* proteinuria as well as those with renal transplants or systemic disease affecting the kidneys.

In the long run it would be enormously helpful to have better tools to identify those women who are going to do well – so they need not be concerned and not require highly medicalised pregnancies – and those women who will do badly, perhaps against current risk predictions.[16] The advent of new biomarkers for pre-eclampsia might herald a new era for identifying high-risk women in specific populations such as those with CKD but further research is required.

References

1. Imbasciati E, Gregorini G, Cabiddu G, Gammaro L, Ambroso G, Del Giudice A, *et al.* Pregnancy in CKD stages 3 to 5: fetal and maternal outcomes. *Am J Kidney Dis* 2007;49:753–62.
2. Coresh J, Byrd-Holt D, Astor BC, Briggs JP, Eggers PW, Lacher DA, *et al.* Chronic kidney disease awareness, prevalence, and trends among U.S. adults, 1999 to 2000. *J Am Soc Nephrol* 2005;16:180–8.
3. Coresh J, Astor B, Sarnak MJ. Evidence for increased cardiovascular disease risk in patients with chronic kidney disease. *Curr Opin Nephrol Hypertens* 2004;13:73–81.
4. Fischer MJ. Chronic kidney disease and pregnancy: maternal and fetal outcomes. *Adv Chronic Kidney Dis* 2007;14:132–45.
5. Smith MC, Moran P, Ward MK, Davison JM. Assessment of glomerular filtration rate during pregnancy using the MDRD formula. *BJOG* 2008;115:109–12.

6. Holt JL, Mangos GJ, Brown MA. Measuring protein excretion in pregnancy. *Nephrology (Carlton)* 2007;12:425–30.
7. Cooper WO, Hernandez-Diaz S, Arbogast PG, Dudley JA, Dyer S, Gideon PS, *et al.* Major congenital malformations after first-trimester exposure to ACE inhibitors. *N Engl J Med* 2006;354:2443–51.
8. EBPG Expert Group on Renal Transplantation. European best practice guidelines for renal transplantation. Section IV: Long-term management of the transplant recipient. IV.10. Pregnancy in renal transplant recipients. *Nephrol Dial Transplant* 2002;17(Suppl 4):50–5.
9. McKay DB, Josephson MA, Armenti VT, August P, Coscia LA, Davis CL, *et al.* Reproduction and transplantation: report on the AST Consensus Conference on Reproductive Issues and Transplantation. *Am J Transplant* 2005;5:1592–9.
10. Sifontis NM, Coscia LA, Constantinescu S, Lavelanet AF, Moritz MJ, Armenti VT. Pregnancy outcomes in solid organ transplant recipients with exposure to mycophenolate mofetil or sirolimus. *Transplantation* 2006;82:1698–702.
11. Stratta P, Canavese C, Quaglia M. Pregnancy in patients with kidney disease. *J Nephrol* 2006;19:135–43.
12. Jones DC, Hayslett JP. Outcome of pregnancy in women with moderate or severe renal insufficiency. *N Engl J Med* 1996;335:226–32.
13. Goshorn, J, Youell TD. Darbepoetin alfa treatment for post-renal transplantation anemia during pregnancy. *Am J Kidney Dis* 2005;46:e81–6.
14. Blowey DL, Warady BA. Outcome of infants born to women with chronic kidney disease. *Adv Chronic Kidney Dis* 2007;14:199–205.
15. Bar J, Ben-Rafael Z, Padoa A, Orvieto R, Boner G, Hod M. Prediction of pregnancy outcome in subgroups of women with renal disease. *Clin Nephrol* 2000;53:437–44.
16. Karumanchi SA, Lindheimer MD. Preeclampsia and the kidney: footprints in the urine. *Am J Obstet Gynecol* 2007;196:287–8.

3

Chapter 3

Chronic kidney disease in pregnancy: patterns of care and general principles of management

Mark A Brown

Basic principles of antenatal care

Management of the pregnant woman with chronic kidney disease (CKD) ideally begins prior to pregnancy to allow time for appropriate counselling regarding the potential risks and likely outcomes not only of the pregnancy but for the woman postpartum. Attitudes have changed over the past 20–30 years and CKD is no longer seen as an automatic contraindication to pregnancy.[1] Nevertheless, the data used to counsel women today are generally those derived from a few key studies published more than 10 years ago,[2–10] summarised clearly in two key reviews.[11,12]

Controversy remains as to whether the primary underlying renal disorder affects the pregnancy outcome or, more likely, the outcome is dependent upon the baseline level of renal function, with the possible exception of systemic lupus erythematosus (SLE). In either case, maternal hypertension is a significant adverse factor;[13] live births now occur in 64–98% of pregnancies depending upon the degree of renal impairment and the presence or absence of hypertension.

On occasion, women with CKD have an accelerated course towards dialysis, either during pregnancy or postpartum.[7] In women with advanced renal failure, this possibility should be discussed before conception in the context of possible pre-emptive transplantation, which is usually associated with a better chance of having a successful pregnancy.

The key principles of antenatal care in women with chronic renal disease are:

- measurement, interpretation and management of hypertension
- measurement, interpretation and management of changes in glomerular filtration rate (GFR)
- measurement, interpretation and management of proteinuria, including nephrotic syndrome
- consideration of the primary underlying renal disease and its specific problems
- identification of abnormalities of renal tubular function

- identification and management of urinary tract infection
- clinical assessment and maintenance of volume homoeostasis
- consideration of appropriate 'renal' and antihypertensive medications throughout pregnancy
- identification of superimposed pre-eclampsia
- assessment of fetal wellbeing.

Hypertension

Blood pressure normally falls by the end of the first trimester of pregnancy as part of a vasodilator response, accompanied by an increase in cardiac output and stimulation of the renin–angiotensin system.[14] Most women with CKD will not exhibit this fall in blood pressure and many will undergo an increase in blood pressure as the pregnancy progresses. Factors mediating this progression are unclear, given that in normal pregnancy the majority of vascular factors favour dilation of blood vessels; although circulating renin and aldosterone concentrations are increased, there is typically some refractoriness to the vascular effects of pressor substances. Whether this refractoriness is lost in women with underlying chronic renal impairment is unknown. Pregnancy is accompanied by significant volume expansion, which under normal circumstances does not induce hypertension.[14] However, in the context of chronic renal impairment outside of pregnancy there is often an inability to excrete a sodium load with accompanying hypertension and it is likely that this mechanism is partly involved in the development of hypertension in these women during pregnancy. Regardless of the cause, persistence of hypertension is an adverse factor in pregnancy outcome[15] and it is therefore imperative that considerable attention is paid to the blood pressure of women with CKD during their antenatal care.

Measurement of blood pressure has traditionally been done by mercury sphygmomanometry but this is slowly being replaced by a range of automated blood pressure recorders. It is probable that most of the automated blood pressure recorders used in routine clinical practice have not been validated for use in pregnancy. Even those that have been tested and have received appropriate grading from the British Hypertension Society (BHS)[16] or the Association for the Advancement of Medical Instrumentation (AAMI)[17] are not necessarily accurate in an individual pregnant woman. Where possible, blood pressure should still be recorded using mercury sphygmomanometry, recording the phase 5 sound as the true diastolic pressure.[18] Hypertension is generally defined as a blood pressure above 140/90 mmHg and in pregnancy treatment is generally reserved for blood pressures above this level. However, it is important to remember that the target blood pressure for most women with chronic renal impairment is below 130/80 mmHg and there is a question whether a period of 40 weeks or so of blood pressures above this level could lead to progressive renal impairment after the pregnancy. This remains unknown to date.

Most women with chronic renal impairment, particularly those with proteinuria above 1 g/day, will be receiving angiotensin-converting enzyme (ACE) inhibitors or angiotensin II receptor blockers (ARBs) before pregnancy. These must be discontinued, preferably before pregnancy and certainly once pregnancy is diagnosed, owing to increased risks of fetal growth restriction, oligohydramnios, neonatal renal failure and probably cardiac and neurological development abnormalities.[19,20] Suitable antihypertensives include methyldopa, labetalol, oxprenolol, hydralazine, prazosin and nifedipine. Fear of using antihypertensives in pregnancy can be associated with poorer pregnancy outcomes, at least in women with renal transplants.[21] Target blood pressures should probably be in the region of 110–140/80–90 mmHg, seeking to preserve maternal renal function while not lowering the blood pressure so far as to reduce uteroplacental perfusion. There is no solid research to allow us to know what the ideal blood pressure is in these women but it is prudent to commence antihypertensives if blood pressure is above 140/90 mmHg.

It is also important to appreciate that blood pressure will often rise significantly soon after delivery; therefore, blood pressure measurement must be just as diligent in the early postpartum period as during pregnancy.

Glomerular filtration rate

The GFR should rise by about 40% during normal pregnancy, typically apparent by the end of the first trimester. One study has suggested that failure to increase GFR is associated with miscarriage.[22]

Under experimental conditions, ensuring both adequate hydration and urine output, GFR is measured as either creatinine clearance or inulin clearance. From a practical point of view, clinicians rely on serum creatinine as the main measurement of GFR during pregnancy. Measurement of creatinine clearance requires 24 hour urine collection, which is cumbersome and even when conducted diligently may be inaccurate because of ureteric dilation, which results in pooling of urine and an incomplete collection. Cystatin C has been used to measure GFR during pregnancy[23] together with beta-2 microglobulin. Cystatin C correlated weakly with 24 hour creatinine clearance but less well than serum creatinine in one study[24] and beta-2 microglobulin correlated weakly with serum creatinine in another.[25] However, there are problems with both measurements and serum creatinine remains the main tool for assessing GFR during pregnancy.

The Modification of Diet in Renal Disease (MDRD) formula is now used widely outside of pregnancy[26] but does not work during pregnancy[27] and has never been recommended for this purpose. Similarly, the Cockcroft–Gault formula[28] has also not been validated; this formula depends on body weight as a reflection of muscle mass and body weight changes considerably during pregnancy, not because of changes in body mass but largely as a result of volume expansion, maternal fat and the fetus.

For practical purposes, a serum creatinine above 90 µmol/l is considered abnormal for pregnancy, reflecting impaired GFR. A serum creatinine above 130 µmol/l means that the pregnant woman carries substantial fetal and maternal hypertensive and renal impairment risks throughout her pregnancy; problems may also develop in some women at lower serum creatinine levels.

Proteinuria and nephrotic syndrome

In the nonpregnant woman, daily protein excretion is generally less than 150 mg/day, consisting of up to 20 mg/day albumin with the remainder being other proteins, often of tubular origin.[29] Albumin excretion during normal pregnancy appears to be unchanged but total protein excretion is increased across all trimesters with an upper limit of excretion around 300 mg/day. The mechanisms of this increased excretion are unclear but appear to relate to increased glomerular porosity[30] rather than to substantial changes in glomerular haemodynamics.

Evidence has shown that soluble fms-like tyrosine kinase 1 (sFlt1) production is increased from the placenta in pregnancies complicated by pre-eclampsia and that this production may predate the clinical appearance of the disorder.[31] It is clear from animal experiments that sFlt1 may reduce levels of vascular endothelial growth factor (VEGF) resulting in disrupted glomerular endothelial cells, loss of endothelial cell fenestrations in the glomerulus and significant proteinuria.[32] To date, no such studies have been undertaken in women with primary renal disease during their pregnancy but it is possible that such women who develop superimposed pre-eclampsia have changes in glomerular structure and renal function as a result of sFlt1 and perhaps other angiogenic factors such as endoglin. This is an area for future research.

There has been a shift in nephrology practice outside of pregnancy to measure urinary protein excretion as the spot urine protein/creatinine ratio (PCR) instead of 24 hour urinary protein excretion. However, examination of source studies leading to this conclusion reveals often poor agreement between a single PCR and 24 hour urinary protein excretion. Lane *et al.*[33] showed that while there was statistically significant correlation between the spot PCR and 24 hour urinary protein excretion, agreement between predicted and actual 24 hour urinary protein excretion was poor for protein excretion above 1 g/day. On the other hand, spot PCR provided good threshold values which discriminated between protein excretions above or below excretion rates of 300 mg/day, 500 mg/day, 1 g/day and greater than 3 g/day.

Urinalysis alone is a poor predictor of protein excretion in pregnancy.[34,35] Use of spot PCR in pregnancy has become a popular and reasonably reliable method of determining whether protein excretion is abnormal, i.e. above 300 mg/day,[36] and is most often needed to diagnose the presence of pre-eclampsia. There have been no studies to date testing whether serial spot PCR during pregnancy in a woman with renal disease is a reliable method of predicting changes in 24 hour urinary protein excretion in that woman. While it is likely that this would be the case, 24 hour urine protein excretion remains the gold standard for assessing true changes in protein excretion during pregnancy within an individual woman. A practical approach is to measure 24 hour urinary protein and creatinine excretion at the original visit and determine the PCR from that collection, as a way of 'validating' the PCR in that woman. Subsequent PCR will provide a guide to changes in her protein excretion although it needs to be acknowledged that this is a guide only.

Even where there is a true change in protein excretion during pregnancy in women with underlying renal disease, there are very few therapeutic options available apart from ensuring blood pressure control. ACE inhibitors and ARBs or aldosterone antagonists cannot be used during pregnancy, although diltiazem can be used and may have a small benefit.[37] There is thus no great imperative to keep measuring 24 hour urinary protein excretion in these women, other than to detect nephrotic syndrome. Some advocate increasing protein excretion as a marker of superimposed pre-eclampsia in women with underlying renal disease, although no studies have been able to confirm this and protein excretion may increase in these women either owing to appropriate increases in glomerular filtration or progression of the underlying primary renal disease or suboptimal blood pressure control. In other words, an increase in urinary protein excretion should highlight the need for the clinician to look for features of pre-eclampsia but by itself is not sufficient to make a diagnosis of superimposed pre-eclampsia. Moreover, proteinuria is not felt to be an independent predictor of adverse pregnancy outcome and should not be used by itself as an indicator for delivery.[38]

Benign proteinuria is sometimes observed during pregnancy, where an otherwise healthy pregnant woman is found to have increased protein excretion, usually detected first by urinalysis and subsequently by a spot PCR, in the absence of any other feature of pre-eclampsia or hypertension and with a normal serum creatinine, i.e. normal

GFR. In some cases this may represent *de novo* orthostatic proteinuria while others appear to be just a benign increase in protein excretion during normal pregnancy that generally returns to normal after pregnancy. It is unlikely that such women have any later propensity to significant renal disease but this remains unknown. The main management issue is that urinalysis is reassessed 3–6 months postpartum in these women and appropriate nephrological assessment undertaken if this is persistent, above 500 mg/day.

The most common cause of nephrotic syndrome during pregnancy is pre-eclampsia but nephrotic syndrome during pregnancy is also a problem for women with underlying primary glomerular disease. Serum albumin normally falls during pregnancy, partly owing to volume expansion, but values below 30 g/l should raise suspicion of the development of nephrotic syndrome. A spot urine PCR above 230 mg/mmol signifies a strong likelihood that protein excretion is above 3 g/day[33] and 24 hour urinary protein and creatinine should then be measured to confirm this. These women will generally have oedema although this is a poor diagnostic sign during pregnancy as it accompanies two-thirds of normal pregnancies. There is little point in measuring serum cholesterol, usually a component of the nephrotic syndrome, as this is increased during normal pregnancy.

In pre-eclampsia without underlying CKD, retrospective studies show that proteinuria above 5 g/day, or even 10 g/day, is not associated with any worse outcome than in those women with lesser degrees of proteinuria.[39] Chan *et al.*[40] addressed this question using spot PCR and found that, although there was an association between maternal and fetal risks and the PCR in proteinuric pre-eclampsia, no reliable discriminant value could be found above which risks were truly increased within this group. There was some evidence that a spot PCR above 900 mg/mmol (about 10 g/day), or above 500 mg/mmol if also over the age of 35 years, might indicate significantly greater risks. Regardless of the predictive worth of proteinuria in pre-eclampsia, confirmation of true nephrotic syndrome in pregnancy is important as it allows recognition of the other aspects of this syndrome that may accompany the heavy proteinuria and be important to the pregnancy. These include loss of vitamin D-binding protein, transferrin, immunoglobulins, antithrombin 3 (also accompanied by increased hepatic synthesis of clotting factors) and a propensity for intravascular volume contraction in severe cases. The net result of these changes includes calcium deficiency, iron deficiency, increased likelihood of infection, venous thromboembolism and reduced uteroplacental blood flow with fetal growth restriction or death[41] and sometimes reduced renal blood flow with worsening renal function. Treatment requires oral calcium, vitamin D and iron supplementation and subcutaneous heparin for thrombosis prophylaxis as well as ensuring adequate fetal growth and amniotic fluid by ultrasound and reassessment of maternal serum creatinine on a regular basis. Low-molecular-weight heparin (LMWH) is suitable if GFR is near normal, i.e. above 60 ml/minute, a safe serum creatinine level to use LMWH being below 110 μmol/l. Where nephrotic syndrome occurs early in pregnancy and heparin is commenced at that point, it is prudent to add vitamin D for prophylaxis against subsequent osteoporosis, although there are as yet no controlled trials to test the benefit of this practice and, unlike for unfractionated heparin, there is no evidence that LMWH causes osteoporosis.

Follow-up of proteinuria after pregnancy is important not only in women with known CKD but also in women who have had pre-eclampsia. Bar *et al.*[42] found that 42% had albuminuria 3–5 years after delivery, signifying either underlying renal disease before the pregnancy or renal damage consequent upon pre-eclampsia. Most would not find such a high figure in usual clinical practice but the clear message is that women with early onset or severe pre-eclampsia should be assessed several months postpartum to ensure underlying renal disease is excluded.

The primary underlying renal disease and its specific problems

Management of specific renal diseases are addressed in other chapters in this book. However, it is integral to proper antenatal care of women with underlying renal disease to consider the nuances of the underlying primary disorder. The most common renal diseases predating pregnancy in this age group are primary glomerulonephritis (usually immunoglobulin A (IgA) nephropathy or focal and segmental glomerulosclerosis (FSGS)), reflux nephropathy, diabetic nephropathy and adult polycystic kidney disease. Long-term follow-up of childhood IgA nephropathy showed that later pregnancy was complicated by hypertension in half the cases and preterm birth in one-third,[43] but these outcomes are not specific to this form of nephropathy. While lupus nephritis is not a common cause of end-stage renal failure overall, it is a disorder with a large preponderance towards young women and, as such, is another renal disease commonly seen by obstetric medicine physicians. In general, women with SLE should have quiescent disease prepregnancy to offer the best chance of a successful pregnancy outcome.[44]

The basic principles of care in this group include:

- detection of deterioration in GFR and its extent
- midstream urine culture at the beginning of pregnancy, then on two or three other occasions even in the absence of symptoms to assess for underlying urinary tract infection (particularly in those with reflux nephropathy)
- good control of blood sugar and blood pressure to offset the disadvantage of not being able to use ACE inhibitors or ARBs in diabetic nephropathy
- use of appropriate immunosuppression when required in lupus nephritis, as well as determining whether the woman has anticardiolipin antibodies or lupus anticoagulant or has the anti-SSA/B antibodies with a propensity for fetal atrioventricular (AV) node disorders.

Inherited renal disorders are likely to have been diagnosed prior to the pregnancy and the specific implications of this for the offspring will have been discussed. The most common such renal disorder is adult polycystic kidney disease with an autosomal dominant inheritance; IgA nephropathy and reflux nephropathy are not inherited by specific Mendelian traits but tend to co-segregate within families and the pregnant woman needs to be aware of this. While still uncommon, disorders such as Alport's syndrome and familial hyperuricaemic nephropathy[45] occur in this age group and appropriate counselling needs be provided before and during pregnancy.

Assessment of renal tubular function

There are substantial changes in renal physiology during pregnancy that are largely centred on changes in renal blood flow and GFR. There are subtle changes in renal tubular function that include decreased proximal tubular glucose reabsorption, probably mediated through a volume expansion effect, leading to glycosuria in many women without reflecting diabetes. Normal pregnant women have a mixed respiratory alkalosis and metabolic acidosis with an increased urinary pH. Studies have shown the anion gap in pregnancy to be slightly lower than that postpartum.[46]

Tubular catabolism of albumin is probably normal as the fractional excretion of albumin is unchanged in pregnant compared with nonpregnant women.[47] The very large increase in filtered sodium is offset by increased tubular reabsorption, largely through resistance to atrial natriuretic peptide and increased renin and aldosterone production causing distal nephron sodium retention with accompanying potassium secretion and a tendency for low normal serum potassium levels.[48] While there is a resetting of plasma osmolality about 10 mosm/kg below normal, renal concentrating and diluting abilities are intact.[49]

The clinical implications for women with primary renal disease are as follows. Those with glomerular disorders such as primary glomerulonephritis or lupus nephritis are unlikely to have significant changes in renal tubular function but are more likely to have exaggerated sodium retention if GFR is reduced. Those with disorders affecting the tubulo-interstitial system such as reflux nephropathy, medullary cystic disease and polycystic kidney disease may have a propensity to sodium loss and thus experience volume contraction and fetal growth restriction, or occasionally impaired urinary concentrating ability, which exaggerates the propensity for volume contraction.

However, from a practical point of view, changes in renal tubular function in women with underlying primary renal disorders are rarely of clinical consequence during pregnancy. Three pregnancies have been reported in two women with type 1 renal tubular acidosis: all developed hypertension and mild renal impairment but had good pregnancy outcomes.[50] Measurement of serum sodium, potassium and bicarbonate together with creatinine is generally sufficient to ensure significant tubular dysfunction has not been missed in women with underlying CKD during pregnancy.

Plasma uric acid is commonly measured as a potential marker of pre-eclampsia, although it is not clear that this practice has any value today. In renal transplant patients in particular, where urate excretion is influenced by both tubular function and drugs such as ciclosporin, there is no point in measuring uric acid during such pregnancies. Uric acid undergoes reabsorption in the proximal tubule then secretion followed by post-secretory reabsorption and its excretion therefore can be influenced at several points along the nephron. Elevated plasma urate has been suggested as being pathogenic[51] or else a marker of renal vasoconstriction. In one small study, pre-eclamptic women receiving probenecid had lower serum uric acid and creatinine (but no difference in creatinine clearance) and higher platelet counts than women in a control group, but pregnancy outcomes were similar.[52] Consequently, a baseline uric acid level is only useful so that an elevated level is not interpreted by others later in pregnancy as indicating pre-eclampsia; serial measurement of uric acid in women with CKD is not of much help in clinical management.

Urinary tract infection

It is generally accepted that urine culture at the commencement of pregnancy is a cost-effective means of detecting asymptomatic bacteriuria, which should be treated in all pregnant women. This is of greater importance in women with underlying renal disease as they appear to be more predisposed to urine infection,[53,54] and this includes women who have had successful surgical correction of vesicoureteric reflux in childhood.[55] Ascending urine infection, or infection which leads to bacteraemia, may precipitate a decline in renal function with subsequent fetal risks of impaired growth or preterm birth, as well as increased risk of preterm rupture of membranes.

A reasonable approach is to ensure that all women with underlying renal disease have a routine urine culture at the commencement of pregnancy. Women with a history of prior urine infections or surgical correction of a urinary tract anomaly, those taking immunosuppressive drugs, including renal transplant recipients, and those with impaired GFR should have further routine cultures done at around 24, 28 and 32–34 weeks of gestation. Assuming an initial uninfected sample, the remainder of women should have repeat urine cultures performed only if they develop symptoms of urinary tract infection or if routine urinalysis demonstrates new onset pyuria or nitrites.

Organisms responsible for urinary tract infection during pregnancy are generally the same as in nonpregnant women, with *Escherichia coli* being the predominant organism. Renal ultrasound is generally not indicated unless for some reason renal imaging has never been undertaken or if the infection fails to respond to initial antibiotic treatment. Normal ureteric and renal pelvic dilation will be seen and the temptation to decompress the urinary tract with nephrostomy should be resisted unless there is generalised sepsis and/or deteriorating GFR failing to respond to intravenous antibiotics.

There are no controlled trials to determine the optimum management of urinary tract infection in women with underlying renal disease during pregnancy. Conventional practice is to treat the initial infection for approximately 1 week and thereafter maintain a low dose of antibiotics, e.g. cefalexin 250 mg each night. This should be continued until shortly after delivery to avoid episodes of pyelonephritis with its fetal and maternal risks.

Clinical assessment and management of volume homoeostasis

Adequate intravascular volume is essential to preservation of GFR and, therefore, a good pregnancy outcome for mother and baby regardless of the underlying renal disorder. However, it is particularly difficult to assess maternal volume homoeostasis clinically during pregnancy. Typical clinical signs used in nonpregnant women, such as oedema, are of little value in assessing volume homoeostasis during pregnancy. For this reason, the haematocrit should be measured in women with underlying CKD as part of the full blood count at the initial first-trimester visit, together with serum albumin. Both measures should fall slightly as pregnancy progresses. A rise in either value strongly suggests intravascular volume contraction, although there is no discriminant value above which it is certain that volume depletion is definite.[56] Conversely, a significant fall in either value does not necessarily mean excessive volume expansion because the haematocrit depends on other factors, such as the ability to maintain adequate red cell production, and serum albumin may fall in patients with nephrotic syndrome who in turn may have reduced intravascular volume. In practice, even if volume excess has occurred, provided that there is no respiratory compromise and that blood pressure can be controlled, this is a more favourable situation to preserve maternal renal function and fetal growth than if there is volume depletion.

There are no controlled trials to show whether intravascular volume expansion with intravenous fluids is of benefit or risk in women with underlying renal disease during pregnancy. Studies in pre-eclamptic women have shown no convincing benefit or adverse outcomes,[57] although analyses of women having pulmonary oedema in association with pre-eclampsia generally point towards over-vigorous intravascular fluid replacement. Therefore, when there is concern about fetal growth or deteriorating GFR in women with CKD, it is prudent to check the change in haematocrit and albumin from baseline. If these suggest reduced intravascular volume, then a trial of intravenous normal saline of no more than 1 litre per day under observation in hospital is a reasonable clinical approach, based on first principles alone.

Appropriate use of medications for treatment of renal disease in pregnancy

Specific medications for specific renal diseases and hypertension management are considered in separate chapters. However, this is an important aspect of antenatal care and some general principles apply.

As discussed above, control of blood pressure is imperative to successful pregnancy outcome in women with underlying renal disease. Antihypertensives to avoid include ACE inhibitors and ARBs,[58] in view of their fetal risk, and atenolol, which has been associated with fetal growth restriction.[59] Diuretics are also best avoided but may be necessary in some pregnant women when there is obvious fluid overload.

Cephalosporins, amoxicillin, trimethoprim and nitrofurantoin are safe to use for treatment of urine infection during pregnancy, although trimethoprim can induce hyperkalaemia in some women and is best avoided in the first trimester as it could theoretically antagonise folate. Quinolones and aminoglycosides are best avoided, although gentamicin is sometimes necessary in the presence of severe pyelonephritis with associated systemic sepsis as the benefits of treating the sepsis in this setting outweigh any potential fetal risk of the aminoglycoside.

Recombinant erythropoietin is routinely advocated to correct anaemia during pregnancy in women with chronic renal impairment but it is important to remember that in some women it may worsen blood pressure control[60] and more frequent blood pressure measurement is needed.

The 'usual' immunosuppressive drugs are generally considered safe in the transplant patient[61] and women with lupus nephritis or other connective tissue disorders may also require immunosuppressive drugs during pregnancy. In general, prednisolone, azathioprine, ciclosporin and hydroxychloroquine are safe to use; tacrolimus has been associated with neonatal hyperkalaemia[62] but recent data suggest it is probably safe overall;[4] mycophenolate is associated with embryo toxic effects and cyclophosphamide with congenital abnormalities. Although cyclophosphamide has been used successfully in occasional cases of *de novo* lupus nephritis occurring in pregnancy,[63] this is an extreme situation and should only be done by a nephrologist and after fully explaining the risks to the mother.

The Paris collaborative trial has confirmed that aspirin is of benefit in preventing pre-eclampsia, although approximately 56 women require treatment to prevent one case.[64] Few studies have examined the prophylactic benefit of aspirin in women with underlying renal disease. However, these studies suggest that aspirin reduces the likelihood of developing pre-eclampsia in women with underlying CKD, with the number needed to treat being 9–57 to prevent pre-eclampsia and 42–357 to prevent perinatal death.[65]

The effects of low doses of aspirin, (up to 150 mg/day) on renal function are quite minimal and in general this is a safe approach, particularly for women who have had early-onset severe pre-eclampsia and/or fetal loss. Therefore, women with CKD, including transplant recipients, should receive low-dose aspirin beginning in the first trimester to help optimise maternal and fetal outcomes.

Identification of superimposed pre-eclampsia

Pre-eclampsia is a placental disorder of unknown aetiology that has several predisposing risk factors, one of which is CKD. There appears to be a genetic predisposition and possibly an altered maternal immune adaptation to the pregnancy with resultant changes in oxidative stress, exaggerated inflammatory response of pregnancy and more recently recognised changes in angiogenic factors. The maternal organ systems mostly affected are the kidney, liver and brain with accompanying systemic hypertension and sometimes thrombocytopenia. Decreased fetal blood flow and/or oxygen and nutrient transfer lead to fetal growth restriction and in some cases intrauterine fetal death. The maternal renal effects include a reduction in renal blood flow, increased sodium and uric acid reabsorption, reduced circulating renin and aldosterone concentrations, proteinuria and impaired GFR.[66] Women who begin pregnancy with impaired renal function have an increased risk of developing pre-eclampsia.

It is apparent that the development of superimposed pre-eclampsia in a woman with underlying renal impairment will lead to a worsening of renal function, exaggerated hypertension and proteinuria with risks of nephrotic syndrome, short-term and long-term risks to maternal renal function as well as increased risks for fetal growth restriction, preterm birth and perinatal mortality. However, it is very difficult to diagnose superimposed pre-eclampsia in a woman who begins her pregnancy with renal impairment and/or proteinuria. An increase in blood pressure, decline in GFR or increasing protein excretion can all be due to progression of the underlying renal disorder rather than superimposed pre-eclampsia and, as yet, there is no diagnostic test to distinguish between these two scenarios. However, when these features are accompanied by neurological signs such as hyper-reflexia with clonus or by abnormal liver transaminases or new-onset thrombocytopenia (except in SLE where this may be an autoimmune phenomenon) then it is likely that superimposed pre-eclampsia has developed.

In many ways this is an academic distinction as clinicians caring for women with underlying renal disease should be vigilant for these changes in all cases, leading to increased surveillance not only of the mother but also of fetal wellbeing (see below). The indications for delivery in women with superimposed pre-eclampsia are broadly the same as those in women with progressive underlying renal disease, i.e. inability to control blood pressure, deteriorating GFR with no reversible component, neurological abnormalities, progressively deteriorating thrombocytopenia, increasing liver transaminases or failure of fetal growth.

Therefore, clinicians should not worry too much about distinguishing superimposed pre-eclampsia from progressive underlying renal disease but rather focus on being vigilant throughout pregnancy for any of the above situations that would necessitate delivery.

Assessment of fetal wellbeing

Traditional assessment of fetal wellbeing has depended upon a fetal morphology scan at around 20 weeks of gestation followed by regular ultrasound scans to assess fetal growth and amniotic fluid index as well as Doppler studies of umbilical artery blood flow. The introduction of routine blood tests at 12 weeks of gestation, such as human chorionic gonadotrophin and alpha-fetoprotein, in combination with measurement of placental morphology and uterine artery pulsatility index at 20 weeks of gestation has provided a good negative predictive test for adverse fetal outcome in women with high-risk pregnancies.[67] While these studies are not specific for women with underlying renal disease, these women have high-risk pregnancies and a clinical approach such as this may provide some reassurance to them as they are understandably very concerned about their pregnancy outcomes. The positive and negative predictive values of these tests have yet to be studied in women with primary underlying renal disease.

Pregnancy-associated plasma protein A (PAPP-A) is now recognised as a marker of vascular damage and blood levels decrease after successful renal transplantation but rise as chronic vascular changes occur in the transplant kidney.[68] It has not yet been tested for this role in renal transplant patients during pregnancy but higher levels may signify renal as well as placental abnormality. This is a possible area for future research.

Models of antenatal care

Women with underlying renal disease in pregnancy are best managed jointly by an obstetrician and renal or obstetric medicine physician in conjunction with a specialist midwife. It is imperative that the obstetrician has an understanding of maternal renal disease in pregnancy and that the physician has an understanding of the possible fetal issues which may occur. Ideally, these women's pregnancies are managed through a high-risk pregnancy clinic or a day assessment unit.

An appropriate schedule of visits for these 'at risk' pregnancies is as follows.

- From 12 weeks to 28 weeks of gestation, four-weekly visits to the obstetrician and to the nephrologist should alternate so that the pregnant woman is seen fortnightly.
- Thereafter until delivery, visits to the obstetrician and nephrologist should be fortnightly, alternating so that the pregnant woman is seen weekly.
- Following delivery, routine obstetric review at 6 weeks postpartum is required but nephrology review should occur within the first 4 weeks as impairment of renal function may occur even after delivery in women with underlying renal disease.

Appropriate testing of renal function in these women is as follows.

- During the initial visit at 12 weeks of gestation, tests should be: full blood count (haemoglobin, haematocrit, platelet count), serum creatinine and electrolytes, uric acid, liver function, midstream urine culture and 24 hour urinary protein and creatinine if proteinuria is apparent on dipstick testing. The PCR can be calculated from the 24 hour urine collection and used as a baseline. Fetal surveillance includes measurement of human chorionic gonadotrophin and alpha-fetoprotein together with a nuchal translucency scan.
- Women with baseline normal GFR do not require further blood tests until around 24 weeks of gestation; those with abnormal GFR at baseline require a full blood count, creatinine and electrolytes, liver function and spot urinary PCR every 4 weeks.
- Midstream urine culture should be repeated routinely at approximately 24, 28 and 32–34 weeks of gestation in those at risk of further infections, as highlighted above.
- Fetal assessment in those with impaired GFR and/or heavy proteinuria should include ultrasound for uterine artery pulsatility index and placental morphology at 20 weeks, then for fetal growth, blood flow and amniotic fluid index monthly from 24 weeks of gestation.

Conclusion

Clinicians and pregnant women are limited by the paucity of published guidelines dedicated to the management of renal disease in pregnant women (see www.patient.co.uk/showdoc/40000296/, www.cari.org.au/Pregnancy.pdf or Wiggins and Harvey[69]) and specific guidelines should be developed to assist clinicians and pregnant women in this area.

While these pregnancies are certainly high risk compared with that in a normal pregnant woman, it is important for clinicians to remember that, provided a diligent approach such as that recommended above is taken, the final pregnancy outcome in most cases is successful for both mother and baby. For this reason, it is appropriate that the clinicians managing a pregnant woman with underlying renal disease take a positive approach to the pregnancy, at all times emphasising the need for diligence and assessment for potential complications, but highlighting that the end result in most cases will be good, which will in turn help to relieve some of the stress that accompanies pregnancy for these women.

References

1. Lindheimer MD, Davison JM, Katz AI. The kidney and hypertension in pregnancy: twenty exciting years. *Semin Nephrol* 2001;21:173–89.
2. Jungers P, Chauveau D. Pregnancy in renal disease. *Kidney Int* 1997;52:871–85.
3. Jones DC. Pregnancy complicated by chronic renal disease. *Clin Perinatol* 1997;24:483–96.
4. Hou S. Pregnancy in chronic renal insufficiency and end stage renal disease. *Am J Kidney Dis* 1999;33:235–52.
5. Jungers P, Chauveau D, Choukroun G, Moynot A, Skhiri H, Houillier P, *et al.* Pregnancy in women with impaired renal function. *Clin Nephrol* 1997;47:281–8.
6. Jungers P, Houillier P, Chauveau D, Choukroun G, Moynot A, Skhiri H, *et al.* Pregnancy in women with reflux nephropathy. *Kidney Int* 1996:50:593–9.
7. Jones DC, Hayslett JP. Outcome of pregnancy in women with moderate or severe renal insufficiency. *New Engl J Med* 1996;335:226–32.
8. Lindheimer MD, Katz AS. *Kidney Function and Disease in Pregnancy*. Philadelphia: Lea & Febiger; 1977. p. 146–87.
9. Holley JL, Bernardini J, Quadric KH, Greenberg A, Laifer SA. Pregnancy outcomes in a prospective matched control study of pregnancy and renal disease. *Clin Nephrol* 1996;45:77–82.
10. Imbasciati E, Gregorino G, Cabiddu G, Gammaro L, Ambroso G, Del Giudice A, *et al.* Pregnancy in CKD stages 3 to 5: fetal and maternal outcomes. *Am J Kidney Dis* 2007;49:753–62.
11. Lindheimer MD, Katz AI. Gestation in women with kidney disease: prognosis and management. *Baillieres Clin Obstet Gynaecol* 1994;8:387–404.
12. Lindheimer MD, Greenfeld JP, Davison JM. Renal disorders. In: Barron WM, Lindheimer MD, editors. *Medical Disorders in Pregnancy*. St Louis: Mosby; 2000. p. 39–70.
13. Ramin SM, Vidaeff AC, Yeomans ER, Gilstrap LC. Chronic renal disease in pregnancy. *Obstet Gynecol* 2006;108:1531–9.
14. Gallery EDM, Brown MA. Volume homeostasis in normal and hypertensive human pregnancy. *Baillieres Clin Obstet Gynaecol* 1987;1:835–51.
15. Chakravarty EF, Colon I, Langen ES, Nix DA, El-Sayed YY, Genovese MC, *et al.* Factors that predict prematurity and preeclampsia in pregnancies. *Am J Obstet Gynecol* 2005;192:1897–904.
16. O'Brien E, Petrie J, Littler W, de Swiet M, Padfield PL, O'Malley K, *et al.* The British Hypertension Society Protocol for the elevation of automated and semi-automated blood pressure measuring devices with special reference to ambulatory systems. *J Hypertens* 1990;8:607–19.
17. White WB, Berson AS, Robbins C, Jamieson MJ, Prisant LM, Roccella E, *et al.* National standard for measurement of resting and ambulatory blood pressure with automated sphygmomanometers. *Hypertension* 1993;21: 504–9.
18. Brown MA, Buddle ML, Farrell TJ, Davis G, Jones M. Randomised trial of management of hypertensive pregnancies by Korotkoff phase IV or phase V. *Lancet* 1998;352:777–81.
19. Cooper WO, Hernandez-Diaz S, Arbogast PG, Dudley JA, Dyer S, Gideon PS, *et al.* Major congenital malformations after first-trimester exposure to ACE inhibitors. *New Engl J Med* 2006;354:2443–51.
20. Serreau R, Luton D, Macher MA, Delezoide AL, Garel C, Jacqz-Aigrain E. Developmental toxicity of the angiotensin II type 1 receptor antagonists during human pregnancy: a report of 10 cases. *BJOG* 2005;112:710–12.
21. Galdo T, Gonzalez F, Espinoza M, Quintero N, Espinoza O, Herrera S, *et al.* Impact of pregnancy on the function of transplanted kidneys. *Transplant Proc* 2005;37:1577–9.

22. Davison JM, Noble MCB. Serial changes in 24 hour creatinine clearance during normal menstrual cycles and the first trimester of pregnancy. *Br J Obstet Gynaecol* 1981;88:10–17.
23. Akbari A, Lepage N, Keely E, Clark HD, Jaffey J, MacKinnon M, *et al.* Cystatin C and beta trace protein as markers of renal function in pregnancy. *BJOG* 2005;112:575–8.
24. Moodley J, Gangaram R, Khanyile R, Ojwang PJ. Serum cystatin C for assessment of glomerular filtration rate in hypertensive disorders of pregnancy. *Hypertens Pregnancy* 2004;23:309–17.
25. Ben- Haroush A, Bardin R, Erman A, Hod M, Chen R, Kaplan B, *et al.* Beta2-microglobulin and hypertensive complications in pregnant women at risk. *Clin Nephrol* 2002;58:411–16.
26. Levey AS, Bosch JP, Lewis JB, Greene T, Rogers N, Roth D. A more accurate method to estimate glomerular filtration rate from serum creatinine: a new prediction equation. Modification of Diet in Renal Disease Study Group. *Ann Intern Med* 1999;130:461–70.
27. Smith MC, Moran P, Ward MK, Davison JM. Assessment of glomerular filtration rate in pregnancy using the MDRD formula. *BJOG* 2008;115:109–12.
28. Cockcroft DW, Gault MH. Prediction of creatinine clearance from serum creatinine. *Nephron* 1976;16:31–41.
29. Roberts M, Lindheimer MD, Davison JM. Altered glomerular permselectivity to neutral dextrans and heteroporous membrane modelling in human pregnancy. *Am J Physiol* 1996;270:F338–43.
30. Milne JE, Lindheimer MD, Davison JM. Glomerular heteroporous membrane modelling in third trimester and post-partum before and during amino acid infusion. *Am J Physiol Renal Physiol* 2002:282:F170–5.
31. Levine RJ, Lam C, Qian C, Yu KF, Maynard SE, Sachs BP, *et al.* Soluble endoglin and other circulating antiangiogenic factors in preeclampsia. *New Engl J Med* 2006;355:992–1005.
32. Baumwell S, Karumanchi SA. Pre-eclampsia: clinical manifestations and molecular mechanisms. *Nephron* 2007;106:c72–81.
33. Lane C, Brown M, Dunsmuir W, Kelly J, Mangos G. Can spot urine protein/creatinine ratio replace 24 h urine protein in usual clinical nephrology? *Nephrology (Carlton)* 2006;11:245–9.
34. Gangaram R, Ojwang PJ, Moodley J, Maharaj D. The accuracy of urine dipsticks as a screening test for proteiuria in hypertensive disorders of pregnancy. *Hypertens Pregnancy* 2005;24: 117–23.
35. Phelan LK, Brown MA, Davis GK, Mangos G. A prospective study of the impact of automated dipstick urinalysis on the diagnosis of pre-eclampsia. *Hypertens Pregnancy* 2004;23:135–2.
36. Cote AM, Brown MA, Lam EM, von Dadelzen P, Firoz T, Liston RM, Magee LA. The urinary spot protein/creatinine ratio is a reasonable diagnostic test for proteinuria in hypertensive pregnancy: A systematic review. *BMJ* (in press).
37. Khandelwal M, Kumanova M, Gaughan JP, Reece EA. Role of diltiazem in pregnant women with chronic renal disease. *J Matern Fetal Neonatal Med* 2002;12:408–12.
38. Airoldi J, Weinstein L. Clinical significance of proteinuria in pregnancy. *Obstet Gynecol Surv* 2007;62:117–24.
39. Newman MG, Robichaux AG, Stedman CM, Jaekle RK, Fontenot MT, Dotson T, *et al.* Perinatal outcomes in preeclampsia that is complicated by massive proteinuria. *Am J Obstet Gynecol* 2003;188:264–8.
40. Chan P, Brown MA, Simpson JM, Davis G. Proteinuria in pre-eclampsia: how much matters? *BJOG* 2005;112:280–5.
41. Basgul A, Kavak ZN, Sezen D, Basgul A, Gokaslan H, Cakalagaoglu F. A fare case of early onset nephrotic syndrome in pregnancy. *Clin Exp Obstet Gynecol* 2006;33:127–8.
42. Bar J, Kaplan B, Wittenberg C, Erman A, Boner G, Ben-Rafael Z, *et al.* Microalbuminuria after pregnancy complicated by pre-eclampsia. *Nephrol Dial Transplant* 1999;14:1129–32.
43. Ronkainen J, Ala-Houhala M, Autio-Harmainen H, Jahnukainen T, Koskimies O, Merenmies J, *et al.* Long-term outcome 19 years after childhood IgA nephritis: a retrospective cohort study. *Pediatr Nephrol* 2006;21:1266–73.
44. Germain S, Nelson-Piercy C. Lupus nephritis and renal disease in pregnancy. *Lupus* 2006;15:148–55.
45. Simmonds HA, Cameron JS, Goldsmith DJ, Fairbanks LD, Raman GV. Familial juvenile hyperuricaemic nephropathy is not a rare genetic metabolic purine disease in Britain. *Nucleosides Nucleotides Nucleic Acids* 2006;25:1071–5.

46. Akbari A, Wilkes P, Lindheimer M, Lepage N, Filler G. Reference intervals for anion gap and strong ion difference in pregnancy: a pilot study. *Hypertens Pregnancy* 2007;26:111–119.
47. Brown MA, Wang M-X, Buddle ML, Calton MA, Cario GM, Zammit VC, *et al.* Albumin excretory rate in normal and hypertensive pregnancy. *Clin Sci* 1994;86:251–5.
48. Brown MA, Sinosich MJ, Saunders DM, Gallery EDM. Potassium regulation and progesterone aldosterone interrelationships in human pregnancy: a prospective study. *Am J Obstet Gynecol* 1986;155:349–53.
49. Davison JM, Sheills EA, Philips PR, Lindheimer MD. Serial evaluation of vasopressin release and thirst in human pregnancy. Role of human chorionic gonadotrophin in the osmoregulatory changes of gestation. *J Clin Invest* 1988;81:789–806.
50. Rowe TF, Magee K, Cunningham FG. Pregnancy and renal tubular acidosis. *Am J Perinatol* 1999;16:189–91.
51. Kang DH, Finch J, Nakagawa T, Karumanchi SA, Kanellis J, Granger J, *et al.* Uric acid, endothelial dysfunction and pre-eclamisia: searching for a pathogenetic link. *J Hypertension* 2004;22:229–35.
52. Schackis RC. Hyperuricaemia and preeclampsia: is there a pathogenic link? *Med Hypotheses* 2004;63:239–44.
53. Trevisan G, Ramos JG, Martins-Costa S, Barros EJ. Pregnancy in patients with chronic renal insufficiency at Hospital de Clinicas of Porto Alegre, Brazil. *Ren Fail* 2004;26:29–34.
54. Schwartz MA, Wang CC, Eckert LO, Critchlow CW. Risk factors for urinary tract infection in the post-partum period. *Am J Obstet Gynecol* 1999;181:547–53.
55. Bukowski TP, Betrus GG, Aquilina JW, Perimutter AD. Urinary tract infections and pregnancy in women who underwent antireflux surgery in childhood. *J Urol* 1998;159:1286–9.
56. Brown MA, Zammit VC, Mitar DM. Extracellular fluid volumes in pregnancy-induced hypertension. *J Hypertens* 1992;10:61–8.
57. Duley L, Williams J, Henderson-Smart DJ. Plasma volume expansion for treatment of pre-eclampsia. *Cochrane Database Syst Rev* 1999;(4):CD001805.
58. Bass JK, Faix RG. Gestational therapy with an angiotensin II receptor antagonist and transient renal failure in a premature infant. *Am J Perinatol* 2006;23:313–17.
59. Podymow T, August P. Hypertension in pregnancy. *Adv Chronic Kidney Dis* 2007;14:178–90.
60. Kashiwagi M, Breymann C, Huch R, Huch A. Hypertension in a pregnancy with renal anemia after recombinant human erythropoietin (rhEPO) therapy. *Arch Gynecol Obstet* 2002;267:54–6.
61. Bar J, Stahl B, Hod M, Wittenberg C, Pardo J, Merlob P. Is immunosuppression therapy in renal allograft recipients teratogenic: A single-center experience. *Am J Med Genet* 2003;116:31–6.
62. Jain A, Venkataramanan R, Fung JJ, Gartner JC, Lever J, Balan V. *et al.* Pregnancy after liver transplantation under tacrolimus. *Transplantation* 1997;64:559–65.
63. Kart Koseoglu H, Yucel AE, Kunefeci G, Ozdemir FN, Duran H. Cyclophosphamide therapy in a serious case of lupus nephritis during pregnancy. *Lupus* 2001;10: 818–20.
64. Askie LM, Duley L, Henderson-Smart DJ, Stewart LA, PARIS Collaborative Group. Antiplatelet agents for prevention of pre-eclampsia: a meta-analysis of individual patient data. *Lancet* 2007;369:1791–8.
65. Coomarasamy A, Honest H, Papaioannou S, Gee H, Khan KS. Aspirin for prevention of pre-eclampsia in women with historical risk factors: a systematic review. *Obstet Gynecol* 2003;101:1319–32.
66. Brown MA, Whitworth JA. The kidney in hypertensive pregnancies – victim and villain. *Am J Kidney Dis* 1992;20:427–42.
67. Toal M, Chan C, Fallah S, Alkazaleh F, Chaddha V, Windrim RC, *et al.* Usefulness of a placental profile in high-risk pregnancies. *Am J Obstet Gynecol* 2007;196:363.e1–7.
68. Kalousova M, Bartosova K, Zima T, Skibova J, Teplan V, Viklicky O. Pregnancy-associated plasma protein A and soluble receptor for advanced glycation end products after kidney transplantation. *Kidney Blood Press Res* 2007;30: 31–7.
69. Wiggins KL, Harvey KS. A review of guidelines for nutrition care of renal patients. *J Ren Nutr* 2002;12:190–6.

Chapter 4
Midwifery issues

Kylie Watson

Introduction

Do midwives have a defined role and responsibility in the provision of care for women with a high-risk diagnosis such as renal disease in pregnancy? And if they do have a distinct role, then what is it? All women need a midwife, some will need doctors too, and this has been highlighted as a guiding principle for modern maternity services in the recently published *Maternity Matters*.[1] The role of the midwife has its traditions in care for women and infants experiencing normal pregnancy and birth and detecting deviations from this; however, the role of the midwife is increasingly changing and adapting to new ways of working.[2] No matter how complicated or high risk a pregnancy is deemed to be, the distinct and unique contribution that midwifery can make to the care of these women in the childbirth continuum cannot be overestimated.

This chapter focuses on midwifery issues in caring for women with renal disease in pregnancy and includes topics on perceptions and definitions of risk, defining 'normal', continuity of care, women's and midwives' experiences, and the distinct role that midwifery has. A brief case study will also be used to examine the midwifery role. Many of the discussions in this chapter are not only relevant to care of women with renal disease in pregnancy but may extend to care of all women experiencing high-risk pregnancies.

The label of 'risk'

The majority of women with pre-existing or antenatally identified renal disease are likely to be viewed as high risk and their care will be managed accordingly, often under the responsibility of an obstetrician and/or physician and with many more visits to the antenatal clinic and robust care plans formulated. For some women this will be a comfort – their care is managed, someone else is in control of their pregnancy and responsibility can be handed over to the medical experts. This may be particularly pertinent for women who have had difficulty conceiving or who have previously lost a pregnancy. For others, this label will add to stress and anxiety about the pregnancy and also about the unborn baby. Loss of control in decision making can also be frightening and lead to feelings of powerlessness and inadequacy as a woman and mother-to-be.[3] It is not surprising that women with complicated pregnancies may view their risks as higher than those without,[4] but the perception and level of this risk may not always be congruent with that of the health professionals providing the care.[4,5]

Most women experience some level of anxiety and uncertainty about a pregnancy and need to be given space and freedom to articulate this and for these feelings to be viewed as a normal part of the childbearing process. For women experiencing pregnancies labelled as high risk, the elevated levels of anxiety and concern also need to be considered with all professionals providing care, in order that both the perceived and the real levels of risk are clear and defined. The challenge for midwifery is to help the woman, and those around her, focus on the normal aspects of her pregnancy among this mêlée of uncertainly and anxiety. This in turn can lead to empowerment of the woman and her abilities to achieve the best outcome for her and her baby alongside and in partnership with the professionals caring for her.

What is 'normal'?

The Royal College of Midwives defines normal childbirth as one where a woman commences, continues and completes labour physiologically at term.[6] Midwives are viewed as the experts and guardians of this process. For women with renal disease in pregnancy, and indeed any other medical condition that deems them high risk, their pregnancy may involve increased fetal surveillance, medication and antenatal hospitalisation.[7] They may be induced or have a preterm birth, and are more susceptible to the cascades of medical intervention their diagnosis prescribes. However, all women will have normal needs that can only be met by a midwife. The role of the midwife in caring for women in these situations is to focus on the normal experiences that can exist for each woman and indeed that exist in each pregnancy whether high risk or not. These may include a focus on normal physiological changes in pregnancy, normal fetal growth and movement, preparing for the baby and breastfeeding, and discussions about expectations and realities for labour and birth that may increase chances of a vaginal birth without unnecessary interventions. The definitions and the goalposts of what is normal may change for women and midwives caring for them. A fluidity surrounding what is normal and what is not may evolve. There is some evidence that midwives who have sound knowledge and clinical experience surrounding medical complications in childbirth are able to raise the limit for what they consider normal without compromising safety or the recognition of acute situations.[8]

Continuity of care

Continuity of care (in this instance also including continuity of carer, one-to-one midwifery concepts and caseload midwifery) may be defined as 'a continuing relationship that allows the woman and her midwife to get to know each other and develop a relationship of trust over time'[9] generally involving care for pregnancy, labour and birth, and the postnatal period. Much has been written about this concept.[10–14] A Cochrane review by Hodnett[14] stated that there were clear benefits to be found for women from continuity of care. These benefits included reduced antenatal admissions, fewer drugs for pain relief in labour and increased attendance at antenatal classes. Of interest is that it was not clear from the Cochrane review whether the benefits were due to greater continuity of care or to midwifery care. Continuity of care from medical providers may also confer great benefit. The intricacies of caseload midwifery have also been explored and clear benefits identified.[15,16] For women with renal disease in pregnancy or experiencing high-risk pregnancies, the many advantages of continuity of midwifery care should be made available to them and this is an area that needs further investigation and research. The development of specialist midwife posts or specialist midwife caseloading teams that can provide continuity of care for women experiencing high-risk pregnancies should be encouraged and may lead to reduced anxiety and stress for women[17] as well as improved outcomes.

Women's and midwives' experiences

While very little literature exists specifically on the experiences of women with renal disease in pregnancy, there is a small amount of literature surrounding women's and midwives' experiences of high-risk and complicated pregnancies.[3,8,18] Women labelled as high risk often have the same needs and expectations of midwifery care as other women. In a phenomenological study of women's experiences of complicated childbirth, Berg and Dahlberg[18] identified several themes surrounding the women's experiences. Women expressed a desire to be recognised, seen and respected as a unique individual; a requirement that surely every woman entering a pregnancy deserves and should receive. For those experiencing a high-risk pregnancy, such as those with renal disease, there may be a tendency, however, to focus primarily on the disease and its process rather than on the woman who has the medical problem. When encountering several practitioners over the course of a pregnancy and birth, there may also be the risk of women feeling like part of the institution rather than as a distinct individual. This is where midwifery input is crucial and time can be given to the woman to focus on everything else *but* the medical condition: to focus on her as a pregnant woman. Other themes identified as important to the women in this study were trust and confidence in caregivers, sincere verbal communication and dialogue, and having control over the situation. By having a degree of control, even if this means making the decision to relinquish control to a health practitioner, the resultant feeling of shared responsibility may lead to enhanced feelings of capability and self-esteem.

The views of midwives caring for women at high obstetric risk or who have obstetric complications have also been explored.[8] For midwives in Berg and Dahlberg's work,[8] the essence of their midwifery care for women experiencing high-risk pregnancies was described as 'a struggle for the natural process'. With most midwives' expertise being centred on the normal process, there can be difficulties in focusing on this in a complicated pregnancy as the need to be continually aware of the medical and obstetric interventions can override autonomous decision making. This leads to midwives seeking to find a balance between medical and midwifery models of care ensuring the woman is at the centre of the process and that professional autonomy is maintained. Some may argue that midwives working with high-risk women experience a marginalisation of their role[8] and relinquish some of their professional autonomy to medical colleagues, in effect becoming obstetric handmaidens.[19] There are several reasons why this is not true. There are degrees of professional autonomy that exist for midwives depending on individual circumstances, the environment the midwife is working in and the degree of autonomy the midwife chooses to exercise.[20] However, the key to midwives acting as autonomous practitioners lies in the Nursing and Midwifery Council Code of Professional Conduct, which states that midwives are personally accountable for their practice.[21] In essence this means that every decision to act that a midwife makes is made within the context of her own sphere and boundaries of professional activity. In addition, advice given by others, including medical colleagues, can be accepted or rejected as midwives are ultimately accountable for the care that they provide.[22] Bromley[20] identifies three ways in which professional autonomy can be maintained for midwives providing care for women experiencing high-risk pregnancies, including those with renal disease. These are:

1. having a firm grounding in normal midwifery and recognising normal physiological processes within obstetric complications
2. contributing to unit guidelines, policies and procedures
3. taking part in education that increases knowledge surrounding obstetric and medical complications.

By having a thorough knowledge of the medical and obstetric process, midwives' own feeling of security and safety increases thus allowing a focus on normal processes and giving confidence to challenge non-evidence-based and unnecessary interventions.[3,8] Increased knowledge will also foster mutual respect between members of the multidisciplinary team and contribute to positive and collaborative working relationships.

The role of the midwife

The following aspects of care can be viewed as essential to the midwifery role in caring for women with renal disease in pregnancy as well as those experiencing other high-risk medical conditions. Some of these aspects are not mutually exclusive and there may be some overlap with care provided by other members of the multidisciplinary team.

Promoting normality in situations that allow it

Midwifery expertise lies in the normal physiological processes of pregnancy and childbirth that exist for all women, no matter how complicated their pregnancy. By promoting and fostering normality in appropriate situations, the midwives can enhance the childbearing woman's confidence in her own abilities as a woman and mother-to-be, and inappropriate interventions can be avoided. Midwifery time in the antenatal period can be spent on nonmedical issues that may include facilitating antenatal education, discussing infant feeding and ensuring support networks are in place following the birth. Many women with severe renal disease may enter a pregnancy assuming that they will need to have a caesarean section and may be surprised when this is not the case. Antenatal education is crucial in ensuring that women are prepared for labour and birth, particularly if this is not what they had envisaged initially. Intrapartum care can incorporate tenets of active birth such as supporting non-pharmacological pain-relief methods, adopting mobile and upright positions even when there is a need for continuous fetal monitoring, and ensuring the birth environment contributes to fostering normal processes. This may include creating a home-like environment with the use of dim lighting, beanbags and birthing balls, ensuring that maintaining privacy is of utmost importance, and ensuring that unnecessary interruptions and interventions are avoided.

Promoting women's autonomy

Government reports including the *National Service Framework*[23] and *Maternity Matters*[1] highlight the need and importance for women to have real choice in their care and to be involved in decision making about all aspects of care. Midwives also have a statutory requirement and professional responsibility to promote women's autonomy.[21,24] This may be more difficult to protect in the high-risk or emergency setting, but it is the responsibility of the midwife to ensure that women are making informed decisions about the care provided.

Interpreting the medical picture

Midwifery skill can often lie in the ability to interpret complex situations and explain procedures and concepts in lay terms. Midwives may be more readily accessed than their medical colleagues and are often the first port of call for women who have questions about their care.

Acting as an advocate

One of the guiding principles in midwifery practice is to act as an advocate for women. For women who have a disability or communication difficulties, advocacy skills may be required to a greater extent. For some women with severe renal disease or other high-risk complications, their vulnerability increases and autonomy decreases[20] and a midwife acting as an advocate can be essential. Practising midwifery within an obstetric framework is not always easy though and Warriner[25] speaks of midwives being forced into the role of arbitrator rather than advocate – struggling to find balance between personal and institutional policy. The midwifery role as an advocate for women, both individually and as a group, needs to be supported.

Recognising and dealing with social and emotional needs

For midwives this may simply mean spending time with women listening to their anxieties and concerns. For women admitted to antenatal wards for prolonged periods of time, the constant support and presence of a known midwife can be invaluable.

Facilitating communication between all members of the multidisciplinary team

Women with renal disease will often have a large number of practitioners involved in their care. If the woman is to be placed at the centre of this care, communication between all members is paramount. Midwives can often be the link between the woman and other members of the team and ensure all are kept informed of current situations.

Promoting and facilitating breastfeeding where possible

It is widely accepted that breast milk is the best form of nutrition for newborns and the World Health Organization recommends exclusive breastfeeding for 6 months with introduction of complementary foods and continued breastfeeding thereafter.[26] For women with significant renal disease or those who may have a complicated drug therapy regimen following renal transplant, the risks to the newborn, particularly from immunosuppressants, should be weighed against the significant benefits of breastfeeding. Indeed for women with renal disease who are more likely to deliver preterm, the protective effects of breastfeeding against infections such as gastroenteritis should be discussed. There is a small amount of recent literature in the area of immunosuppressants and breastfeeding.[27,28] Midwives can ensure that women have access to the up-to-date literature and are given the opportunity to speak to neonatologists or other health professionals that can advise accordingly on an individual basis. If breastfeeding is not possible then the benefits of skin-to-skin contact following birth and other bonding-promoting activities can be encouraged.

Case study

The following case study illustrates how a midwifery role may function within a multidisciplinary team. Only brief medical details have been included.

Woman A was a 22-year-old white Mediterranean primigravida with an unplanned pregnancy. She lived with her partner and was a non-smoker.

Her medical history was of end-stage renal failure secondary to antineutrophil cytoplasmic antibody (ANCA)-positive vasculitis. She received a cadaveric renal transplant in 1996. She had stable graft function with a serum creatinine of 110–130 μmol/l. She had been a poor attender for follow-up prior to pregnancy. She also had asthma. She was taking the following medication: prednisolone 5 mg daily, azathioprine 75 mg daily and ciclosporin 100 mg daily.

Booking was completed at 10 weeks of gestation by a midwife. A full history was taken and the plan of care for pregnancy discussed, which included making the woman aware of all names of members in the multidisciplinary team, expected frequency of visits and scans. The 24 hour contact details for the midwifery team were given. The woman had the following appointments:

- 12 weeks – obstetric consultant/physician appointment
- 16 weeks – midwifery visit
- 18 weeks – renal consultant appointment
- 21 weeks – obstetric consultant/physician appointment.

The woman was seen every fortnight, with alternating visits between midwife and consultant. She booked to attend antenatal classes starting at 32 weeks, and infant feeding was discussed.

At 30 weeks she was admitted to the antenatal ward for investigation of rising creatinine (207 μmol/l). She was seen daily by the renal team, on-call obstetric consultants and midwives known to the woman. The midwife facilitated attendance at an antenatal education day workshop as an inpatient. She was seen by a neonatologist to discuss preterm delivery risks and breastfeeding.

The woman remained normotensive and non-proteinuric, but was given three pulses of 1 g methylprednisolone for presumed rejection. She was discharged 2 weeks after admission when the serum creatinine had stabilised.

She received continued antenatal care from midwives and consultants until 36 weeks and 4 days. The birth plan was discussed at length with midwives after a decision was made to aim for vaginal birth.

Membranes spontaneously ruptured at 36 weeks and 4 days. She was admitted for augmentation. The plan from the medical team was for oxytocin but once the midwife had examined the woman and found that the cervix was unfavourable she discussed with the obstetrician whether 2 mg prostaglandin could be given instead. Prostaglandin was given, and then oxytocin and an epidural (at the woman's request) were given 6 hours later. In labour the woman received care from midwives known to her.

The woman had a normal vaginal birth of a live female infant weighing 2040 g. Mother and baby were discharged on day 3 with the baby fully breastfed. She was visited at home by known midwives and follow-up appointments for mother and infant were arranged and communicated to the woman by the midwife.

Conclusion

This chapter has outlined the distinct role that midwives have in caring for women with renal disease in pregnancy. The label of 'risk' has been discussed as has the concept of 'normal'. Several components of the role of the midwife in caring for women with renal disease in pregnancy have been identified. Midwifery has its foundations in the normal birth process but the profession's expertise is crucial in the multidisciplinary care of women with renal disease in pregnancy. Midwifery skills are unique and essential in ensuring women get the best possible care. Focusing on the woman as an individual and increasing confidence in her abilities as a woman and her impending role as a mother will lead to improved outcomes for all.

References

1. Department of Health. *Maternity Matters: Choice, Access and Continuity of Care in a Safe Service.* London: Department of Health; 2007.
2. Royal College of Midwives. *Refocusing the Role of the Midwife: Position Statement.* London: Royal College of Midwives; 2006.
3. Berg M. A midwifery model of care for childbearing women at high risk: genuine caring in caring for the genuine. *J Perinat Educ* 2005;14:9–21.
4. Gupton A, Heaman M, Cheung LW. Complicated and uncomplicated pregnancies: women's perception of risk. *J Obstet Gynecol Neonatal Nurs* 2001;30:192–201.
5. Lindsay P. Creating normality in a high-risk pregnancy. *Pract Midwife* 2006;9:16–19.
6. Royal College of Midwives. *Normal Childbirth: Position Statement.* London: Royal College of Midwives; 2004.
7. Germain S, Nelson-Piercy C. Lupus nephritis and renal disease in pregnancy. *Lupus* 2006;15:148–55.
8. Berg M, Dahlberg K. Swedish midwives' care of women who are at high obstetric risk or who have obstetric complications. *Midwifery* 2001;17:259–66.
9. Page L. One-to-one midwifery: restoring the 'with woman' relationship in midwifery. *J Midwifery Womens Health* 2003;48:119–25.
10. Warren C. Exploring the value of midwifery continuity of carer. *B J Midwifery* 2003;11:S34–7.
11. Saultz J. Defining and measuring interpersonal continuity of care. *Ann Fam Med* 2003;1:134–43.
12. Haggerty JL, Reid RJ, Freeman GK, Starfield BH, Adair CE, McKendry RM. Continuity of care: a multidisciplinary review. *Br Med J* 2003;327:1219–21.
13. Sandall J. Choice, continuity and control: changing midwifery, towards a sociological perspective. *Midwifery* 1995;11:201–9.
14. Hodnett ED. Continuity of caregivers for care during pregnancy and childbirth. *Cochrane Database Syst Rev* 2002;(1):CD000062.
15. North Staffordshire Changing Childbirth Research Team. A randomised study of midwifery caseload care and traditional 'shared-care'. *Midwifery* 2000:16:295–302.
16. Benjamin Y, Walsh D, Taub N. A comparison of partnership caseload midwifery care with conventional team midwifery care: labour and birth outcomes. *Midwifery* 2001;17:234–40.
17. Homer C, Farrell T, Davis G, Brown M. Women's worry in the antenatal period. *Br J Midwifery* 2002;10:356–60.
18. Berg M, Dahlberg K. A phenomenological study of women's experiences of complicated childbirth. *Midwifery* 1998;14:23–9.
19. Livingston C. High-risk pregnancies. *Br J Midwifery* 2004;12:744.
20. Bromley A. Autonomous practice: a critical investigation. In: Billington M, Stevenson M, editors. *Critical Care in Childbearing for Midwives.* Oxford: Blackwell Publishing; 2007. p. 19–29.
21. Nursing and Midwifery Council. *The NMC Code of Professional Conduct: Standards for Conduct, Performance and Ethics.* London: NMC; 2004.
22. Marshall JE. Autonomy and the midwife. In: Raynor MD, Marshall JE, Sullivan A, editors. *Decision Making in Midwifery Practice.* Edinburgh: Churchill Livingston; 2005.

23. Department of Health. *National Service Framework for Children, Young People and Maternity Services.* London: Department of Health; 2004.
24. Nursing and Midwifery Council. *Midwives Rules and Standards.* London: NMC; 2004.
25. Warriner S. Midwives: advocates or arbitrators? *Br J Midwifery* 2003;11:532–3.
26. World Health Organization. *The Optimal Duration of Exclusive Breastfeeding: Report of and Expert Consultation.* Geneva: WHO; 2002.
27. Sau A, Clarke S, Bass J, Kaiser A, Nelson-Piercy C. Azathioprine and breastfeeding: is it safe? *BJOG* 2007;114;498–501.
28. Gardiner SJ, Begg EJ. Breastfeeding during tacrolimus therapy. *Obstet Gynecol* 2006;107(2 Pt 2):453–5.

5

Chapter 5

Postpartum follow-up of antenatally identified renal problems

Liz Lightstone

Introduction

Some renal problems are more likely to be diagnosed in pregnancy than others. Urinary abnormalities will almost always be detected as a result of the near universal application of urinary dipstick testing throughout pregnancy. Renal dysfunction without associated urine abnormalities may be less likely to be diagnosed as the biochemical profile is not part of routine booking blood work. However, serum creatinine is usually measured in women who present with urine abnormalities, hypertension/pre-eclampsia and/or recurrent urine infections as well as unexplained severe anaemia. Thus pregnancy provides an opportunity to identify women with hitherto undiagnosed or new-onset kidney problems. How these women should be followed up postpartum depends on the presentation and the severity.

There are some basic principles that should be followed. All women found to have a renal problem need to have a renal diagnosis made, ideally during pregnancy but certainly postpartum where that is not practical. For instance, during pregnancy this may be a simple matter of the woman having a renal ultrasound that demonstrates scarred kidneys from recurrent urinary tract infections (UTIs) and hypertension, confirming the diagnosis of reflux nephropathy. In other circumstances diagnosis might not be confirmed during pregnancy because of the requirement for tests that pose an unacceptable risk to the mother or baby, for example certain forms of imaging. A woman who presents with modest proteinuria in early pregnancy with no hypertension, with normal function and with no markers of systemic disease would not warrant a renal biopsy during pregnancy as diagnosis will not alter management. However, if the proteinuria persists postpartum, then she may well merit biopsy to determine diagnosis and prognosis, not least for future pregnancies.

So all women found to have a kidney problem during pregnancy need to be made aware of the need for postpartum diagnostic tests and follow-up. They need to be advised of its significance, which in turn depends on the diagnosis, the stage of kidney disease and the level of associated hypertension and/or proteinuria. Follow-up plans should be made well before delivery when events may overtake the woman and the need for postpartum follow-up may be overlooked.

Follow-up plans

All women with *de novo* renal disease should be followed up at least once postpartum in order to:

- evaluate baseline proteinuria and function when not pregnant
- ensure appropriate diagnostic tests are requested
- most importantly, ensure a proper care pathway is identified that is clear both to the woman and to her primary care physician.

This first follow-up appointment would normally be with a nephrologist or an experienced obstetric physician able to make a suitable diagnostic and prognostic evaluation. Importantly, medications can be reviewed and optimised with respect to renoprotection, especially institution of therapy with angiotensin-converting enzyme (ACE) inhibitors or angiotensin II receptor blockers (ARBs).

The scenario to be avoided is that of a woman who presents with end stage renal failure and who volunteers that she was noted to have hypertension and proteinuria in each of her pregnancies a few years previously but was never seen postpartum nor advised that she had significant kidney disease or that she needed any follow-up. It is always tragic to consider that she may have had preventable renal failure and at the very least missed opportunities for risk factor management and pre-emptive transplantation.

Who should follow up the woman?

A nephrologist should be the first port of call postpartum for all women with significant proteinuria (protein/creatinine ratio (PCR) above 100 mg/mmol or 24 hour urine protein above 1 g) that presented early in pregnancy and persists postpartum. Additionally all women with persistent proteinuria after pre-eclampsia need to be evaluated by a nephrologist – the pre-eclampsia may have been the first manifestation of underlying renal disease and, while proteinuria can persist for some months post pre-eclampsia, it is important to monitor its decline to ensure that renal function has returned to normal and that blood pressure is well controlled. Such women do sometimes require a renal biopsy to exclude other causes of proteinuria if the proteinuria does not resolve completely, although in some cases this may take more than 6 months.

All women who are found to have abnormal renal function in pregnancy (and bearing in mind that glomerular filtration rate (GFR) rises and serum creatinine falls significantly in women with normal kidney function during pregnancy) should have their renal function checked soon after delivery and again at 6 weeks postpartum. If the abnormalities persist they too should be referred to a nephrologist. If the renal impairment was clearly associated with severe pre-eclampsia and resolves rapidly postpartum then it may well not be necessary to refer. Conversely, if their renal function was unstable towards the end of pregnancy, for example with a rapid rise in creatinine or proteinuria, then the woman should be seen and assessed very soon postpartum and again within 2 weeks. Women can lose all their renal function in a matter of weeks after delivery in certain conditions, particularly where serum creatinine was already significantly raised, and a blanket policy of seeing everyone 6 weeks postpartum will miss such women.[1] Similarly, delivery may have been expedited to allow safe renal biopsy and diagnosis in a woman suspected of having active nephritis, such as that associated with systemic lupus erythematosus (SLE). These women need to be aware before delivery that the nephrologists wish to expedite a diagnosis as soon as is practical and safe postpartum. The key is not letting the woman disappear back into the community before follow-up plans have been established, documented and communicated to the woman, her family and all relevant medical and nursing personnel. It is often difficult to persuade a mother who perhaps has a vulnerable preterm baby that she also needs to be looked after and investigated. However, it is important to do so.

In other settings it is reasonable to refer women back to their GPs for continuing care but with advice about monitoring and referring to clinical practice guidelines.[2–4] These women would include those found to have minimal proteinuria or isolated microscopic haematuria and to have normal or mildly elevated blood pressure and impaired renal function, i.e. stage 1 and 2 chronic kidney disease (CKD). These women should have a renal ultrasound scan to exclude structural abnormalities (and indeed are likely to have had this done in pregnancy) and to have postpartum assessments of proteinuria, haematuria and renal function. Similarly, women found to have anatomical evidence of reflux nephropathy (scarred/dysplastic kidneys) and recurrent UTIs but with normal or mildly impaired function can be monitored by their GPs. These women need to be advised that they have kidney abnormalities which put them at higher risk of developing high blood pressure and possibly cardiovascular disease.[3,4] They should be advised to stop smoking as it is an independent risk factor for progression of kidney disease regardless of contributing to cardiovascular risk. Regular follow-up by their GP is needed to review their blood pressure, kidney function and urine dipstick abnormalities. The threshold for treating their blood pressure would be lower than in women with normal kidney function. Many women who had normal blood pressure prepregnancy can develop sustained hypertension during pregnancy and postpartum. The two most important determinants of progression of kidney failure, regardless of underlying disease, are blood pressure control and degree of proteinuria. Thus women need to be advised of the importance of monitoring and treating proteinuria and hypertension – if both are present, the ideal first-line agent would be an ACE inhibitor or an ARB. The need for follow-up should be explained to GPs at the time of discharge from obstetric follow-up. Importantly, it is also worth giving some guidance as to when referral back to a nephrologist would be warranted. This would be if proteinuria rises significantly, renal function deteriorates or hypertension becomes difficult to manage.

Some women who are found to have kidney disease in pregnancy might also be under the care of other hospital physicians for long-term conditions. The most notable of these is diabetes. Diabetic nephropathy is now the most common cause of renal failure in the UK and is rising rapidly owing to the epidemic of type 2 diabetes. Some women will present with type 2 diabetes for the first time in pregnancy and they may already have complications such as retinopathy and nephropathy. It is imperative that such women are firmly embedded in a good diabetic care pathway postpartum to slow their progression to end stage.[5] Furthermore, the physicians looking after their diabetes need to be aware of changes in their renal state during pregnancy as risk factor management will need optimising postpartum. Women with type 1 diabetes are likely to be under the care of a diabetic service already but may have been lost to follow-up during adolescence. Postpartum reassessment allows the opportunity to ensure continuing follow-up.

Women with a connective tissue disease may have had a renal flare for the first time in pregnancy and need long-term renal follow-up. Close communication with their rheumatologist or GP will be required postpartum and immunosuppression will need to be reviewed and optimised. These women need to be kept under close surveillance postpartum as they can flare and progress rapidly. They are often reluctant to start immunosuppression during pregnancy or when breastfeeding. It is important that the diagnosis is confirmed with a renal biopsy and clear discussions are held at an early stage postpartum about the risks of not treating active nephritis.[6]

Newly diagnosed kidney disease with a heritable component

Women need to be informed not only about how their kidney disease might impact on future pregnancies but also how it might affect their new baby. Many renal diseases have a heritable component and this may be difficult to acknowledge for the first time during pregnancy. Postpartum review allows a full discussion of the implications for the woman and her child. For instance, a woman in her mid-20s may well be unaware she has adult polycystic kidney disease (APKD) – she is likely to have normal function, may have 1+ blood only on urine dipstick and may have no family history. However, she is very likely to develop significant hypertension early on in pregnancy, is at higher risk of pre-eclampsia and, because of minor urine abnormalities, will end up having a renal ultrasound that confirms the diagnosis. It is somewhat shocking to discover one has a heritable renal disease at any time but more so when pregnant. These women need to understand what the disease means for them, the risk it poses to their offspring (a one in two chance of inheriting APKD which is autosomal dominant) and when it is likely to manifest in them (young adulthood at the earliest). Sometimes the discussions are harder – a woman may present with microscopic haematuria but with the history of kidney disease among the men in her family; it is likely she is a carrier for an X-linked condition known as Alport syndrome in which affected boys often require dialysis/transplantation by their late teens. They also develop sensorineural deafness. Such women may well request genetic counselling as well as consideration of screening of their male offspring.

As mentioned in Chapter 2 on prepregnancy advice, vesicoureteric reflux (VUR) is commonly diagnosed in pregnancy as women who may have been entirely asymptomatic prepregnancy develop recurrent UTIs, modest proteinuria and hypertension. Vesicoureteric reflux has a strong heritable component and is probably autosomal dominant in a large number of cases. Women found to have reflux nephropathy should thus be advised that their children are at risk of developing the same condition and that, if diagnosed early, it may be prevented. Their GP should be advised to refer the child to a paediatrician for screening. The problem is how best to screen. Ultrasound of an infant will not detect reflux or scarring, and in the newborn scarring would not have occurred so an isotope scan would be premature. The only useful diagnostic test in an infant is a micturating cystourethrogram (MCUG), which is invasive but much easier in an infant than in older children. If a diagnosis of reflux is made in the mother, then she should be advised that her infant should be screened in the newborn period with MCUG. If she has older children who have not been screened, then they could have renal ultrasound and they should only need more invasive tests if this is abnormal. Others argue that not all reflux is bad and it does not necessarily lead to UTIs and scarring. Some feel that only the higher grades of VUR with dilated ureters need diagnosing and treating. Therefore, it may be that getting a 'good' ultrasound in a baby at about 3 months of age or in older children and with them well hydrated at the time may be all that is needed. While there is clearly debate among paediatricians as to the best way to diagnose and manage reflux, the responsibility of the obstetricians and physicians who make the diagnosis in the mother is that she should be made aware that her children need early review by a paediatrician.[7]

Conclusion

Pregnancy provides an opportunity to identify women with renal disease, but this opportunity is wasted if they are not appropriately followed up postpartum.[8] The key to safe long-term care is to empower the women. Ideally, they should be given information pamphlets explaining the basic facts about kidney disease and the importance of making a diagnosis and monitoring function, blood pressure and urine abnormalities. Above all, they need to be advised to attend for regular follow-up. In the first instance, all women identified with a renal problem in pregnancy need a postpartum review in hospital to establish stability of function/proteinuria (or not), to ensure appropriate diagnostic tests have been done or are planned, and to give some advice about future pregnancy. At the postpartum outpatient appointment it is crucial to define who will follow up the woman thereafter. Where disease is mild and stable this can be in primary care, but where there are diagnostic dilemmas, significant disease or inherited conditions this should be with a nephrologist.

References

1. Jones DC, Hayslett JP. Outcome of pregnancy in women with moderate or severe renal insufficiency. *N Engl J Med* 1996;335:226–32.
2. Royal College of General Practitioners. *Introducing eGFR. Promoting Good CKD Management.* London: RCGP [www.renal.org/eGFR/resources/eGFRnatInfoLflt0406.pdf].
3. Joint Specialty Committee of the Royal College of Physicians, Renal Association. *Concise UK CKD Guidelines.* London: RCP; 2005 [www.renal.org/eGFR/eguide.html].
4. Royal College of Physicians of Edinburgh. *Consensus Statement on Management of Early CKD, February 2007.* Royal College of Physicians of Edinburgh; 2007 [www.renal.org/CKDguide/consensus.html].
5. Landon MB. Diabetic nephropathy and pregnancy. *Clin Obstet Gynecol* 2007;50:998–1006.
6. Molad Y, Borkowski T, Monselise A, Ben-Haroush A, Sulkes J, Hod M, *et al.* Maternal and fetal outcome of lupus pregnancy: a prospective study of 29 pregnancies. *Lupus* 2005;14:145–51.
7. Gargollo PC, Diamond DA. Therapy insight: What nephrologists need to know about primary vesicoureteral reflux. *Nat Clin Pract Nephrol* 2007;3:551–63.
8. Thomas MC. Caring for Australians with Renal Impairment (CARI). The CARI guidelines. Prevention of progression of kidney disease: early detection of patients with kidney disease. *Nephrology (Carlton)* 2007;12 Suppl 1:S37–40.

Section 3

Chronic kidney disease

6

Chapter 6
Pregnancy and dialysis

Liam Plant

Introduction

For women treated by dialysis for end-stage renal disease (ESRD), pregnancy is an uncommon event.[1–7] Although pregnancy outcomes have improved[5–7] since the first reported case in 1971,[8] miscarriage, stillbirth, preterm birth and neonatal death remain substantial risks. Strategies (such as 'enhanced' dialysis regimens) to improve fetal outcomes are, themselves, not without the potential to cause harm.[9,10] Furthermore, experience in managing these patients is sporadic. This is reflected in the nature of much of the published literature, which predominantly[10–16] consists of small case series (incorporating all the potential bias of these) with non-systematic review of other published series. Pregnancy in such women, whether treated by haemodialysis or peritoneal dialysis, thus poses a formidable challenge to renal physicians, obstetricians, neonatologists, dialysis nurses and dieticians.

Incidence of pregnancy

No prospective survey that corrects for patterns of contraception use, sexual activity and other relevant issues on the incidence of pregnancy in women on dialysis has been conducted. Insight is offered from three large studies of variable methodology. A comprehensive national survey[1] in Belgium of 1472 dialysis-treated women of childbearing age reported an incidence of pregnancy (extending beyond the first trimester) of 0.3 per 100 patient-years. A larger survey[2] of 6230 women aged 14–44 years indicated that about 2% became pregnant over a 4 year period. However, this survey was based on responses received from fewer than 50% of all dialysis units in the USA. A Japanese survey[3] in 1996 suggested that 0.44% of 38 889 women treated by dialysis became pregnant. Giatras *et al.*[6] reviewed 120 identified cases published between 1971 and 1998. In almost half of these, pregnancy occurred during the first 2 years of dialysis treatment. Fewer than 5% of reported cases occurred in women on dialysis for more than 10 years.

It is reasonable to conclude that pregnancy is an extremely uncommon event in any individual dialysis unit, particularly when one reflects that dialysis units treat a population in which male gender, older age and multiple comorbidity are the predominant demographics. One could speculate (extrapolating from the above) that a dialysis unit with 200 people under treatment might anticipate having to care for a pregnant woman no more often than once every 3–10 years. Alternatively, one could anticipate that pregnancy will occur in about 1 in 200 women of childbearing potential treated by dialysis. Clearly, the accumulation of individual unit expertise is difficult at frequencies such as these.

The patient group under treatment at Cork University Hospital in September 2007 (Table 6.1) illustrates this. A total of 218 patients with ESRD were treated by dialysis. Of these, 28 (13% or 45 per million population) were women aged between 15 and 50 years. Twenty-four of these were listed for renal transplantation and 24 (85%) were known to be sexually active. Based on the projections estimated above, one might anticipate a pregnancy once every 8 years (although a cluster might also occur).

This group may be contrasted with those ESRD patients with a functioning renal transplant. Out of 232 such patients, 46 (20%) were women between the ages of 15 and 50 years and 40 (87%) of these were known to be sexually active. Non-systematic data collection over the previous 5 years recorded ten pregnancies (eight successful) in those with a functioning transplant compared with two pregnancies (neither successful) in those treated by dialysis.

Pregnancy is more common and more successful after transplantation,[7] and it may be that patients are best counselled to wait for this to occur. It may also be pertinent to reflect on possible future consequences of continuing investigations into the causes of diminished fertility in women on dialysis. There is little doubt that sexual dysfunction is common in this group and may not be accorded the same attention from healthcare professionals as other problems. Nutritional status, anaemia, fatigue, psychosocial problems and disturbances in hypothalamic–pituitary–gonadal function all contribute.[17] Strategies addressing these may in future be followed by an increased incidence of conception.

Outcome of pregnancy

In the absence of a systematic format for reporting on pregnancy outcomes in women on dialysis, the following summary conclusions (Table 6.2) seem robust: the proportion of pregnancies ending with a surviving infant has increased over time,[5–7] and is higher if conception has occurred before the need to initiate dialysis.[1,2,5]

Table 6.1. Women with end-stage renal disease with the potential to become pregnant in a catchment population of 620 000 (Cork University Hospital, September 2007)

	Woman aged 15–50 years	Sexually active	Transplant listed
Dialysis (*n* = 218)	28 (13%)	24 (85%)	24 (85%)
Transplant (*n* = 232)	46 (20%)	40 (87%)	–

Table 6.2. Pregnancies in women on dialysis concluding with a surviving infant (selected series)

Study	Pregnancies	Comment	Surviving infant
Giatras *et al.* (1998),[6] HD and PD	*n* = 49	Reported 1971–90	57%
	n = 55	Reported 1991–98	71%
Bagon *et al.* (1998),[1] HD	*n* = 15 total	Conceived on dialysis	50%
		Conceived before starting dialysis	80%
Okundaye *et al.* (1998),[2] HD and PD	*n* = 184	Conceived on dialysis	40%
	n = 57	Conceived before starting dialysis	74%
Toma *et al.* (1999),[3] HD	*n* = 172	Data from 79 pregnancies only	49%

HD = haemodialysis; PD = peritoneal dialysis

Other series[4,11–13,15,16] report a success rate of 50–70%. More recent series[10,14] report even better outcomes, but caution in generalisation should be maintained because of the very small size of these series with the attendant potential for reporting bias. In all these series, doubt may be expressed that miscarriage, particularly in the first trimester, may not be as reliably captured as later events. Many studies are probably best viewed as reporting outcomes in *identified* pregnancies that have progressed beyond the first trimester, with a strong focus on *later* fetal outcomes.

The survey of Okundaye *et al.*,[2] which used a detailed questionnaire, found that, in 184 women who conceived when already on dialysis, first-trimester miscarriage occurred in 25% of pregnancies. An additional 17% experienced second-trimester miscarriage. The rate from conception may, therefore, be less than the more hopeful figures presented.

In addition, the following summary conclusions seem reasonable (in that they 'make sense' and are supported by some observational case series):

- Extending total hours of haemodialysis to more than 20 hours per week is associated with an increase in the proportion of pregnancies ending with a surviving infant, possibly for reasons discussed below.[1,2,4,9]
- There is no compelling data set[2,4] to support a systematic difference in outcomes between women treated by haemodialysis or by peritoneal dialysis (although such comparisons as are reported tend to compare peritoneal dialysis with standard-intensity haemodialysis, rather than with the intensified haemodialysis regimens now more widely employed).

Complications of pregnancy

Women on dialysis are prone to the complications of pregnancy and the complications of ESRD. Added to this is the risk that changes in renal replacement therapy regimens, designed to improve pregnancy outcomes, may introduce new treatment-related complications. The complication that probably has the strongest impact on fetal outcomes remains the increased risk of preterm birth and low birthweight (LBW).

Pregnancy concludes at or before 37 weeks of gestation in 85%[6] to 100%[1] of cases. In a range of case series[2,4,6] the mean duration of gestation at delivery was 32–33 weeks, even in modern series[10,15] with aggressive dialysis regimens. Average birthweight was 1.5–1.7 kg.[1,2,4,6,10,15] Although fetal growth restriction is reported, the principal reason[6] for LBW has been preterm birth with weight appropriate to the duration of gestation. The principal factors contributing to this include:

- *maternal hypertension, especially if severe, or pre-eclampsia supervenes*: typical reported frequencies include hypertension in up to 80% of cases,[2] exceeding 170/110 mmHg in 17%.[4] Pre-eclampsia[4] supervenes in 11% of cases: the diagnosis/definition of this is difficult in these women, most of whom are already hypertensive or who may already have proteinuria or be anuric.
- *an increased frequency of polyhydramnios:* polyhydramnios is reported in almost all series, ranging from 18%[6] to 40%[11] and 60%[1] of pregnancies. The reason for this is unclear. A number of theories have been advanced, although none has the benefit of a robust scientific validation. These include the possible osmotic effects of raised maternal urea concentration on fetal urine production. There is no doubt, and it has been demonstrated,[18] that amniotic fluid volume closely follows maternal fluid volume in women treated by haemodialysis.

Additional dialysis therapy-induced factors might include:

- *acute shifts in maternal fluid volume status:* this may lead to polyhydramnios, as above. However, decreases may lead to oligohydramnios or otherwise compromise uteroplacental and fetal perfusion. It has been reported[19] that the umbilical artery pulsatility index and the fetal heart rate both exhibit substantial variation after a dialysis treatment; this effect has not been seen in other cases[6,20] with more deliberately applied strategies to minimise treatment-induced fluid shifts.
- *dialysis-induced hypotension:* this is a risk in nonpregnant patients also and exhibits considerable overlap with disturbances in maternal fluid volume status. Once again, it is the disturbance in uteroplacental and fetal perfusion that is important.
- *dialysis-induced reductions in serum progesterone:* it has been speculated that dialysis-induced falls in progesterone might be responsible for preterm labour. However, its response to dialysis exhibits a patient-specific variability in which there is little demonstrable association with uterine contractions.[21]

The occurrence of preterm labour can reflect any combination of the above factors and it is in seeking to minimise their impacts that contemporary strategies have been developed to deal with pregnancies in women having dialysis treatment.

Strategies that may optimise pregnancy outcomes

Information sharing and counselling

Dialysis units should provide systematic information on reproductive health issues to all women, supplemented as needed by more focused counselling.[22] Sharing information with women should allow them to make informed choices with regard to pregnancy. Given the difficulties associated with managing pregnancy in women on dialysis and that outcomes are considerably better following successful renal transplantation,[7,22] all suitable patients should be activated on the waiting list for transplantation at the earliest opportunity. In an ideal world, deferring pregnancy until after successful transplantation seems a prudent option. In reality, patients become pregnant in a sporadic fashion and not usually after 'careful reflection' on the inherent risks. The uptake of reproductive health services may be less extensive than desired, even when freely available.[23]

Early diagnosis and rapid activation of a multidisciplinary care plan

The hormonal diagnosis of pregnancy may depend upon blood rather than urine samples. Furthermore, pregnancy may not even be suspected until it is well advanced (this cadre of women are frequently amenorrhoeic, and they and their medical advisers may be under the illusion that they 'can't get pregnant'). Late diagnosis of pregnancy is probably common. A culture in which proper attention is paid to reproductive health issues should promote good practice in suspecting, evaluating and confirming pregnancy at an early stage. Early diagnosis allows early review and adjustment of medications, formulation of a multidisciplinary care plan and implementation of the arrangements necessary to delivery it.[6,7] The series reported by Haase *et al.*[10] details the kind of systematic protocol for dialysis management that informs current practice. In this particular series,[10] haemodiafiltration was used; similar protocols employing haemodialysis[6,14,15,24] have been reported. The multidisciplinary team will include renal physicians, dialysis nurses, dieticians, obstetricians with expertise in high-risk pregnancy, midwives and neonatologists.

Changes in dialysis regimen

It is well recognised in nonpregnant haemodialysis patients that better control of fluid volumes,[25] blood pressure[25] and small solute clearances[26] is achieved with more frequent (5–7 times per week) treatments than with more traditional (3 times per week) regimens. This observation, in common with a construct that 'more physiological' renal replacement therapy seems 'logical', has continued to influence practice that had already begun to move in this direction following multiple observations[1,2,4,9] that successful pregnancies were more common with regimens delivering more than 20 of hours haemodialysis.

It is difficult to be prescriptive, but it seems reasonable to deliver as much haemodialysis as the woman can be persuaded to tolerate (because of distance from the care centre, problems with vascular access or personal tolerance) and the local resources can deliver. At a minimum it should exceed 20 hours per week and should be delivered at a frequency greater than thrice weekly (although 5–7 treatments per week is more desirable). Typically, the use of more biocompatible dialysers is selected.[6,10,14,15] Strategies designed to minimise intradialytic events need to be deployed. Setting a kinetic target for urea removal may be helpful.[10]

If haemodiafiltration is available, it may be used in place of haemodialysis. The prescription should be decided upon early in the course of pregnancy and it should be continuously reviewed in light of clinical developments. It is important to match locally available technologies and competencies to achieve the best outcome. The reported experiences of individual series may be helpful in informing such choices.[10,11,13–15]

There are fewer cases reported[9,11] that have been managed by peritoneal dialysis, but in these the dialysate volume is typically increased.[27] There will be more of a limitation to this than applies to increasing haemodialysis hours. The potential for peritonitis is an additional risk factor for these women.

Changes in fluid balance management

Fluid balance management is of particular importance in anuric patients and is intimately integrated with the dialysis regimen. Better control of salt and water balance, achieved with more frequent haemodialysis/haemofiltration, should improve control of hypertension, allowing less use of antihypertensive agents and protecting mother and fetus from the dangers of uncontrolled hypertension.[6,9,10,24]

Perhaps of greater importance is the minimisation of maternal fluid volume shifts that may be mirrored by changes in amniotic fluid volume or uteroplacental perfusion with the attendant hazards of polyhydramnios or oligohydramnios/diminished fetal perfusion, respectively.[6,18–20] Daily treatment with more limited ultrafiltration volumes offers the optimal potential to minimise these shifts. Appropriate monitoring of amniotic fluid volume and uteroplacental circulation may assist achievement of these objectives.[6,20]

Weight gain is an integral component of pregnancy and the target post-treatment dry weight needs to be adjusted on a continuing basis. An adequately nourished woman can be expected to gain 1.0–1.5 kg in the first trimester. Subsequent weight gain of about 0.45 kg per week[6] (although it may be much more variable in individual women[10]) occurs until delivery. Careful continuing clinical examination balancing nutritional status, blood pressure and amniotic fluid volume to customise this target weight gain is essential.

Correction of potential problems due to more frequent dialysis

This change in dialysis regimen is not without potential hazard. Weekly assessment of electrolyte levels may reveal a variety of potential problems. Such regimens may lead to hypophosphataemia and total body phosphate depletion, which may require the introduction of phosphate into the dialysate.[28] A similar problem may develop with potassium balance, requiring an increased potassium concentration in the dialysate.[6]

The progesterone-induced hyperventilation of pregnancy may lead to a respiratory alkalosis without the normal renal compensatory mechanisms. This may lead to a persistent alkalosis (particularly if emesis is an additional feature of the pregnancy) if dialysate bicarbonate concentration is not reduced.

Changes in calcium metabolism are features of pregnancy: digestive absorption of calcium increases, as does hypercalciuria. These changes are associated with increases in calcitriol, hyperparathyroidism and parathyroid hormone-related protein (PTH-rP).[6] Dialysis patients have hyperparathyroidism and are frequently prescribed calcium-containing phosphate binders. This multifactorial potential for hypercalcaemia may require a reduction in dialysate calcium concentrations.

Typically, dialysis patients have normal/high serum magnesium concentrations. In the absence of urinary excretion, there is a real potential to induce iatrogenic hypermagnesaemia if standard-dose magnesium infusions are used as a tocolytic or in the treatment or prevention of eclampsia.

Ensuring good maternal nutrition

More frequent dialysis allows a reduction/removal of the dietary and fluid restrictions that are standard with less intense regimens.[6,10] Nutritional supervision should be provided by a trained dietician,[29] with promotion of a caloric intake of up to 3000 kcal/day and an increase in dietary protein intake to up to 1.8 g/kg/day.[6,10] Water-soluble vitamins, particularly folic acid, need generous supplementation (especially as these will be lost with the more intensive regimens). Many protocols also incorporate supplementation of trace minerals.[30]

Intensified anaemia management

Anaemia management needs to be intensified.[6,27] Requirements for exogenous erythropoietin increase[6] (often to doses greater than 300 iu/kg/week[10]). The large molecular size of erythropoietin makes it unlikely to cross the placenta;[31] there are no erythropoietin receptors on the human placenta.[32] In this circumstance, it is unlikely that the fetus is harmed at doses used in clinical practice. Despite more aggressive management, some women in reported series have required supplementary red cell concentrate transfusions.

Iron loss is increased in haemodialysis and oral absorption is not enhanced. Maintaining adequate iron stores to support optimal erythropoiesis usually requires parenteral supplementation.[30]

It is important to maintain good extracorporeal-circuit anticoagulation during dialysis. There may be a need for an increased dose of heparin, particularly if low-molecular-weight heparin (LMWH) is used. Frequent circuit clotting and loss of blood will not help anaemia management.

Fetal and maternal monitoring

The optimal frequency and form of monitoring is unclear.[6,10,20] However, regular fetal ultrasonography is needed to detect fetal growth restriction and changes in amniotic fluid volume. Regular monitoring of maternal blood pressure with serial assessments of uterine–umbilical artery blood flow (with Doppler velocimetry) and continuous fetal heart-rate tracings may be performed before, during and after each dialysis session. Some authors suggest that such fetal heart-rate monitoring should be performed during each dialysis from about 25 weeks until delivery.[10]

Conclusion

The most important aspect of management is fastidious attention to detail by a competent multidisciplinary team. Those focusing on the renal replacement therapy need to achieve excellence in the many elements detailed above. Obstetricians and midwives will need to perform far more frequent assessments of maternal and fetal wellbeing than with more standard cases and they will face many challenges in tocolysis, emergency deliveries and related issues. Neonatologists are almost guaranteed the birth of preterm LBW infants.

Pregnancy outcomes have improved over the past 30 years, at least in those pregnancies continuing beyond the first trimester. However, there are no data to suggest that one can now become complacent. Even with very fastidious implementation of strategies such as those detailed above, preterm birth and other problems remain almost universal.

This is a rare challenge for individual renal units. The reported experiences above can help formulate a local policy to be implemented when the event does occur. In particular, recognition of the potential that precipitous preterm labour may occur in the dialysis unit, ensuring immediate access to a delivery pack and establishing emergency contact numbers for the midwife, obstetrician and neonatologist are important precautions that need to be taken by the renal team.

Renal units, in conjunction with obstetric units, should formulate a protocol for the management of women receiving or starting dialysis in pregnancy to be activated when a patient on dialysis becomes pregnant. It would seem reasonable to base this upon the strategies reported from case series published since 2000 (modified as necessary to match local resources and competencies).

References

1. Bagon JA, Vernaeve H, De Muylder X, Lafontaine JJ, Martens J, Van Roost G. Pregnancy and dialysis. *Am J Kidney Dis* 1998;31:756–65.
2. Okundaye I, Abrinko P, Hou S. Registry of pregnancy in dialysis patients. *Am J Kidney Dis* 1998;31:766–73.
3. Toma H, Tanabe K, Tokumoto T, Kobayashi C, Yaqisawa T. Pregnancy in women receiving renal dialysis or transplantation in Japan: a nationwide survey. *Nephrol Dial Transplant* 1999;14:1511–16.
4. Chan WS, Okun N, Kjellstrand CM. Pregnancy in chronic dialysis: a review and analysis of the literature. *Int J Artif Organs* 1998;21:257–68.
5. Levy DP, Giatras I, Jungers P. Pregnancy and end-stage renal disease – past experience and new insights. *Nephrol Dial Transplant* 1998;13:3005–7.
6. Giatras I, Levy DP, Malone FD, Carlson JA, Jungers P. Pregnancy during dialysis: case report and management guidelines. *Nephrol Dial Transplant* 1998;13:3266–72.
7. Hou S. Historical perspective of pregnancy in chronic kidney disease. *Adv Chronic Kidney Dis* 2007;14:116–18.
8. Confortini P, Galanti G, Ancona G, Giongo A, Bruschi E, Lorenzini E. Full term pregnancy and successful delivery in a patient on chronic haemodialysis. *Proc Eur Dial Transplant Assoc* 1971;8:74–80.
9. Hou S. Pregnancy in dialysis patients: where do we go from here? *Semin Dial* 2003;16:376–8.

10. Haase M, Morgera S, Bamberg C, Halle H, Martini S, Hocher B, *et al.* A systematic approach to managing pregnant dialysis patients – the importance of an intensified haemodiafiltration protocol. *Nephrol Dial Transplant* 2005;20:2537–42.
11. Romao JE, Luders C, Kahhale S, Pascoal IJ, Abensur H, Sabbaga E, *et al.* Pregnancy in women on chronic dialysis. A single-center experience with 17 cases. *Nephron* 1998;78:416–22.
12. Nakabayashi M, Adachi T, Itoh S, Kobayashi M, Mishina J, Nishida H. Perinatal and infant outcome of pregnant patients undergoing chronic hemodialysis. *Nephron* 1999;82:27–31.
13. Chao AS, Huang JY, Lien R, Kung FT, Chen PJ, Hsieh PC. Pregnancy in women who undergo long-term hemodialysis. *Am J Obstet Gynecol* 2002;187:152–6.
14. Eroglu D, Lembet A, Ozdemir FN, Ergin T, Kazanci F, Kuscu E, *et al.* Pregnancy during haemodialysis: Perinatal outcome in our cases. *Transplant Proc* 2004;36:53–5.
15. Moranne S, Samouelian V, Lapeyre F, Pagniez D, Subtil D, Dequiedt P, *et al.* Pregnancy and hemodialysis. *Nephrologie* 2004;25:287–92.
16. Malik DH, Al-Harbi A, Al-Mohaya S, Dohaimi H, Kechrid M, Shetaia MS, *et al.* Pregnancy in patients on dialysis – experience at a referral centre. *J Assoc Physicians India* 2005;53:937–41.
17. Anantharam P, Schmidt RJ. Sexual function in chronic kidney disease. *Adv Chronic Kidney Dis* 2007;14:119–25.
18. Brost BC, Newman RB, Fries M, Calhoun BC. The effects of hemodialysis on total intrauterine volume. *Ultrasound Obstet Gynecol* 1996;8:34–6.
19. Oosterhof H, Navis GJ, Go JG, Dassel ACM, De Jong PE, Aarnoudse JG. Pregnancy in a patient on chronic haemodialysis: fetal monitoring by Doppler velocimetry of the umbilical artery. *Br J Obst Gynaecol* 1993;100:1140–1.
20. Malone FD, Craigo SD, Giatras I, Carlson J, Athanassiou A, D'Alton ME. Suggested ultrasound parameters for the assessment of fetal well-being during chronic hemodialysis. *Ultrasound Obstet Gynecol* 1998;11:450–2.
21. Brost BC, Newman RB, Hendricks SK, Droste S, Mathur RS. Effect of hemodialysis on serum progesterone level in pregnant women. *Am J Kidney Dis* 1999;33:917–19.
22. Watnick S. Pregnancy and contraceptive counselling of women with chronic kidney disease and kidney transplants. *Adv Chronic Kidney Dis* 2007;14:126–31.
23. Kerkhoff BA, O'Connor TC, Plant WD, Higgins JR. Poor uptake of reproductive health screening services by renal transplant recipients. *Ir Med J* 2006;99:78–80.
24. Moranne S, Samouelian V, Lapeyre F, Pagniez D, Subtil D, Dequiedt P, *et al.* A systematic approach to managing pregnant dialysis patients – the importance of an intensified haemodiafiltration protocol. *Nephrol Dial Transplant* 2006;21:1443.
25. Nesrallah G, Suri R, Moist L, Kortas C, Lindsay RM. Volume control and blood pressure management in patients undergoing quotidian haemodialysis. *Am J Kidney Dis* 2003;42 Suppl 1:13–17.
26. Suri R, Depner TA, Blake PG, Heidenheim AP, Lindsay RM. Adequacy in quotidian haemodialysis. *Am J Kidney Dis* 2003;42 Suppl 1:42–8.
27. Reddy SS, Holley JL. Management of the pregnant chronic dialysis patient. *Adv Chronic Kidney Dis* 2007;14:146–55.
28. Hussain S, Savin V, Piering W, Tomasi J, Blumenthal S. Phosphorus-enriched hemodialysis during pregnancy: Two case reports. *Hemodial Int* 2005;9:147–52.
29. Brookhyser J, Wiggins K. Medical nutrition therapy in pregnancy and kidney disease. *Adv Renal Replace Therapy* 1998;5:53–63.
30. Grossman SD, Hou S, Moretti MI, Saran S. Nutrition in the pregnant dialysis patient. *J Renal Nutr* 1993;3:56–66.
31. Schneider H, Malek AR. Lack of permeability of the human placenta for erythropoietin. *J Perinat Med* 1995;23:71–6.
32. Pekonen F, Rosenlof K, Rutanen EM, Fyhrquist F. Erythropoietin binding sites in human fetal tissues. *Acta Endocrinol* 1987;116:561–7.

Chapter 7

Pregnancy and the renal transplant recipient

Sue Carr

The first successful birth in a renal transplant patient was in 1958, although it was not reported until 1963.[1] Now the literature contains over 14 000 reported pregnancies worldwide (Figure 7.1)[2] and approximately 2% of women of childbearing age with a renal transplant will become pregnant.[3]

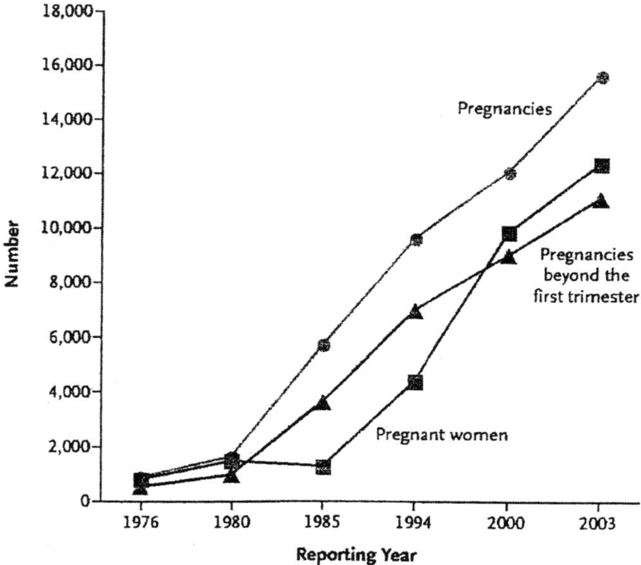

Figure 7.1. Pregnancies in kidney transplant recipients reported worldwide; the circles represent the numbers of pregnancies reported worldwide in kidney transplant recipients during the indicated year; the numbers include therapeutic terminations, miscarriages, ectopic pregnancies and stillbirths; the squares represent the numbers of female transplant recipients reported to have been pregnant during that year, again including all outcomes; the triangles represent the numbers of pregnancies beyond the first trimester reported in the literature during the indicated year; the data are from the National Transplantation Pregnancy Registry in the USA, the European Dialysis and Transplant Association Registry and the UK Transplant Pregnancy Registry; reproduced with permission from McKay and Josephson[2]

Timing of pregnancy

Fertility and the ability to conceive rapidly improve within a few months of successful renal transplantation.[2,4,5] In order to avoid pregnancy early post-transplant, it is important that appropriate contraceptive advice is given to women before transplantation.[2,6,7]

Published guidelines[4,8] advise women to defer pregnancy for 12–24 months following a renal transplant (Box 7.1). Recent studies have reported favourable pregnancy outcomes 12 months post-transplant[9] and the American Society of Transplantation guidelines state that in women with a stable renal transplant, who are at low risk of complications, pregnancy may be considered at 12 months (Box 7.2).[4] The optimal timing of pregnancy is probably between 12 months and 5 years post-transplant. However, some women who do not fulfil the recommendations regarding preferred timing of pregnancy will accidentally conceive or decide to conceive and then the situation has to be assessed on an individual basis.

Box 7.1. Criteria for considering pregnancy in renal transplant recipients; MMF = mycophenolate mofetil; reproduced with permission from European Best Practice Guidelines Expert Group on Renal Transplantation[8]

1. Good general health for about 2 years after transplantation.
2. Good stable allograft function [serum creatinine < 177 µmol/l (2 mg/dl), preferably < 133 µmol/l (< 1.5 mg/dl)].
3. No recent episodes of acute rejection and no evidence of ongoing rejection.
4. Normal blood pressure or minimal antihypertensive regimen (only one drug).
5. Absence of or minimal proteinuria (< 0.50 g/day).
6. Normal allograft ultrasound (absence of pelvicalyceal distension).
7. Recommended immunosuppression:
   - prednisone < 15 mg/day
   - azathioprine ≤ 2 mg/day
   - ciclosporin or tacrolimus at therapeutic levels
   - MMF and sirolimus are contraindicated
   - MMF and sirolimus should be stopped 6 weeks before conception is attempted.

Box 7.2. Criteria on which to determine the timing of pregnancy following renal transplant; American Society of Transplantation guidelines; reproduced with permission from McKay *et al.*[4]

Basis on which to determine timing of pregnancy:

- no rejection in the past year
- adequate and stable graft function (e.g. creatinine < 1.5 mg/dl but true GFR needs to be defined in prospective studies) or no or minimal proteinuria (level needs to be defined)
- no acute infections that might impact fetus
- maintenance immunosuppression at stable dosing

Special circumstances that impact on recommendations:

- rejection within the first year (consider further graft assessment – biopsy and GFR)
- maternal age
- comorbid factors that may impact pregnancy and graft function
- established medical noncompliance

Pregnancies outside the guidelines need to be evaluated on a case-by-case basis. In general these considerations could be met at 1 year post-transplant based on individual circumstances.

Effects of pregnancy on the renal transplant recipient

In normal pregnancy, the glomerular filtration rate (GFR) increases by approximately 50% owing to increased renal plasma flow (45% by 9 weeks and 70% in mid-pregnancy). This results in a fall in serum creatinine (SCr) by 45–70 μmol/l, which persists throughout normal pregnancy. In renal transplant patients, a similar increase in GFR has been reported during pregnancy, the magnitude of which is dependent upon prepregnancy renal function.[10–12] Fischer *et al.*[9] reported the increase in GFR in pregnancy to be similar in both azathioprine- and ciclosporin-treated patients although the prepregnancy creatinine was lower in azathioprine-treated women (Figure 7.2).

Renal function during and after pregnancy

The UK Transplant Pregnancy Registry (UKTPR), US National Transplantation Pregnancy Registry (NTPR) and numerous recent single-centre studies have investigated the effect of pregnancy on renal allograft function (Table 7.1).[9,13–27]

In general, most[9,14,17,19,23,27,28] but not all[21,24,25] studies report no significant deleterious effect of pregnancy on graft function.

In general, SCr levels at conception and during pregnancy were lower in azathioprine-treated women compared with ciclosporin-treated women. SCr levels of greater than 133 μmol/l were reported in 14% versus 24% of azathioprine- and ciclosporin-treated women, respectively.[9,29]

Fischer *et al.*[9] reported outcomes following 81 renal transplant pregnancies. There was no significant deterioration in renal function (mean creatinine 115 μmol/l at conception and 119 μmol/l postpartum) and no difference in graft survival at 10 years in female transplant recipients who became pregnant, or between women treated

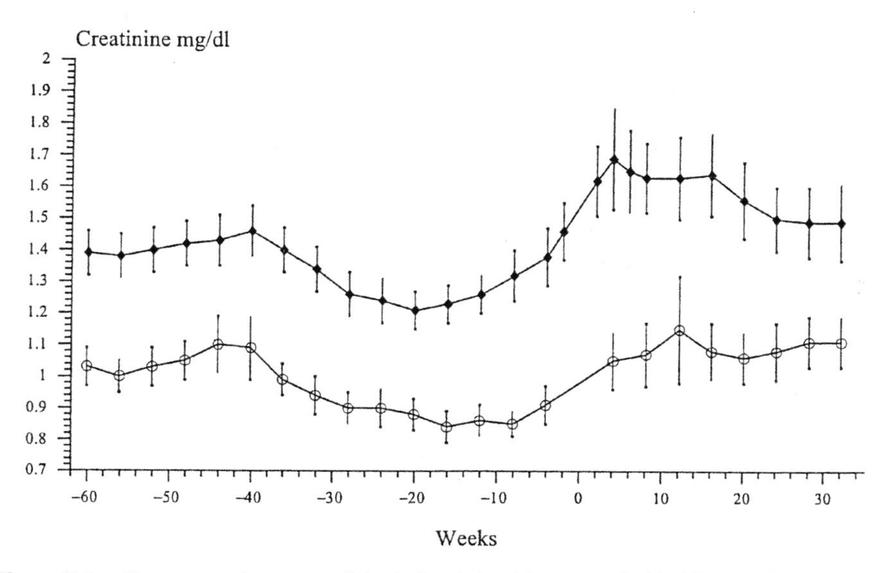

Figure 7.2. Time course of serum creatinine in the study subjects treated with ciclosporin (n = 41, thick line) and azathioprine (*n* = 40, thin line) before (–60 to –40 weeks), during (–40 to 0 weeks) and after (0 to 30 weeks) delivery; reproduced with permission from Fischer *et al.*[9]

Table 7.1. Studies on the effect of pregnancy on graft and patient survival

Study	Country	Time	Patients (pregnancies)	Study type	Patient survival	Graft survival	Renal function and proteinuria	Hypertension (pre-eclampsia)
Rahamimov *et al.*[23]	Israel	1983–98	39 (69)	Retrospective case–controlled	84.8% 15 year follow-up No difference from controls	61.6% (controls 68.7) Follow-up median 14 years 13% graft failure within 2 years No difference from controls No acute rejection	No data	44% (15%)
Thompson *et al.*[25]	UK	1976–2001	24 (48) Mean time post transplant 6.5 years	Retrospective case note review compared with registry data (outcomes in 27–30 pregnancies that progressed)		3.3% graft loss at 3 years No acute rejection	20% had persistent graft dysfunction more than 6 months postpartum Effect most marked was creatinine > 155 µmol/l Proteinuria 9 patients 0.4 g/day prepregnancy 1.37 g/day third trimester 0.47 g/day 3–6 months postpartum	77% (29%)
Miniero *et al.*[20]	Italy	1987–2002	96 (52 in kidney transplant)	Retrospective survey by questionnaire				16% onset 58.2% term
Yongwon *et al.*[27]	South Korea	Up to 2000	36 (47)	Retrospective review			No changes in serum creatinine	28%
Fischer *et al.*[9]	Germany		81 (81)	Case–control study matched with female transplant recipients who had not become pregnant	10 year patient survival 93.4% versus 89% in controls No relation to pregnancy	10 year graft survival 62.5% versus 67% in controls	Mean creatinine at conception 119 µmol/l Mean creatinine postpartum 119 µmol/l	
Crowe *et al.*[14]	UK		29 (33)			All patients with creatinine > 200 µmol/l required dialysis within 2 years	Proteinuria 0.45 g/day conception to 1.11 g/day at delivery resolved to baseline at 3 months	
Samela *et al.*[30]	Finland	1971–91	22 (29)	38 matched female controls		10 year graft survival 69 versus 100 % in control group ($P < 0.005$)		

Study	Country	Time	Patients (pregnancies)	Study type	Patient survival	Graft survival	Renal function and proteinuria	Hypertension (pre-eclampsia)
Gutiérrez *et al.*[17]	Spain	1976–2004	35 (43)			87.5% functioning graft at 53 months	Creatinine 93 µmol/l prepregnancy and 102.5 µmol/l postpartum 85.7% no proteinuria postpartum, remainder mild mean 0.6 g/24 hours	64% (37.5%)
Keitel *et al.*[19]	Brazil	1977–2001	41 (44)		No difference in patient survival	No difference long-term graft survival	Median creatinine 88 µmol/l before pregnancy and 111 µmol/l 6 months postpartum 30% had creatinine > 133 µmol/l 37% > 0.5 g/day proteinuria	66% (20.4%, 1 maternal death)
Pour-Reza-Gholi *et al.*[22]	Iran	1984–2004	60 living donor (74) 17.5% of pregnancies were in first year and 4 patients in first 3 months	Telephone interview Controls matched female transplant patients		No difference in 1, 3, 5 and 10 year graft survival pregnant patients versus controls 6.7% acute rejection, all had failed pregnancy	Creatinine at conception < 133 µmol/l 64 patients, 69% had no increase 4 patients (creatinine 133–265 µmol/l) had significant rise in creatinine and 1 needed dialysis	
Cruz Lemini *et al.*[15]	Mexico	N/A	60 (75)				Creatinine > 133 µmol/l at conception was associated with delivery before 34 weeks	45.3%
Yildirim and Uslu[26]	Turkey	1998–2005	17 (20)	Retrospective review		No acute rejection	Creatinine > 133 µmol/l associated with preterm delivery	
Kurata *et al.*[57]	Japan	1984–2003	42 (53)	Case–control study			38% had creatinine > 133 µmol/l Hypertension, proteinuria and creatinine > 133 µmol/l were predictors of preterm delivery	
Galdo *et al.*[16]	Chile	1982–2002	30 (37)	Retrospective notes review		13.5% acute rejection	Creatinine (umol/l): baseline 105, delivery 127, 1 year postpartum 122, significant $P = 0.02$, $P = 0.004$, respectively	(19%)
Hooi *et al.*[18]	Malaysia	1984–2001	72 (46)		10 year patient survival 94%	10 year graft survival 83% No acute rejection	Mean creatinine prepregnancy 113 µmol/l 12 months postpartum 119 µmol/l	38% (15%)

with azathioprine or ciclosporin during pregnancy. Similarly, Crowe *et al.*[14] reported stable renal function during pregnancy and up to 1 year postpartum in 33 pregnancies. Keitel *et al.*,[19] in a study from Brazil, reported no significant rise in creatinine following pregnancy and no difference in long-term graft survival following pregnancy in 44 transplant recipients, although over 30% of women in the study had creatinine levels above 133 μmol/l.

However, several studies have reported less favourable outcomes. The UKTPR reported an increased SCr postpartum when the SCr was greater than 150 μmol/l before pregnancy ($P = 0.04$).[24] Thompson *et al.*[25] performed a retrospective case note review and compared outcomes with registry data. It was evident that 20% of women experienced a permanent decline in renal function that persisted up to 6 months postpartum. This effect was most marked in women with prepregnancy SCr level greater than 155 μmol/l.

Previously, Samela *et al.*[30] reported reduced graft survival in 69% of transplant recipients who had been pregnant versus no graft failures in matched female controls at 10 years ($P < 0.005$), a highly unusual outcome, it has to be said, related to flaws in definitions and study design.

Galdo *et al.*[16] in a recent single-centre report of 37 renal transplant pregnancies in Chile reported a significant decline in renal function from mean SCr 105 μmol/l at baseline to 127 μmol/l at delivery and 122 μmol/l at 1 year postpartum ($P = 0.02$ and $P = 0.004$, respectively). In Brazil, Oliveira *et al.*[21] also found that 44% of women had a decline in renal function during pregnancy or postpartum.

A study from Iran reported outcomes for 74 pregnancies in recipients of living donor kidneys with good renal function in 64/74 cases (creatinine below 133 μmol/l). Sixty-nine percent had no decline in renal function but nine had significant deterioration in renal transplant function. However, 17.5% of pregnancies in this study were within 12 months of renal transplantation and had a poor outcome.[22]

These studies indicate a considerable variation in renal transplant outcomes in different centres around the world. As a general rule renal transplant patients with significantly impaired prepregnancy renal function are more likely to suffer a pregnancy-related decline in renal function.

In a previous analysis of NTPR data, Armenti *et al.*[31] had reported that women with prepregnancy creatinine above 177 μmol/l all needed dialysis 2 years postpartum. This has been discussed in a review by Stratta *et al.*[28] who concluded that renal prognosis following pregnancy was determined by prepregnancy creatinine level (less than 133 μmol/l) as well as time post-transplant.

In summary, as of 2007, it is generally accepted that there is no need to alter optimistic counselling practices in women with good graft function.

Effects of multiparity and multiple pregnancies

The European Dialysis and Transplant Association (EDTA) registry reported that 14% of 820 women had a second pregnancy following a successful first pregnancy between 1967 and 1990. Repeated pregnancy did not seem to adversely affect graft function provided that graft function was good at the onset of pregnancy.[32]

The NTPR reported the outcome of multiple pregnancies (ten sets of twins, four sets of triplets) in 13 women from a cohort of 458 renal transplant recipients.[33] Five of the multiple pregnancies were conceived using assisted conception techniques. The pregnancies were complicated by hypertension in 77% of cases, pre-eclampsia in 29% and infection in 25%. Mean SCr at beginning or prepregnancy was on average 133 μmol/l with a rise to a mean of 150 μmol/l postpartum. In this group the mean gestational age was 33 weeks and birthweights were low at 1736 g. Seven of the 13 women were followed up, two of which experienced reduced graft function and one returned to dialysis.

Differential diagnosis of deteriorating renal transplant function during pregnancy

Renal transplant dysfunction may develop for many reasons during a pregnancy and it is important to establish the underlying cause, which may be multifactorial. Table 7.2 lists the types of transplant dysfunction and their possible causes. Investigation of acute graft dysfunction in pregnancy requires the following investigations.

1. Biochemistry: urea and electrolytes, liver function tests and glucose. Urate may be raised in patients with a diagnosis of pre-eclampsia but urate levels may be increased by calcineurin inhibitors (CNIs) and are difficult to interpret in a transplant patient. Lactate dehydrogenase (LDH) may be raised in a woman with haemolysis and may aid diagnosis of HELLP syndrome (haemolytic anaemia, elevated liver enzymes and low platelet count).
2. Full blood count, platelet count and a blood film to exclude schistocytes and microangiopathic haemolytic anaemia.
3. Quantification of urinary protein excretion: 24 hour urine protein collection or protein/creatinine ratio (PCR).
4. Immunology screen: autoantibodies, dsDNA antibodies, complement levels C3 C4, antineutrophil cytoplasmic antibodies (ANCA). In women with systemic lupus erythematosus (SLE) lupus anticoagulant and anticardiolipin antibodies should be estimated.
5. Ciclosporin or tacrolimus levels.
6. Urine culture to exclude infection.

Table 7.2. Differential diagnosis of renal transplant dysfunction in pregnancy

Type of renal transplant dysfunction	Possible causes to consider
Pre-renal	Hypovolaemia and/or hypotension due to vomiting, haemorrhage (postpartum or antepartum) or sepsis (often due to acute pyelonephritis)
	Vasoconstriction – especially associated with pre-eclampsia (may be exacerbated by ciclosporin)
Intrarenal transplant	Acute tubular necrosis due to prolonged pre-renal factors
	Microangiopathy – in pre-eclamptic syndromes, severe hypertension (or rarely *de novo* haemolytic uraemic syndrome)
	Acute interstitial nephritis – diuretics, antibiotics
	Acute rejection
	Calcineurin inhibitor nephrotoxicity
	Viral infections – polyoma virus, cytomegalovirus infection
	Recurrent glomerular disease or *de novo* glomerulonephritis
Post-renal	Hydronephrosis of transplant kidney due to calculi, polyhydramniotic uterus or, rarely, exaggerated physiological dilation of transplant kidney

7. Ultrasound scan: diagnosis of urinary tract obstruction may be difficult as urinary tract dilation is a feature of normal pregnancy.
8. Renal transplant biopsy may be considered when acute rejection or recurrent or *de novo* glomerular disease is suspected. This should be performed after pre- and post-renal causes have been excluded and when clotting and platelet counts are normal (many patients will be receiving aspirin, which should be discontinued).

Risk of acute rejection

The immunological changes that occur in pregnancy may protect against acute rejection.[2,28] Overall, the reported incidence of acute rejection during pregnancy is low and the consensus from the literature is that acute rejection rates in pregnancy are no higher than in nonpregnant patients.[23,25,28]

However, Galdo *et al.*[16] reported a 13.5% incidence of acute rejection in 37 renal transplant pregnancies in Chile, which was similar to a previous report from NTPR in which Armenti *et al.*[29] found an incidence of 14.5% in 115 ciclosporin-treated mothers. In addition, a single-centre study in Iran[22] reported a 6.7% incidence of acute rejection, which was universally associated with poor pregnancy outcomes. In this study, 17.5% of women became pregnant within 1 year post transplant, when risk of rejection is high.

The American Society of Transplantation (AST) and the European Best Practice Guidelines (EBPG) Expert Group on Renal Transplantation guidelines recommend deferring pregnancy for 12–24 months to reduce the risk of acute rejection and other problems that are frequently associated with the early months following renal transplantation.[4,8]

Fluctuation in CNI levels during pregnancy may be an additional predisposing factor for acute rejection, with Fischer *et al.*[9] reporting that ciclosporin levels can fall during pregnancy necessitating a 33% increase in dose after 20 weeks of gestation. However, the authors found a sharp increase in levels postpartum and doses had to be reduced to avoid toxicity (Figure 7.2). Careful attention should thus be given to monitoring CNI levels during pregnancy and the puerperium.

The treatment of acute rejection in pregnancy has been reviewed by several authors.[4,8] In general, treatment with corticosteroids is reported to be safe.[2,4,8] However, there are limited data regarding the use of monoclonal antibodies, iOKT3, antithymocyte globulin (ATG) or basiliximab or daclizumab. The AST guidelines advise intravenous immunoglobulin, which has been used extensively in pregnancy, but ATG and rituximab should be avoided in pregnancy.[4]

Hypertension

In early pregnancy, peripheral vascular resistance decreases, leading to lower blood pressure that then gradually rises in the later stages of pregnancy. Some renal transplant patients may require a reduction in antihypertensive mediation in early pregnancy but the majority will be hypertensive and require increased treatment in later pregnancy.

The NTPR reported that 47–73% of renal transplant patients were hypertensive during pregnancy and recent reports have endorsed this.[2,29] The UKTPR[24] reported 69% of women with treated hypertension prepregnancy and a further 8% were commenced on treatment during pregnancy. Yongwon *et al.*[27] reported a lower incidence of hypertension (28%) in pregnant transplant patients and an Italian study[20] reported hypertension in only 16% of pregnant transplant patients at booking, increasing to 58.2% at term.

Several studies have reported the incidence of hypertension to be higher in ciclosporin-treated mothers (51.7%).[9,29]

The risk of superimposed pre-eclampsia is high in this population and may be exacerbated further by CNIs.[2,29]

Registry reports and recent studies have indicated that the incidence of pre-eclampsia was between 15% and 58% in this group (Table 7.1). However, the diagnosis of pre-eclampsia can be difficult in renal transplant patients as blood pressure often rises in the second trimester, women with renal transplant often have pre-existing proteinuria, and urate levels are increased by CNIs. In addition, renal transplant recipients may have other comorbid factors such as diabetes or SLE, increasing the risk of pre-eclampsia further.

Hypertension is an important determinant of pregnancy outcome in the renal transplant patient. Studies have reported an association with preterm delivery and the UKTPR found hypertension to be associated with poorer long-term graft survival in women with SCr above 150 μmol/l.[2,24]

Proteinuria

A pregnant renal transplant patient may have underlying chronic allograft nephropathy or recurrent glomerular disease associated with proteinuria in early pregnancy. In addition, discontinuation of angiotensin-converting enzyme (ACE) inhibitor therapy before or at conception may lead to a rise in baseline proteinuria. In general, renal transplant patients experience an increase in pre-existing proteinuria during pregnancy especially in the third trimester,[11,14,25] which returns to baseline at 3–6 months. Forty percent of women developed up to 2–3 g proteinuria/day in the third trimester even in the absence of superimposed pre-eclampsia.[34]

Thompson *et al.*[25] found an increase in proteinuria from 0.4 g/day prepregnancy to 1.37 g/day in the third trimester which returned to baseline levels 3–6 months postpartum. Similarly, Crowe *et al.*[14] reported a rise in proteinuria from 0.45 g/day to 1.11 g/day at delivery which returned to baseline at 3 months.

Pregnancy is associated with increased thromboembolic risk[35] and the presence of proteinuria may exacerbate this risk further, especially in women with other risk factors for thromboembolic disease, such as smoking, obesity and previous DVT.[36,37] In addition, renal transplant patients have been reported to have an acquired hypercoagulable state especially in the first 6 months post transplant.[38,39] Some authors have reported that the thromboembolic risk is increased in ciclosporin-treated patients owing to changes in platelet function and alterations in the coagulation cascade.[39]

The risk of thromboembolic disease must be carefully assessed in a pregnant renal transplant patient with proteinuria and be balanced against risks of prophylactic anticoagulation. Consideration should also be given to the underlying renal disease, which may further increase the thromboembolic risk, for example the presence of antiphospholipid antibodies in women with SLE.

Obstetric outcomes following pregnancy in renal transplant recipients

Registry data show that good renal function and normal or well-controlled blood pressure are the most important factors for a favourable obstetric outcome. A review of the obstetric outcomes in 7110 pregnancies between 1961 and 2000 concluded that SCr below 125 µmol/l was an important prognostic factor (Table 7.3).[3]

Perinatal mortality

In previously published studies, the perinatal mortality has always been higher than that in the general population.[28] In the 1980s in the USA, perinatal mortality was 3% in the renal transplant population and 1.3% in the general population.[28] Ten years later this had improved and was reported to be 2.8% in renal transplant patients and 0.58% in the general US population.[40]

Recent studies of transplant pregnancies worldwide have reported live birth rates of between 43.2% and 84% (Table 7.4). The low live birth rate reported in the study of Pour-Reza-Gholi *et al.*[22] from Iran appeared to be due to the high proportion of pregnancies occurring in the first 3–12 months post transplant and associated high incidence of acute rejection in this subgroup.

Armenti *et al.*[41] reported a lower live birth rate in tacrolimus-treated women compared with ciclosporin-treated women. However, the pregnancies reported may have occurred at the time when tacrolimus therapy was mainly used in women with highest immunological risk and as rescue therapy following acute rejection.

Table 7.3. Influence of renal allograft function on pregnancy outcome; reproduced with permission from Davison and Bailey[3]

Serum creatinine	Complicated pregnancy	Successful outcome	Long-term obstetric problems
≤ 125 µmol/l (1.4 mg/dl)	30%	97%	7%
≥ 125 µmol/l (1.4 mg/dl)	82%	75%	27%

Estimates are based on data from 7110 pregnancies in 5370 women (1961–2000) that attained at least 28 weeks of gestation

Table 7.4. Studies on fetal outcomes in kidney transplant recipients

Study	Miscarriage (%)	Therapeutic termination of pregnancy (%)	Stillbirth (%)	Neonatal death	Live birth (%)
UK Transplant Pregnancy Registry 1994–2001[24]	11	6	2	2	79 (and 1 infant died before 3 months)
Armenti *et al.*[13]	12–24	1–8	1–3	1–2	76
Rahamimov *et al.*[23]	20				55
Thompson *et al.*[25]				6%	69
Miniero *et al.*[20]	29				68
Yongwon *et al.*[27]	4 miscarriage	18			
Gutiérrez *et al.*[17]	21	23			65.6 successful outcome
Keitel *et al.*[19]	14	23	3.2 fetal death		61.4 successful outcome
Pour-Reza-Gholi *et al.*[22]	24		9.5		43.2
Cruz Lemini *et al.*[15]		15 abortions			84
Galdo *et al.*[16]	19				
Hooi *et al.*[18]					63
Oliveira *et al.*[21]				1 (prematurity)	

Preterm birth

Rates of preterm birth are high particularly in women with hypertension.[24] The incidence of preterm birth is also increased by the high incidence of urinary tract infection in renal transplant patients,[12,28] the effects of CNIs[2,9,29] and the increased incidence of pre-eclampsia in these women.[2,29] The timing of delivery is often influenced by the medical and obstetric team and may be hastened by the presence of severe hypertension, deteriorating graft function or fetal growth restriction (Table 7.5).

The incidence of preterm birth has varied widely from 26% to 60% in recently reported studies from a range of populations around the world. The average gestational age when reported was 35–37 weeks (Table 7.5).

Sibanda *et al.*[24] reported a 50% incidence of preterm birth in renal transplant patients compared with 7% in the general population. Women with hypertension and SCr above 150 μmol/l were at particularly high risk of preterm birth.

Fetal growth

Infants of transplant recipients are often preterm and frequently have lower birthweight. Recent studies have reported the incidence of low birthweight babies to be 19–54% (average 42%) and the incidence of very low birthweight (less than 1500 g) to be 11–17.8%.[25,29]

In addition to the effects of preterm birth, several authors have reported an association between ciclosporin use and low birthweight infants. The NTPR reported significantly lower birthweights in infants of ciclosporin-treated mothers (2250 g versus 2505 g, $P = 0.03$),[8,29,31] Some studies have reported an association between low birthweight and hypertension and impaired renal function (SCr above 130 μmol/l).[24]

Delivery

The transplanted kidney rarely causes obstetric problems and is not injured by vaginal delivery. In recent studies the incidence of caesarean section varied from 34% in South Korea[27] to 91% in an Italian study[20] (Table 7.5).

Table 7.5. Studies on obstetric outcomes for kidney transplant recipients

Study	Preterm birth before 37 weeks (mean gestation)	Low birthweight less than 2500 g (mean weight)	Lower segment caesarean section
Sibanda *et al.*[24]	50% (35.6 weeks)	54% (2316 g)	64% (90 elective)
Armenti *et al.*[13]	52–54% (35–36 weeks)	46–50% (2378–2493 g)	46–55%
Rahamimov *et al.*[23]	60%	52%	
Thompson *et al.*[25]	56% (34.9 weeks)	41%, associated creatinine > 133 μmol/l	59%
Miniero *et al.*[20]	42% (36.1 weeks)		91%
Yongwon *et al.*[27]	25.5% (36.9 weeks)	40% (2260 g)	34%
Gutiérrez *et al.*[17]	29%	33%	46%
Keitel *et al.*[19]	36.4%	(2195 g)	
Pour-Reza-Gholi *et al.*[22]	7.22 months		
Cruz Lemini *et al.*[15]	37 weeks	19%	
Galdo *et al.*[16]	56% (30 weeks)	(2463 g)	55%
Hooi *et al.*[18]	35%		37%
Oliveira *et al.*[21]	38.4%	30%	61.5%

Caesarean section should only be performed for specific obstetric reasons and the most frequent indications are preterm problems, pre-eclampsia and deteriorating renal function. Sibanda *et al.*[24] reported that 83% of preterm infants were born by caesarean section, labour was induced in 12%, and only 5% were born by spontaneous delivery.

Outcomes in children of renal transplant patients

The children of transplant recipients are frequently born preterm or suffer fetal growth restriction and are of low birthweight (Table 7.6).[40,42–45] This leads to an increased risk of developmental and neurodevelopmental problems in later life. It is important that women understand the implications and risks facing a small and/or preterm baby and this should be addressed when advice is given before pregnancy or in early pregnancy.

In addition, the children of transplant patients are exposed to immunosuppressive and other medications in pregnancy, which may affect their long-term outcomes. Concerns regarding late effects of exposure to CNIs *in utero* were originally raised by Tendron-Franzin *et al.*[46] following experiments in an animal model.

Immunological

The long-term effects of *in utero* exposure to immunosuppressive agents are unknown. Some authors have hypothesised that immunological abnormalities may be induced in the fetus.[2,28] In animal studies, administration of CNIs during pregnancy resulted in abnormal T cell development and had a profound effect on the fetal immune system. Data in humans are limited but one study showed children of immunosuppressed women had low B cell numbers and another reduced T and B cells at birth, which normalised in a few months.[47,48] One case report of a child with multiple autoimmune problems[49] raised concerns regarding the induction of autoimmune disease in later life but subsequent reports have shown no increased incidence above the general population.[2]

The response of neonates to routine childhood vaccinations may alter following exposure to ciclosporin *in utero* and may be better delayed until after 6 months of age.[47]

Renal

Concerns have been expressed by Cochat *et al.*[50] that children exposed to immunosuppressants *in utero* may be at theoretical risk of renal impairment owing to fetal growth restriction (associated with reduced nephron number and oligomeganephronia) and fetal nephrotoxicity. However, despite the animal data, preliminary results in children are encouraging.[2]

Paediatric neurodevelopment

A small number of studies have reported outcomes in the offspring of renal transplant recipients (Table 7.6).[40,42–45] A study of 20 children (age 3–13 years) exposed to ciclosporin and azathioprine in pregnancy identified no differences in global, verbal or performance IQ or in language skills compared with controls.[42]

McKay and Josephson[2] highlighted the outcome of several studies which reported that small numbers of children suffered from sensorineural deafness and behavioural disorders.

As the number of babies born to transplant recipients grows, it is important to collect further prospective data on the outcome of children in the longer term.

Table 7.6. Neurodevelopment of children exposed to immunosuppressive agents *in utero*

Study	Number of children	Immunosuppressive drugs	Follow-up	Outcome	Other
Nulman *et al.*[42]	20 (3–13 years)	Ciclosporin and azathioprine		No difference in IQ or language skills	
Willis *et al.*[43]	48 (56% preterm)		5.2 years		
Stanley *et al.*[45]	175 (4 months to 12 years, 71 at school)	Ciclosporin	Telephone interview 4 months to 12 years	Mean gestation 34 weeks: 16% developmental delays (mean gestation < 33 weeks: 48% developmental delays, especially language) 14% of the children in the study needed educational support versus 11% of children in US public schools 1.7% major disabilities	97% mothers high school graduates Mean gestation 36 weeks
Sgro *et al.*[40]	44		Case–control 3 months to 11 years	3 developmental or learning disabilities	Born 34, 34, 38 weeks
Coscia *et al.*[44]	249	Ciclosporin	Questionnaires, case notes, telephone calls Mean age 11 years Mean length of follow-up 9.2 years	5.2% attention deficit hyperactivity disorder (6–7% general population) 4% neurocognitive defects 4% structural malformations	Mean gestation 36 weeks, birthweight 2554 g

Fertility issues in renal transplant patients

In view of the high reported rate of therapeutic termination of pregnancy within the renal transplant population (1–23%) in recent studies, (Table 7.4), it is very important that women are given appropriate contraceptive advice prior to or immediately following transplantation.[2,7] Hooi *et al.*[18] reported 54% of pregnancies in transplant patients in Malaysia were unplanned and Lessan-Pezeshki *et al.*[6,7] reported 48% of transplant pregnancies were unplanned and 93.8% of these women were not using any specific contraception.

Both reversible and irreversible methods of contraception can be considered, but the approach has to be tailored to the needs of the individual woman or couple.

Reversible methods of contraception in a renal transplant patient include:

- *Progestogen-only contraception*: This mode of contraception, which has no adverse medical effects in renal transplant patients, can be delivered in several forms, including mini-pill, injections, implants (duration 3 years) and the progestogen-releasing intrauterine device (duration 5 years). Progestogen-only mini-pills are not particularly reliable but newer preparations give a longer (12 hour) window between doses. It is important to advise the woman of the risk and/or possible implications of irregular menstrual bleeding or amenorrhoea.
- *Oral contraception*: In a renal transplant patient with well-controlled blood pressure and without risk factors for thromboembolic disease, it is appropriate to use a low-dose combined pill (maximum 30 µg of estrogen). It is advised to avoid third-generation progestogens in view of the increased risk of heart disease and thromboembolism. This form of contraception would not be appropriate for women with significant proteinuria or nephrotic syndrome. The advantage of this form of contraception is that it is reliable and gives good control of the menstrual cycle.
- *Intrauterine contraceptive device (IUCD)*: Copper devices have a duration of action of 5 years and are associated with a slightly increased risk of infection at the time of insertion. This method could be considered for women in a stable relationship with a low risk of pelvic inflammatory disease. IUCDs do not cause menstrual irregularity associated with progestogen-only contraception but they can result in heavier menstruation and do not protect against ectopic pregnancy. In general, immunosuppression reduces the effectiveness of intrauterine devices and increases the risk of intrauterine device-associated infections in transplant recipients.
- *Barrier methods*: These are safe but less reliable and thus women using them should also be advised that they are able to use the morning after pill if they are aware of possible failure of a barrier method.

For irreversible contraception, both male and female renal transplant patients can consider sterilisation procedures but comprehensive pre-sterilisation counselling is mandatory.

Assisted reproduction

The use of assisted reproductive technology has increased and such treatments are now being sought by renal transplant patients who have difficulty conceiving naturally. The rate of infertility was similar to that in the general population (10.4%) in 126 transplanted women in Iran.[7]

The techniques available include ovulation induction, *in vitro* fertilisation and embryo transfer. The outcome of five assisted conception pregnancies were reported within a larger study of 13 multiple pregnancies by Coscia.[33]

There are case reports of successful treatment of male infertility using intracytoplasmic sperm injection for male renal transplant recipients with infertility[51] and successful *in vitro* fertilisation in female transplant recipients.[52,53]

The ethical issues raised regarding fertility treatment in women with organ transplants are discussed in recent reviews.[54,55] See Chapter 13 for further discussion on assisted reproduction for women with renal disease.

Maternal life expectancy following renal transplant pregnancy

When considering pregnancy, a renal transplant patient may seek advice regarding her future prognosis in order to make an informed decision about the future welfare of a child. Indeed, several authors have discussed the ethical dilemmas posed when pregnancy occurs in a mother with a reduced life expectancy.[54,55] Future prognosis in the renal transplant patient is affected by many factors, including graft loss, graft function and the existence of other comorbid factors such as diabetes and hypertension.

Patient survival rates reported in recent mainly single-centre studies are shown in Table 7.1 and were reviewed by McKay and Josephson.[2] Tan *et al.*[56] reported that 10% of transplant patients will die within 7 years postpartum and 50% within 15 years.[28] The average 5 year survival rate of living donor renal transplants was 70–80% and 40–50% in cadaveric donors.[56]

Coscia *et al.*[44] reported follow-up (mean 9.2 years) in 187 women from the NTPR with a mean prepregnancy SCr of 124 μmol/l. At the last follow-up 69% had adequate renal transplant function, 8% poor function, 19% were dialysis dependent and 4% had died.

Unpublished data from the Study in Transplantation Empowering Patients and Practitioners (STEPP) long-term renal transplant outcome study (www.stepp.org.uk) analysing 1992–2001 data from women who had had a transplant (population from six UK transplant centres) showed that women under 40 years with a renal transplant had 80% graft survival at 5 years and 62% at 12 years. In the same population, patient survival was 90% at 11 years 4 months.

Preparation of renal transplant patients for pregnancy

Prepregnancy, antenatal and postpartum care of the renal transplant patient is a complex situation requiring multidisciplinary team care. The renal transplant patient may also have other comorbid conditions that need consideration and management both prepregnancy and during pregnancy. These issues are discussed in detail elsewhere in this book. A simple checklist for the care of the renal transplant patients in the clinic is given in Box 7.3.

Acknowledgement

Thanks to John Bankart, principal statistician for the STEPP study, Department of Epidemiology at Leicester University, for STEPP graft and patient survival data.

Box 7.3. Checklist for the care of pregnant renal transplant patients

1. Prepregnancy or early pregnancy (if no opportunity prepregnancy)

- Rubella vaccination pre-transplant and confirm antibody status
- Stop smoking
- Folic acid
- Discuss medicines in pregnancy:
  - medicines which are contraindicated in pregnancy, e.g. statins, angiotensin-converting enzyme (ACE) inhibitors, angiotensin II receptor blockers (ARBs), mycophenolate mofetil. Plan when to stop and how to convert to a safer alternative if required
  - medications that need to be modified in pregnancy including antihypertensives. Discuss safety of drugs and convert to methyldopa, labetalol or calcium channel blocker
  - consider other medication carefully. Stop bisphosphonates
- Advise about monitoring of calcineurin inhibitor (CNI) levels
- Advise about prevention of urinary tract infections. Plan monthly midstream urine (MSU) sample and consider prophylaxis
- Advise about other conditions: diabetes, systemic lupus erythematosus (SLE), implications in pregnancy including testing for anti-Ro, anti-La, check anticardiolipin antibodies and lupus anticoagulant
- Consider aspirin prophylaxis
- In patients with proteinuria discuss thromboembolic risk associated with increasing proteinuria and need for prophylaxis
- Advise about genetic issues: polycystic kidney disease or chronic pyelonephritis. Baby will need an ultrasound scan (record in maternal notes)
- Discuss Down syndrome testing

2. Antenatal

- Monitor blood pressure
- Monitor CNI levels
- Monthly MSU
- Monitor proteinuria
- Monitor renal function

3. Later pregnancy

- Fetal growth monitoring
- Continue monitoring blood pressure, blood count, biochemistry, protein excretion, urate, platelets
- CNI levels
- MSU
- At 26–28 weeks, consider glucose tolerance test for women treated with tacrolimus

4. Postpartum

- Careful monitoring of fluid balance
- Monitoring of CNI levels to avoid nephrotoxicity
- Advise about breastfeeding and medications – balance between maternal and child factors
- Reintroduce ACE inhibitors after delivery and ARBs after cessation of breastfeeding
- Consider childhood vaccinations
- Arrange ultrasound scan for children of parents with vesicoureteric reflux
- Organise ongoing nephrology follow-up appointments
- Continue low-molecular-weight heparin in heavily proteinuric subjects for up to 6 weeks

References

1. Murray JE, Reid DE, Harrison JH, Merrill JP. Successful pregnancies after human renal transplantation. *N Eng J Med* 1963:269;341–3.
2. McKay DB, Josephson MA. Pregnancy in recipients of solid organs – effects on mother and child. *N Engl J Med* 2006;354:1281–93.
3. Davison JM, Bailey DJ. Pregnancy following renal transplantation. *J Obstet Gynaecol Res* 2003;29:227–33.
4. McKay DB, Josephson MA, Armenti VT, August P, Coscia LA, Davis CL, *et al.* Women's Health Committee of the American Society of Transplantation. Reproduction and transplantation: report on the AST Consensus Conference on Reproductive Issues and Transplantation. *Am J Transplant* 2005;5:1592–9.
5. Hou S. Pregnancy in renal transplant patients. *Adv Ren Replace Ther* 2003;10:40–7.
6. Lessan-Pezeshki M. Pregnancy after renal transplantation: points to consider. *Nephrol Dial Transplant* 2002;17:703–7.
7. Lessan-Pezeshki M, Ghazizadeh S, Khatmani MR, Mahdavi M, Razeghi E, Seifi S, *et al.* Fertility and contraceptive issues after kidney transplantation in women. *Transplant Proc* 2004;36:1405–6.
8. EBPG Expert Group on Renal Transplantation. European best practice guidelines for renal transplantation. Section IV: Long-term management of the transplant recipient. Pregnancy in renal transplant patients. *Nephrol Dial Transplant* 2002;17 Suppl 4:50–5.
9. Fischer T, Neumayer HH, Fischer R, Barenbrock M, Schobel HP, Lattrell BC, *et al.* Effect of pregnancy on long-term kidney function in renal transplant recipients treated with cyclosporine and with azathioprine. *Am J Transplant* 2005;5:2732–9.
10. Hou S, Firanek C. Management of the pregnant dialysis patient. *Adv Ren Replace Ther* 1998;5:24–30.
11. Davison JM. The effect of pregnancy on renal function in renal allograft recipients. *Kidney Int* 1985;27:74–9.
12. Davison JM. Renal disorders in pregnancy. *Curr Opin Obstet Gynecol* 2001;13:109–14.
13. Armenti VT, Radomski JS, Morita M, Gaughan WJ, Hecker WP, Lavelanet A, *et al.* Report from the National Transplantation pregnancy Registry (NTPR): Outcomes of pregnancy after transplantation. In: Terasaki PI, Cecka JM, editors, *Clinical Transplants*. Los Angeles: UCLA Tissue Typing Laboratory; 2004. p. 103–14.
14. Crowe AV, Rustom R, Gradden C, Sells RA, Bakran A, Bone JM, *et al.* Pregnancy does not adversely affect renal transplant function. *Q J Med* 1999;92:631–5.
15. Cruz Lemini MC, Ibargüengoitia Ochoa F, Villanueva González MA. Perinatal outcome following renal transplantation. *Int J Gynaecol Obstet* 2007;96:76–9.
16. Galdo T, González F, Espinoza M, Qunitero N, Espinoza O, Herrera S, *et al.* Impact of pregnancy on the function of transplanted kidneys. *Transplant Proc* 2005;37:1577–9.
17. Gutiérrez MJ, Acebedo-Ribó M, García-Donaire JA, Manzanera MJ, Molina A, González E, *et al.* Pregnancy in renal transplant recipients. *Transplant Proc* 2005;37:3721–2.
18. Hooi LS, Rozina G, Wan-Shaariah MY, Teo SM, Tan CH, Bavanandan S, *et al.* Pregnancy in patients with renal transplants in Malaysia. *Med J Malaysia* 2003;58:27–36.
19. Keitel E, Bruno RM, Duarte M, Santos AF, Bittar AE, Bianco PD, *et al.* Pregnancy outcome after renal transplantation. *Transplant Proc* 2004;36:870–1.
20. Miniero R, Tardivo I, Curtoni ES, Bresadola F, Calconi G, Cavallari A, *et al* Outcome of pregnancy after organ transplantation: a retrospective survey in Italy. *Transpl Int* 2005;17:724–9.
21. Oliveira LG, Sass N, Sato JL, Osaki KS, Medina Pestana JO. Pregnancy after renal transplantation – a five yr single center experience. *Clin Transplant* 2007;21:301–4.
22. Pour-Reza-Gholi F, Nafar M, Farrokhi F, Entezari A, Taha A, Firouzan A, *et al.* Pregnancy in kidney transplant recipients. *Transplant Proc* 2005;37:3090–2.
23. Rahamimov R, Ben-Haroush A, Wittenberg C, Mor E, Lustig S, Gaftrer U, *et al.* Pregnancy in renal transplant recipients: Long term effect on patients and graft survival. A single center experience. *Transplantation* 2006;81:660–4.
24. Sibanda N, Briggs, D, Davison JM, Johnson R, Rudge C. Pregancy after organ transplantation: A report from the UK Transplant Pregnancy Registry. *Transplantation* 2007;83:1301–7.

25. Thompson BC, Kingdon EJ, Tuck Sm, Fernando ON, Sweny P. Pregnancy in renal transplant recipients: the Royal Free Hospital experience. *Q J Med* 2003;96:837–44.
26. Yildirim Y, Uslu A. Pregnancy in patients with previous successful renal transplantation. *Int J Gynaecol Obstet* 2005;90:198–202,
27. Yongwon P, Jaesung C, Younghan K, Changee L, Hyungmin C, Taeyoon K, *et al.* 360 pregnancy outcome in renal transplant recipients: the experience of a single center in Korea. *Am J Obstet Gynecol* 2001;185 Suppl 6:S180.
28. Stratta P, Canavese C, Giacchino F, Mesiano P, Quaglia M, Rosetti M. Pregnancy in kidney transplantation: Satisfactory outcomes and harsh realities. *J Nephrol* 2003;16:792–806.
29. Armenti VT, Ahlswede KM, Ahlswede BA, Jarrell BE, Mortitz MJ, Burke JF. National transplantation Pregnancy Registry – outcomes of 154 pregnancies in cyclosporine-treated female kidney transplant recipients. *Transplantation* 1994;57:502–5.
30. Samela KT, Kyllonen LEJ, Hlomberg C, Gronhagen-Riska C. Imapired renal function after pregnancy in renal transplant recipients. *Transplantation* 1993;56:1372–5.
31. Armenti VT , Gaughan WJ, Dunn SR, Kundu M, Coscia LA, McGrory CH, *et al.* National Transplantation Pregnancy Registry: pregnancy outcomes in female kidney recipients treated with cyclosporine microemulsion (Neoral) or tacrolimus vs. cyclosporine. *Transplantation* 1998;65:S77.
32. Ehrich JH, Loirat C, Davison JM, Rizzoni G, Wittkop B, Selwood NH, *et al.* Repeated successful pregnancies after kidney transplantation in 102 women (Report by the EDTA Registry). *Nephrol Dial Transplant* 1996;11:1314–17.
33. Coscia LA, Cardonick EH, Moritz MJ, Armenti VT. Multiple gestations in female kidney transplant recipients maintained on calcineurin inhibitors [abstract]. *Am J Transplant* 2003:3 Suppl 5;1603:563.
34. Davison JM. Pregnancy in renal allograft recipients: problems, prognosis, practicalities. *Baillieres Clin Obstet Gynaecol* 1994;8:501–25.
35. Greer I. Thrombosis in pregnancy: maternal and fetal issues. *Lancet* 1999;353:1258–65.
36. Royal College of Obstetricians and Gynaecologists. *Thromboembolic Disease in Pregnancy and the Puerperium: Acute Management.* Green-top Guideline No. 28. London: RCOG; 2007 [www.rcog.org.uk/index.asp?PageID=533].
37. British Society for Haematology. Guideleines on the prevention, investigation and management of thrombosis associated with pregnancy. *J Clin Pathol* 1993;46:489–96.
38. Kazory A, Ducloux D. Accquired hypercoagulable state in renal transplant patients. *Thromb Haemost* 2004;91:646–54.
39. Rabelink TJ, Zwaginga JJ, Koomans HA, Sixma JJ. Thrombosis and hemostasis in renal disease. *Kidney Int* 1994;46:287–96.
40. Sgro MD, Barozzino T, Mirghani HM, Sermer M, Moscato L, Akoury H, *et al.* Pregnancy outcome post renal transplantation. *Teratology* 2002;65:5–9.
41. Armenti VT, Radomski JS, Moritz MJ, Branch KR, McGrory CH, Coscia LA. Report from the National Transplantation Pregnancy Registry (NTPR): Outcomes of pregnancy after transplantation. In : Terasaki PI, Cecka JM, editors, *Clinical Transplants.* Los Angeles: UCLA Tissue Typing Laboratory; 2002. p. 121–30.
42. Nulman I, Barrera M, Chitayat D, Koran G. Neurodevelopment in children exposed to ciclosporine and azathioprine following maternal renal transplant: preliminary results. *Clin Pharmacol Ther* 2004;75:74.
43. Willis FR, Findlay CA, Gorrie MJ, Watson MA, Wilkinson AG , Beattie TJ. Children of renal transplant recipient mothers. *J Paediatr Child Health* 2000;36:230–5.
44. Coscia A, Moritz, M, Armenti VT. Long term follow up of the offspring of Sandimmune treated female kidney transplant recipients. World Transplant Congress 2006, 22–27 July 2006, Boston, USA. Abstract 289. p. 164.
45. Stanley CW, Gottlieb R, Zager R, Eisenberg J, Richmond R, Moritz MJ, *et al.* Developmental well-being in offspring of women receiving cyclosporine post-renal transplant. *Transplant Proc* 1999;31:241–2.
46. Tendron-Franzin A, Gouyon J, Guignard J, Decramer S, Justrabo E, Gilbert T, *et al.* Long term effects of *in utero* exposure to cyclosporin A on renal function in the rabbit. *J Am Soc Nephrol* 2004;15;2687–93.

47. DiPaulo S, Schena A, Morrone LF, Manfredi G, Stallone G, Derosa C, *et al.* Immunologic evaluation during the first year of life of infants born to cyclosporine-treated female transplant recipients: analysis of lymphocyte subpopulations and immunoglobulin serum levels. *Transplantation* 2000;69:2049–54.
48. Pilarski LM, Yacyshyn BR, Lazarovits AI. Analysis of peripheral blood lymphocyte populations and immune function from children exposed to ciclosporine or to azathioprine in utero. *Transplantation* 1994;57:133–44.
49. Scott JR, Branch DW, Holman J. Autoimmune and pregnancy complications in the daughter of a kidney transplant patient. *Transplantation* 2002;73:815–16.
50. Cochat P, Decramer S, Robert-Gnansia E, Duborg L, Audra P. Renal outcome of children exposed to cyclosporine *in utero*. *Transplant Proc* 2004;36(2 Suppl):208S–10S.
51. Zeyneloglu HB, Oktem M, Durak T. Male infertility after renal transplantation; achievement of pregnancy after intracytoplasmic sperm injection. *Transplant Proc* 2005;37:3081–4.
52. Tamaki M, Ami M, Kimata N, Tsutsui T, Watanabe Y, Saito T, *et al.* Successful singleton pregnancy outcome resulting from *in vitro* fertilisation after renal transplantation. *Transplantation* 2003;757:1082–3.
53. Case AM, Weissman A, Sermer M, Greenblatt EM. Successful twin pregnancy in a dual-transplant couple resulting from *in-vitro* fertilisation and intracytoplasmic sperm injection. *Hum Reprod* 2000;15:626–8.
54. Davison SN. Ethical considerations regarding pregnancy in chronic kidney disease. *Adv Chronic Kidney Dis* 2007:14:206–11.
55. Ross LF. Ethical considerations related to pregnancy in transplant recipients. *New Engl J Med* 2006;354:1313–16.
56. Tan PK, Tan A, Koon TH, Vathsala A. Effect of pregnancy on renal graft function and maternal survival in renal transplant recipients. *Transplant Proc* 2002;34:1161–3.
57. Kurata A, Maksuda Y, Tanabe K, Hiroshi T, Ohta H. Risk factors for preterm delivery at less than 35 weeks in patients with renal transplant. *Obstet Gynecol Surv* 2007;62:85–7.

8

Chapter 8

Reflux nephropathy in pregnancy

Nigel J Brunskill

Vesicoureteric reflux and reflux nephropathy: epidemiology, pathogenesis and clinical features

One-third of all anomalies detected by routine fetal ultrasonography are congenital abnormalities of the kidney and urinary tract (CAKUT).[1,2] The spectrum of abnormalities seen in individuals with CAKUT is wide and includes ureteric abnormalities (e.g. vesicoureteric reflux (VUR), megaureter and ureterovesical junction obstruction) and kidney abnormalities (e.g. aplastic kidneys, multicystic dysplasic kidneys, hydronephrosis and duplex kidney).

In clinical practice, VUR is the most common manifestation of CAKUT with an incidence in the general population from at least 0.4% to 1.8%.[3–5] Primary VUR results in the retrograde passage of urine from the bladder through the ureter into the upper urinary tract. In the majority, VUR resolves with time and is most often manifest in childhood.[6] There is now clear recognition that this has a familial component. Early segregation analysis pointed to a single dominant gene[7] but more recent evidence points to a polygenic genetically heterogeneous trait with multiple candidate genes affecting males and females equally.[8–12]

Reflux nephropathy is a term that describes coarse unilateral or bilateral renal scarring often found in association with VUR, an appearance previously known as chronic pyelonephritis. However, only a proportion of children with VUR subsequently develop reflux nephropathy. Under the age of 8 years, 26% of children diagnosed with VUR have renal scars, whereas in children 8 years or older 47% have renal scars at the time of diagnosis of VUR.[13] Reflux nephropathy is the most common cause of end-stage renal disease (ESRD) in children and accounts for 10% of all ESRD.[14]

In the majority of affected children the focal scars characteristic of reflux nephropathy develop early in childhood, usually in the setting of severe intrarenal reflux and urinary infection. Some children with VUR, particularly boys, demonstrate small smooth kidneys at birth with histological evidence of renal dysplasia in addition to VUR.[6] Hypertension is common[15] and progressive renal impairment towards ESRD occurs predominantly in those with gross VUR with severe bilateral scarring. The bulk of the initiating injury occurs in early childhood and ESRD may develop thereafter despite the resolution of VUR and in the absence of infection.[16]

Some individuals with VUR and reflux nephropathy are detected through screening programmes in the context of a family history. The commonest clinical presentation of VUR and reflux nephropathy, however, is a complicated urinary tract infection (UTI). The finding of hypertension, proteinuria and/or renal impairment in children and adults may also lead to the subsequent discovery of reflux nephropathy.

Reflux nephropathy in pregnancy

Some asymptomatic and otherwise healthy women with reflux nephropathy may present in pregnancy largely because the antenatal care setting often provides the first opportunity for blood pressure monitoring, urine dipstick analysis and the detection of urinary infection in affected women. Renal scarring and impaired renal function may be detected during subsequent investigation of these abnormal findings. There are several reasons why a maternal diagnosis of reflux nephropathy may affect the outcome of a pregnancy.

Reflux nephropathy and urinary sepsis in pregnancy

Urinary tract infections are one of the most common health problems during normal pregnancy, complicating 8% of pregnancies,[17,18] and women with VUR are at particularly increased risk. Although patients with VUR and reflux nephropathy are prone to UTIs, the reasons are not fully understood. With the combination of physiological dilation of the urinary tract in pregnancy and severe VUR, urinary stasis certainly plays a part.[16]

Given that it is generally accepted that UTIs may hasten renal scar formation, such infections in pregnancy merit treatment on this basis alone. The occurrence of symptomatic UTI in pregnancy is associated with increased risk of preterm rupture of membranes, preterm birth and low birthweight in addition to serious maternal complications such as septic shock.[19] Asymptomatic bacteriuria in pregnancy may be accompanied by similar complications, although this remains controversial.[20] Nonetheless, current consensus suggests that both asymptomatic bacteriuria and UTI in pregnancy should be promptly treated with antibiotics to prevent obstetric and maternal complications.[19,20] In the presence of reflux nephropathy, screening for bacteriuria should be performed regularly. No studies have assessed the optimum timing for such surveillance, although at least once in each trimester has been suggested.[16] If bacteriuria or UTI are detected, then eradication should be achieved using appropriate antibiotics. If urinary sepsis is recurrent, then prophylactic antibiotics should be considered.

Effect of reflux nephropathy on obstetric and maternal outcomes

How renal disease affects pregnancy outcomes has been an issue of interest and debate for 30 years. Based on a number of predominantly retrospective studies, it is currently believed that for pregnancy in the presence of renal disease:

- outcomes are largely dependent on renal function such that if renal functional loss is less than 50% then pregnancy is likely to be successful
- complications such as pre-eclampsia and preterm birth are increased
- poorly controlled hypertension predicts a worse outcome
- the presence of heavy proteinuria is accompanied by increased risks
- renal impairment associated with systemic diseases such as lupus and scleroderma carries a worse prognosis.[21–29]

Several authors have specifically studied the outcome of pregnancies complicated by reflux nephropathy and the results have sometimes been controversial. The series of Katz *et al.*[30] included 26 (out of 121) pregnancies in women with renal biopsy-proven interstitial nephritis probably due to reflux nephropathy, with serum creatinine (SCr) levels less than or equal to 1.4 mg/dl (125 μmol/l). The course of pregnancy and the underlying renal disease in these women did not appear to be different from those with other pathologies.

The Australian group of Becker *et al.*[31] reported pregnancy outcomes in six women with reflux nephropathy, diagnosed according to typical radiological features, who formed part of a subgroup of 20 women with 'moderate' renal failure (SCr of 200–400 μmol/l) among a larger cohort of 184 women with reflux nephropathy under long-term follow-up. Pregnancy was associated with rapid loss of renal function in all six, with four women requiring dialysis within 2 years of delivery. Two babies of mothers with reflux did not survive. The authors suggested that women with reflux nephropathy contemplating pregnancy should be specifically warned of the risk of end-stage renal disease. However, in the French series of 245 pregnancies in 99 women with reflux nephropathy reported by Jungers and colleagues,[32–34] pregnancy outcomes were more favourable and rapidly decreasing renal function was seen only in two hypertensive women with SCr above 200 μmol/l, but not in the majority with better preserved renal function.

Updating the Australian experience, El-Khatib *et al.*[35] presented data from 345 pregnancies in 137 women with unequivocal reflux nephropathy and/or VUR. Over 50% of these pregnancies were complicated. Twenty-six percent of women developed UTI with 6% developing acute pyelonephritis. The rate of fetal loss of 18% in those with SCr above 110 μmol/l was significantly greater than that of 8% in those with SCr below 110 μmol/l at conception. Maternal complications such as pre-eclampsia were greater in the presence of bilateral renal scarring, but persistent VUR had no impact on any pregnancy outcomes. Overall in this study, therefore, the risk of maternal and obstetric complications was predominantly related to the degree of underlying renal impairment and severity of renal scarring.

Jungers *et al.*[36] updated their French series by reporting outcomes in a cohort of 375 pregnancies in 158 women with reflux nephropathy seen over a period of 30 years up to 1994. The diagnosis of reflux nephropathy was carefully established using standard radiological investigations and the presence or absence of persisting VUR was determined in 113 women by micturating cystourethrography (MCUG). In this latter group persistent reflux was present in 43%. Interestingly, the diagnosis of reflux nephropathy was unknown in 56% of these women prior to their first pregnancy and was only revealed after investigation of UTI, proteinuria, hypertension and/or renal impairment. The most common complication was UTI in 22% of pregnancies and was more common and severe in those with persistent VUR but UTI did not appear to have substantial deleterious effects on fetal outcomes. The authors suggested that prospective mothers with VUR and recurrent UTI, particularly pyelonephritis, should consider prophylactic ureteric re-implantation. Maternal renal functional deterioration was observed in 87% of women with prepregnancy SCr above 110 μmol/l compared with only 1.2% of those with prepregnancy SCr below 110 μmol/l. Live births occurred in 92% of pregnancies where prepregnancy SCr was below 110 μmol/l, but in only 63% of pregnancies where prepregnancy SCr was above 110 μmol/l. Fetal loss was much more common in hypertensive mothers. Taking the 30 year cohort as a whole, outcomes generally seemed to show evidence of significant improvement over time and were better when management of pregnancy was intensified and carefully coordinated between obstetricians and nephrologists.

Some studies have suggested that outcomes in pregnancies complicated by glomerular diseases may be less favourable than those complicated by reflux nephropathy.[21,23,24] However, these comparisons are seriously hampered by small numbers of women in such studies.

Screening for VUR

Infants born to mothers with VUR may inherit the same condition. If the maternal diagnosis is apparent during pregnancy, the antenatal ultrasound may be used to detect characteristic changes of reflux nephropathy in the fetus.[16,37] Failing this, the offspring of women with either known VUR or a first-degree relative with VUR should be investigated as soon as possible after birth.[16] In the past, some interest has been shown in screening for bacteriuria in schoolchildren as a potential indicator of underlying VUR, but this is no longer regarded as a practical or useful undertaking.[38]

Conclusion

Reflux nephropathy is relatively common in pregnancy. However, while there are particular problems relating to UTI in pregnancies with reflux nephropathy, these can be adequately treated with standard antibiotics. There is no justification for prospective mothers to undergo MCUG with a view to prophylactic ureteral re-implantation prior to pregnancy. Overall, outcomes of pregnancies with reflux nephropathy appear to be related predominantly to the degree of underlying renal impairment and presence of hypertension rather than the underlying renal disease *per se*. Women with reflux nephropathy should be screened regularly for urinary infection in pregnancy and treated promptly should it occur. The offspring of the women should be screened for VUR.

References

1. Noia G, Masini L, De Santis M, Caruso A. The impact of invasive procedures on prognostic, diagnostic and therapeutic aspects of urinary tract anomalies. In: Cataldi L, Fanos V, Simeoni U, editors. *Neonatal Nephrology in Progress*, Lecce: Agora; 1996, p. 67–84.
2. Pope JCI, Brock JW III, Adams MC, Stephens FD, Ichikawa I. How they begin and how they end: classic and new theories for the development and deterioration of congenital anomalies of the kidney and urinary tract, CAKUT. *J Am Soc Nephrol* 1999;10:2018–28.
3. Kincaid-Smith P, Becker G. Reflux nephropathy and chronic atrophic pyelonephritis: a review. *J Infect Dis* 1978;138:774–780.
4. Bailey R. Vesicoureteric reflux in healthy infants and children. In: Hodson J, Kincaid-Smith P, editors. *Reflux Nephropathy*. New York: Masson; 1979. p. 59–61.
5. Sargent MA. What is the normal prevalence of vesicoureteral reflux? *Pediatr Radiol* 2000;30:587–93.
6. Dillon MJ, Goonasekera CD. Reflux nephropathy. *J Am Soc Nephrol* 1998;9:2377–83.
7. Chapman CJ, Bailey RR, Janus ED, Abbott GD, Lynn KL. Vesicoureteric reflux: segregation analysis. *Am J Med Genet* 1985;20:577–84.
8. Feather SA, Malcolm S, Woolf AS, Wright V, Blaydon D, Reid CJ, *et al.* Primary, nonsyndromic vesicoureteric reflux and its nephropathy is genetically heterogeneous, with a locus on chromosome 1. *Am J Hum Genet* 2000;66:1420–5.
9. Mak RH, Kuo HJ. Primary ureteral reflux: emerging insights from molecular and genetic studies. *Curr Opin Pediatr* , 2003;15:181–5.
10. Woolf AS, Price KL, Scambler PJ, Winyard PJD. Evolving concepts in human renal dysplasia. *J Am Soc Nephrol* 2004;15:998–1007.

11. Murawski IJ, Gupta IR. Vesicoureteric reflux and renal malformations: a developmental problem. *Clinical Genetics* 2006;69:105–17.
12. Lu W, van Eerde AM, Fan X, Quintero-Rivera F, Kulkarni S, Ferguson H, *et al.* Disruption of ROBO2 is associated with urinary tract anomalies and confers risk of vesicoureteral reflux. *Am J Hum Genet* 2007;80:616–32.
13. Smellie J, Edwards D, Hunter N, Normand IC, Prescod N. Vesico-ureteric reflux and renal scarring. *Kidney Int Suppl* 1975;4:S65–72.
14. Bailey R. Vesicoureteric reflux and reflux nephropathy. In: Schrier RW, Gottschalk CW, editors. *Diseases of the Kidney*. 4th ed. Boston: Little, Brown; 1988, p. 747–83.
15. Goonasekera CDA, Dillon MJ. Hypertension in reflux nephropathy. *BJU International* 1999;83:1–12.
16. Lynn K. Vesicoureteral reflux and reflux nephropathy. In: Feehally J, Floege J, Johnson RJ, editors. *Comprehensive Clinical Nephrology*. Oxford: Elsevier Health Sciences; 2007. p. 691–702.
17. Lucas MJ, Cunningham FG. Urinary infection in pregnancy *Clin Obstet Gynecol* 1993;36:855–68.
18. Mikhail MS, Anyaegbunam A. Lower urinary tract dysfunction in pregnancy: a review. *Obstet Gynecol Surv* 1995;50:675–83.
19. Vazquez JC, Villar J. Treatments for symptomatic urianry tract infections during pregnancy. *Cochrane Database Syst Rev* 2003;(4):CD002256.
20. Smaill F, Vazquez JC. Antibiotics for asymptomatic bacteriuria in pregnancy. *Cochrane Database Syst Rev* 2007;(2):CD000490.
21. Imbasciati E, Ponticelli C. Pregnancy and renal disease: predictors for fetal and maternal outcome. *Am J Nephrol* 1991;11:353–62.
22. Jones DC, Hayslett JP. Outcome of pregnancy in women with moderate or severe renal insufficiency. *N Engl J Med* 1996;335:226–32.
23. Jungers P, Chauveau D. Pregnancy in renal disease. *Kidney Int* 1997;52:871–85.
24. Jungers P, Chauveau D, Choukroun G, Moynot A, Skhiri H, Houillier P, *et al.* Pregnancy in women with impaired renal function. *Clin Nephrol* 1997;47:281–8.
25. Davison JM. Renal disorders in pregnancy. *Curr Opin Obstet Gynecol* 2004;13:109–14.
26. Fischer MJ, Lehnerz SD, Hebert JR, Parikh CR. Kidney disease is an independent risk factor for adverse fetal and maternal outcomes in pregnancy. *Am J Kidney Dis* 2004;43:415–423.
27. Franceschini N, Savitz DA, Kaufman JS, Thorp JM. Maternal urine albumin excretion and pregnancy outcome. *Am J Kidney Dis* 2005;45:1010–18.
28. Imbasciati E, Gregorini G, Cabiddu G, Gammaro L, Ambroso G, Del Giudice A, *et al.* Pregnancy in CKD stages 3 to 5: fetal and maternal outcomes. *Am J Kidney Dis* 2007;49:753–62.
29. Lindheimer MD, Davison JM. Pregnancy and CKD: any progress? *Am J Kidney Dis* 2007;49:729–31.
30. Katz AI, Davison JM, Hayslett JP, Singson E, Lindheimer MD. Pregnancy in women with kidney disease. *Kidney Int* 1980;18:192–206.
31. Becker GJ, Ihle BU, Fairley KF, Bastos M, Kincaid-Smith P. Effect of pregnancy on moderate renal failure in reflux nephropathy. *Br Med J (Clin Res Ed)* 1986;292:796–8.
32. Jungers P, Forget D, Henry-Amar M, Albouze G, Fournier P, Vischer U, *et al.* Chronic kidney disease and pregnancy. *Adv Nephrol Necker Hosp* 1986;15:103–41.
33. Jungers P, Forget D, Houillier P, Henry-Amar M, Grunfeld JP. Pregnancy in IgA nephropathy, reflux nephropathy, and focal glomerular sclerosis. *Am J Kidney Dis* 1987;9:334–8.
34. Jungers P, Houillier P, Forget D. Reflux nephropathy and pregnancy. *Baillieres Clin Obstet Gynaecol* 1987;1:955–69.
35. El-Khatib M, Packham DK, Becker GJ, Kincaid-Smith P. Pregnancy-related complications in women with reflux nephropathy. *Clin Nephrol* 1994;41:50–5.
36. Jungers P, Houllier P, Chaveau D, Choukroun G, Moynot A, Skhiri H, *et al.* Pregnancy in women with reflux nephropathy. *Kidney Int* 1996;50:593–609.
37. Blumenthal I. Vesicoureteric reflux and urinary tract infection in children. *Postgrad Med J* 2006;82:31–5.
38. Hansson S, Martinell J, Stokland E, Jodal U. The natural history of bacteriuria in childhood. *Inf Dis Clin North Am* 1997;11:499–512.

9

Chapter 9

Lupus and connective tissue disease in pregnancy

Mike Venning and Mumtaz Patel

There is an increasing understanding of the impact of the presence of lupus nephritis on pregnancy outcome.[1–10] Until recently, relatively little was known about pregnancy in vasculitic diseases, which are less common in women of childbearing age. These include the primary systemic vasculitides with potential for renal involvement: small vessel vasculitides including Wegener's granulomatosis, microscopic polyangiitis, Henoch–Schönlein purpura and Churg–Strauss syndrome. Also included are the medium–large vessel vasculitides such as Churg–Strauss syndrome (which may involve small and medium vessels), polyarteritis nodosa and Takayasu's arteritis.[11] Primary systemic vasculitis is now classified as antineutrophil cytoplasmic antibody (ANCA)-positive (typically Wegener's granulomatosis or microscopic polyangiitis) or ANCA-negative vasculitis, which may blur the distinctions between the classically defined disorders.[12,13] In this chapter the traditional diagnostic terms are retained, as many believe these relate to typically distinct disease entities and these terms are used in the great majority of publications concerning pregnancy.[13,14]

The issues relating to lupus nephritis and vasculitis are discussed, but a review of associated autoantibodies such as antiphospholipid antibodies and the anti-Ro (SSA) and anti-La (SSB) is not included. These autoantibodies need to be screened for and managed according to the separate role they may play. In particular, attention will need to be paid to antiphospholipid syndrome and the neonatal lupus syndromes.

Epidemiology of vasculitic and lupus nephritis

The prevalence of primary systemic vasculitis may be of similar order to that of lupus – the prevalence of lupus in Birmingham, UK, in 1992 was 27.7 per 100 000[15] and the prevalence of primary systemic vasculitis in Norwich, UK, in 1997 was 14.4 per 100 000.[16] Despite this, the age and sex distributions are very different.

The prevalence of lupus in Birmingham was 3.4 per 100 000 in males and 52.0 per 100 000 in females, whereas the prevalence of primary systemic vasculitis in Norwich was 17.0 per 100 000 in males and 12.0 per 100 000 in females.[15,16]

The age distributions are also very different. In 1992–3, only 11% of patients with ANCA-associated renal vasculitis in north-west England were aged less than 40 years,[17] whereas 25–45 % of patients with lupus (depending on racial origin) in Birmingham were aged less than 40 years.[15] These demographic factors would suggest a prevalence ratio of lupus compared with primary systemic vasculitis of 10 : 1 to 15 : 1 in women of childbearing age.

Estimated pregnancy rates

Using the simple assumption of conception at a replacement population birth rate, one can estimate, in a population of 1 million, a birth rate of 5–10 pregnancies/year in women with lupus. Similarly one might estimate 0.5–1 pregnancies/year in women with primary systemic vasculitis. This much lower than expected conception rate in vasculitis explains a significantly smaller clinical experience and the paucity of literature of pregnancy in women with vasculitis.

Two recent studies[18,19] in the north-west of England, both assessing the year 2001, the year of the UK census, emphasise the similar incidence of lupus nephritis to that of renal involvement in primary systemic vasculitis, typically manifesting the histology of pauci-immune necrotising crescentic glomerulonephritis. The incidence of lupus nephritis was 0.41 per 100 000/year with a rate of 0.68 (95% CI 0.40–1.10) in women and 0.09 (95% CI 0.01–0.32) in men. The median age was 38 years (36 in women and 65 in men). The incidence of pauci-immune necrotising crescentic glomerulonephritis was 1.0 per 100 000/year, with median age 67 years and with identical incidence and age distribution in males and females. The incidence in patients aged 65 years or older was 3.2 per 100 000/year. One may conclude that there will be a corresponding order of magnitude greater number of women of childbearing age with lupus nephritis than with renal involvement in primary systemic vasculitis.

Definitions

Renal dysfunction

Renal impairment is defined[20,21] as an estimated glomerular filtration rate (eGFR) below 60 ml/minute/1.73 m^2 or creatinine above 100 μmol/l, whereas in older literature authors on lupus nephritis have used creatinine above 106–125 μmol/l or even 150 μmol/l as thresholds of significant renal dysfunction.[5,22]

Proteinuria

Proteinuric and nephrotic presentations are very rare in vasculitis-associated renal disease, in contrast to lupus. Patients with renal vasculitis will typically present with rapidly progressive glomerulonephritis or with grumbling, remitting–relapsing or subacute variations of this. Proteinuria (with or without haematuria) is more central to the presentation and continuing course of lupus nephritis, whereas haematuria is the characteristic urinary abnormality in vasculitic nephritis.

Agreement is lacking regarding the definition of proteinuria (above 0.3 or above 0.5 g/day or protein/creatinine ratio (PCR) of above 33 or above 55 mg/mmol, respectively).[5,23]

The higher threshold is used in the Euro-Lupus definition.[23] This is also the level at which significant differences in outcome have been demonstrated (see below).[22]

Diagnosis of lupus

Authors generally accept the American College of Rheumatology (ACR) criteria for lupus, particularly in the research setting.[24] There are sometimes complex cases where there is a clinical diagnosis of lupus that does not satisfy the ACR criteria (typically in those patients with negative lupus serology, which may relate (in primary as well as in drug-induced lupus nephritis) to deficiencies of the complement pathways).[25] The development of features of nephritis, however, will usually result in satisfaction of the ACR criteria in these patients.

Diagnosis of vasculitis

A diagnosis of vasculitis requires histological confirmation, although serological evidence, particularly the presence of cytoplasmic-staining c-ANCA or perinuclear/ nuclear-staining p-ANCA, may be sufficient when the clinical presentation is characteristic.[12–14]

Diagnosis of lupus nephritis or vasculitic nephritis

Active nephritis is defined by the presence of haematuria (in lupus typically associated with proteinuria) with at least one of the following: reduced glomerular filtration rate (GFR), salt and water retention or hypertension.[3,6,22] Some authors recommend reliance on the presence of urinary casts, and phase-contrast microscopy with a skilled observer can detect red cell casts and dysmorphic red cells indicating glomerular pathology. The presence of granular casts is non-specific. Most would accept haematuria if present on dipstick testing, but some recommend microscopy: more than 5 rbc/hpf (red blood cell/high power field).[22]

Lupus nephritis more commonly presents with abnormality on urine dipsticks, moderate or nephrotic proteinuria or renal impairment that typically evolves subacutely. In comparison, vasculitic renal involvement is typically characterised by progressive renal dysfunction, often with rapidly progressive glomerulonephritis (RPGN) in which renal decline occurs over days or weeks. Proteinuric renal states, isolated haematuria and stable renal dysfunction are less common in the acute presentation of vasculitis.

The histological classification of lupus nephritis is long established, representing the full spectrum of immune complex renal disease. However, in vasculitis the renal histology is more one-dimensional, with small vessel vasculitides typically presenting as pauci-immune necrotising and crescentic glomerulonephritis (the glomerular manifestation of vasculitis). In the medium and larger vessel vasculitides, an extraglomerular vasculitis or simply regional renal infarction are typical.

Pre-eclampsia or active nephritis?

A major issue is the discrimination between pre-eclampsia and active vasculitic or lupus nephritis. Typical features of active lupus nephritis may include active extrarenal lupus, active urine sediment and active (in particular increasingly abnormal) lupus serology including anti-dsDNA antibodies, low C3 and C4 complement, and sometimes positive Coombs test or antiplatelet antibodies. Le Thi Huong *et al.*[4] described anti-dsDNA antibodies as being better at discriminating lupus nephritis from pre-eclampsia than low C3/C4 complement levels, which may fall with no associated flare in over 50% of cases. Less commonly measured anti-C1q antibodies and evidence of alternative pathway complement activation are also associated with active lupus nephritis. Hypertension may be absent or less severe in women with lupus nephritis.[3,9,22,26]

In the case of the vasculitic disorders, extrarenal disease may be a marker for active renal involvement. Similarly, increasing serological markers such as ANCA may correlate with or precede disease flare.[12–14] The presence of renal impairment is not uncommon in burnt-out disease and this, together with the hypertension which characteristically affects those with polyarteritis nodosa and Takayasu's arteritis, will have a similar adverse effect on pregnancy outcome as in patients with non-inflammatory renal disease.

Occurrence in the first 20 weeks of pregnancy makes pre-eclampsia unlikely.

Disease activity of lupus nephritis or vasculitic nephritis: nephritic/proteinuric flares

The definitions in lupus nephritis by Moroni *et al.*[22] have achieved widespread recognition and are more precise than others that have been used:[10] a *nephritic flare* being an increase in creatinine of at least 30%, with haematuria and generally increased proteinuria; and a *proteinuric flare* being an increase in proteinuria, without modification of plasma creatinine, by 2 g/day or, if baseline proteinuria is above 3.5 g/day, doubling of the proteinuria. (Most authors would accept variation of up to 15–20% in creatinine as within biological/assay variability).

In vasculitis, a renal flare will typically present with renal decline as in a lupus nephritic flare yet, although haematuria is characteristic, proteinuria may be unimpressive.

The Euro-Lupus Nephritis Trial used similar definitions for 'severe' as opposed to 'benign' flares (those not meeting the definition of 'severe' flares).[23] A 'severe' renal flare is:

- a systemic lupus erythematosus (SLE)-related increase in creatinine by 33% or
- recurrence or appearance of a nephrotic state (see above) or
- in patients with baseline proteinuria above 0.5 g/day and below 1 g/day, a three-fold increase in proteinuria if associated with the nephritic features of haematuria and a reduction in C3 complement levels by more than 33% in less than 3 months.

The Euro-Lupus group also included 'severe systemic disease' (see below) as defining a 'severe' renal flare, but this was for therapeutic purposes in the trial and in fact defines a severe non-renal flare.

Extrarenal disease activity in lupus

The most common forms of non-renal disease activity are cutaneous disease, arthritis and haematological disease, particularly thrombocytopenia. Severe flares are considered to include central nervous involvement, lupus pneumonitis or myocarditis, thrombocytopenia below 50×10^9/l, extensive skin or visceral vasculitis and fever.[4,22]

Skin disease is described as occurring in 25–90% of pregnancies and all forms of activity in 15–90%, described in one review as 'around 60%'.[4] Thrombocytopenia has been estimated to occur in 10–40% and severe arthropathy in 20% of pregnancies.[26]

These variable incidences according to different sources reflect different criteria for disease activity.[26] One must also bear in mind the 30% incidence of fibromyalgia in patients with SLE. This may significantly worsen in pregnancy and, together with the back pain of the second and third trimesters, may mimic lupus arthropathy. Similarly, hormone-induced facial blush of pregnancy and melasma may be misdiagnosed as a lupus flare.[26]

Many authors recommend indices of lupus activity such as the Lupus Activity Criteria Count (LACC) or the Systemic Lupus Erythematosus Disease Activity Index (SLEDAI-2K).[6,10] These indices have value in centres with the resources to incorporate their routine use into daily practice but caution is required regarding misclassification by less experienced observers of features such as fibromyalgia and melasma.

The Euro-Lupus definition of significant non-renal flare is: 'central nervous system disease, thrombocytopenia below 100×10^9/l, haemolytic anaemia, lupus pneumonitis or myocarditis, extensive skin vasculitis or serositis not responding to low-dose steroids with nonsteroidal anti-inflammatory drug (NSAID) treatment'.[23]

Extrarenal disease activity in vasculitis

The most common manifestations of vasculitis include the typically purpuric skin rash of small vessel vasculitis, with non-specific features such as malaise, myalgia, arthralgia, fever and sometimes weight loss.[14] Specific features may herald specific disease flares, such as eye, ear or upper respiratory symptoms in Wegener's granulomatosis, asthma exacerbation in Churg–Strauss syndrome and abdominal pain associated with rash and arthralgia in Henoch–Schönlein purpura. In the medium vessel vasculitides, including Churg–Strauss syndrome and polyarteritis nodosa, and in the case of Henoch–Schönlein purpura, a fine purpuric rash is common in the absence of deep organ involvement, for instance accompanying air travel. Any evidence of non-dermatological flare in Henoch–Schönlein purpura and any flare including rash in the other vasculitic disorders should alert the clinician to the possibility of deep organ flare potentially requiring active management. Full clinical and laboratory assessment is likely to be indicated, taking into account the previous manifestation/course of the disease in the individual patient.

Pregnancy and lupus nephritis

Over the past three or four decades, the prospects for successful pregnancy in women with lupus have been more encouraging.[9] The increased risks in mothers with active lupus are recognised.[7,8] Studies from the early 1980s highlight a number of factors recognised to influence outcome in pregnancy with lupus nephritis:[7,8]

- the presence of active lupus nephritis at conception (nephrotic syndrome, creatinine above 130 μmol/l (1.5 mg/dl) or to a lesser extent proteinuria above 0.5 g/day (PCR above 55 mg/mmol)) predicts a worse obstetric outcome
- stable remission of lupus for 6 months or more before conception is associated with an obstetric outcome comparable with that of normotensive gravidas with minor renal disease (even in patients following successful therapy of severe lupus nephritis)
- the isolated cases of maternal death are associated with onset of lupus in pregnancy or active lupus nephritis at conception
- relapse of lupus may be more common during pregnancy than postpartum
- severe renal relapse is associated with disease activity before or during pregnancy, but also has been described 4 months postpartum, in a mother who was in remission before and during pregnancy.

Together with improvements in obstetric and neonatal care, these findings led to a climate in which lupus nephritis was no longer deemed a contraindication to pregnancy. A number of tertiary centres developed managed programmes for the care of mothers with lupus.[1,4,6,9,27] Typical caution in the management of women with lupus nephritis, however, was expressed in 2001 by the Paris Salpêtrière group: 'Pregnancy was contra-indicated when serum creatinine was above 130 μmol/l'.[4] This series described only five of the 32 women studied entering pregnancy with proteinuria in excess of 0.5 g/day, in a setting in which patient autonomy may have been limited by clinical prudence. The Milan group, Moroni *et al.*,[22] reported a series of 70 pregnancies in women with lupus nephritis or who developed lupus nephritis during the pregnancy. Of these 70 pregnancies, six 'with signs of renal activity at the beginning' concluded with therapeutic abortion. Of the 64 remaining pregnancies, the highest plasma creatinine level was 150 μmol/l.

Maternal and fetal outcomes

Renal histological class

A number of authors have addressed the issue of lupus nephritis histological class, which clearly has a close association with disease severity.[10,28,29] Nonetheless, long-term outcomes of lupus nephritis have been shown to correlate with markers of chronic renal damage rather than with histological class, possibly because the glomerular features of lupus nephritis may evolve and change with time and disease activity.[10,29] Most authors would concur that in women with quiescent nephritis at the time of conception, histological class is not associated with pregnancy outcome.[2,4,10] Moroni's group[22] showed no association between histological class and maternal or fetal outcome. On the other hand, based on somewhat limited information on nephritis developing during pregnancy, women with histological class 4 (diffuse proliferative lupus nephritis) may run a more severe course, with classes 1 and 2 representing a lower level of risk.[4,22]

Previous immunosuppression

For lupus nephritis, little information has been presented about the effects of previous immunosuppression, with the exception of the poor prognostic effect of discontinuation of hydroxychloroquine in the months before conception.[26] Prior use of cyclophosphamide was described in 13 of 32 mothers in Le Thi Huong's series[4] without adverse impact on outcome in the setting of 'planned pregnancy'. On the other hand, the authors also described the poor outcome of women recently treated with cyclophosphamide for active nephritis before conception.[4] Clearly the age- and dose-related increased incidence of infertility in women treated with cyclophosphamide needs to be recognised and fully discussed with the woman.[30,31]

Pre-eclampsia

In lupus without renal involvement, the incidence of pre-eclampsia may be 13–35%.[26] Discrimination between pre-eclampsia and active lupus nephritis, as described above, is important and is well discussed by Clowse[26] and by Moroni and Ponticelli,[9] with a key discriminator of pre-eclampsia being abrupt onset. A rise in uric acid is also more characteristic of pre-eclampsia (baseline uric acid may be high with renal impairment) as is a rise in liver function tests.[22,26] Renal biopsy may be helpful as the finding of active nephritis will alter management (see Chapter 16).

Moroni and Ponticelli[9] diagnosed pre-eclampsia in 10% of women entering pregnancy with a diagnosis of lupus nephritis prepregnancy, whereas this rose to 35% of women in whom the first appearance of lupus nephritis was during the pregnancy. Similar results have been reported by others, with a corresponding higher incidence of pre-eclampsia in pregnancies that were 'non-planned' or in women with active lupus nephritis at the time of conception.[4]

Impact of lupus nephritis and renal dysfunction on fetal outcome

Whereas the fetal loss rate in mothers with lupus may be around 20%, the loss rate in women with lupus nephritis is reported at 15–35%, with preterm birth reported between 20–40%, well documented in the review by Moroni and Ponticelli,[9] who again emphasise the importance of disease activity on outcome.

With regard to the impact of renal dysfunction, Moroni and Ponticelli[9] described fetal loss (including stillbirth, neonatal death and miscarriage/spontaneous abortion) in two out of four conceptions with creatinine above 106 μmol/l and loss of three out of five pregnancies with creatinine rising intrapartum to over 133 μmol/l (maximum 354). Julkunen[3] described a fetal loss rate of 50% in women with creatinine over 140 μmol/l and of over 80% with creatinine over 400 μmol/l, stating 'at a creatinine of ≥ 180 μmol/l pregnancy cannot be recommended'.

Other factors present at conception and associated with fetal loss: active nephritis, proteinuria and hypertension

Moroni and Ponticelli[9] documented a historical fetal loss rate of 9–40% in women with lupus nephritis. This was matched in the Guy's series dating back to 1970 with a live birth rate of 81%.[2] In addition to confirming the increased fetal loss rate in women with active nephritis, Moroni, in a study noted for the use of multivariate statistical analysis, demonstrated that proteinuria above 0.5 g/day was associated with risk of fetal loss of 57% compared with 9% in the absence of proteinuria.[22] They quoted an odds ratio of 13.3.

Le Thi Huong[4] and Moroni[22] and colleagues showed that in SLE, in addition to proteinuria and active nephritis, hypertension was a predictor of fetal loss, with an odds ratio of 6.4. This confirmed the non-significant trend noted by Oviasu *et al.*,[2] with 29% fetal loss in hypertensive mothers and 13% fetal loss in mothers with normal blood pressure. Reassuringly, Moroni and colleagues[22] noted no increase in fetal loss in association with renal flares in pregnancy. Their therapeutic approach consisted of 'prompt administration of high dose steroids'.

Many authors stress the importance of prepregnancy planning on fetal outcomes.[4,7,32,33] Outcomes are summarised in tabular form by Le Thi Huong *et al.*,[4] who notes a live birth rate of 75–92% in 'planned' pregnancies, matching the success rate of 91% reported by Jungers *et al.*[7]

Impact of new onset of nephritis or renal flare in pregnancy

Jungers *et al.* in 1982[7] reported only four live births in nine women where initial manifestations of lupus with nephritis developed intrapartum or within 3 months of delivery. Of the nine pregnancies, two led to therapeutic terminations and a further three suffered fetal loss.

In the study by Moroni *et al.*[22] of eight women who developed renal flares in pregnancy on a background of lupus nephritis, one woman died with disseminated intravascular coagulation and sepsis and one ended up on long-term dialysis – further impact on renal function is discussed below.

Extrarenal flares

In lupus without nephritis, the relative risk of flare in pregnancy has been estimated at 7.25 (58% versus 8%); although with rigorous criteria for activity, the associated overall risk of flare may be lower at 15–30%. The risk of flare is increased if there is active lupus in the 6 months before conception. Other factors predisposing to flares include discontinuation of hydroxychloroquine and a previously stormy clinical course with multiple flares.[26] In contrast with Moroni's demonstration of a lack of predictive effect of laboratory markers for renal flares (perhaps because of insufficient power with lower incidence of renal flares), Soubassi *et al.*[5] demonstrated rising antibody levels to DNA in 100% of women with flares and diminished complement levels in 25%.

The timing of lupus flares is variable, but in women without lupus nephritis this seems to be predominantly in the second and third trimesters, with postpartum flares also being common, amounting to some 15–35% of all flares.[1,27] In comparison, postpartum flares may be more common in women with lupus nephritis, in up to 50% of those women experiencing postpartum pregnancy-associated flares.[6]

In women with lupus nephritis the early experience of 81% lupus flares has been followed by progressively better outcomes.[4,5,22,27] Ruiz-Irastorza *et al.*[27] described an absence of effect of pre-existing lupus nephritis on the incidence of pregnancy-associated flares in women with lupus.

Laboratory indices of disease activity

Most authors regard laboratory indices of lupus activity as unreliable but low or falling C3 and C4 complement levels and high or rising levels of anti-dsDNA antibodies may be associated with renal flares. Low or falling C3 and C4 complement levels have been described as associated with poor pregnancy outcome and yet are found in fewer than 50% of women with a clinical lupus flare.[4,5]

Preterm birth

Preterm birth was seen in 11 (28%) of 39 pregnancies that went beyond 23 weeks in the Guy's series (but their definition of preterm was stricter, at 36 weeks rather than the currently accepted 37 weeks).[2] With the 37 week definition, estimates of preterm birth rates in lupus nephritis range from 13% to 53%, mainly around 30%.[4,22,26]

Maternal death

In the series described since 1983, five cases of maternal death are reported. All five women died of sepsis.[4,22,34] In contrast, death is much more common in women with active vasculitis in pregnancy and postpartum.[11,35,36]

Effect of pregnancy on renal outcomes

The 1991 review by Oviasu *et al.*[2] described renal flares in 17% of pregnancies with SLE-nephritis in remission. Moroni *et al.*[22] described renal flares in 9–66% of women according to various authors. Moroni, with multivariate analysis, also determined that the only predictor of renal flare was signs of active nephritis at the beginning of pregnancy (creatinine above 106 μmol/l or proteinuria above 0.5 g/day with haematuria). Laboratory indices (low C3/C4 complement, raised antibodies to DNA, thrombocytopenia) were not predictive of renal flare. Flares occurred in one of 20 pregnancies (5%) with quiescent renal disease and in 12 of 31 pregnancies (39%) with active nephritis.[22] Of the four women in this study with creatinine above 125 μmol/l, two had no renal flare and two had, respectively, a nephritic and a proteinuric flare.

Moroni and colleagues[22] carefully described the impact of antenatal renal flares on renal outcome. Their therapeutic approach to antenatal development of lupus nephritis led to recovery of renal function and proteinuria in all but one of ten women in whom the flare was entirely antenatal; this woman presenting nephrotic and entering partial remission. Three of these women were left with persistent hypertension. More severe outcomes occurred in the other three women whose first presentation of lupus nephritis was antenatal: all three developed proteinuria in the last weeks of pregnancy and progressed postpartum to end-stage renal failure associated with severe extrarenal lupus at 1 week, 2 months and 4 months postpartum, respectively. Two of these three women recovered renal function after 1–2 months and were described as in complete remission a year or so later, the other remaining on dialysis. Thus one of 13 women (7.7%) presenting with *de novo* lupus nephritis in pregnancy ended up on long-term dialysis.[22]

In Moroni's study,[22] of eight women who developed renal flares in pregnancy on a background of lupus nephritis, one woman died with disseminated intravascular coagulation and sepsis and one woman ended up on long-term dialysis. Of six women who developed flares postpartum (all within 4 months), three out of five proteinuric flares developed subsequent to a diagnosis of pre-eclampsia. Four of these five women recovered (complete remission in three, return to baseline proteinuria in one) with treatment, the other had improved proteinuria.

Overall, 27% of women had renal flares, with the previously mentioned death occurring in end-stage renal failure, one other woman in end-stage renal failure (14% of those with flares, 4% overall) and the others were cured by therapy, although hypertension persisted in a minority.[22]

Risk of renal decline

In a 1991 review of eight studies, including their own, Oviasu and colleagues[2] concluded that, in women with lupus nephritis, the risk of pregnancy-associated permanent decline of renal function was 8%. In 2007 Le Thi Huong *et al.*[4] similarly reviewed those and three subsequent series, noting a worsening of renal function in 11–27% of cases. They stressed the low incidence of permanent renal deterioration, documenting a probable improvement in outcome with time and matching the rate of 4% in Moroni's series.[22]

Pregnancy and vasculitic nephritis

There is limited experience of systemic vasculitis and pregnancy, which is summarised in Table 9.1.[11,35,36] The different diseases run very different courses, from the relatively benign course of Henoch–Schönlein purpura, particularly in those with modest renal involvement, to the grim outcomes of women presenting in pregnancy with polyarteritis nodosa.

In systemic vasculitis, Ramsey-Goldman[11] highlighted the severe impact of disease activity on maternal and fetal outcome. The presence of active renal disease is a marker for substantially increased maternal and fetal risk. In ANCA-positive systemic vasculitis, ANCA titres correlate weakly with disease activity (aided somewhat by C-reactive protein levels), yet a rise in ANCA titre may herald relapse. Erythrocyte sedimentation rate (ESR), which is often helpful in monitoring disease activity, is not reliable in pregnancy.[14,35]

In active Takayasu's arteritis and polyarteritis nodosa as well as in most women with Wegener's granulomatosis or Churg–Strauss syndrome, full-dose cyclophosphamide therapy, with steroids, and possibly plasma exchange and/or biological therapies may be indicated to preserve maternal life and wellbeing.

Limited data suggest that in Churg–Strauss syndrome and granulomatous vasculitis control of active disease in advance of pregnancy may lead to satisfactory outcome, with subsequent pregnancy being free from disease activity.[35] In his 2007 review, Seo[35] was clear that pregnancy should take place only after 'prolonged remission has been achieved'.

Maternal death

In contrast with lupus nephritis in which death would appear to be strongly associated with sepsis, death is much more common in women with active vasculitis in pregnancy and postpartum, not infrequently associated with active vasculitis.[11,35,36]

Lupus nephritis and vasculitic nephritis: management

Prepregnancy management

Both in lupus and vasculitis with renal involvement, the risks associated with pregnancy are potentially high, particularly in the setting of active disease or unplanned pregnancy. All clinicians caring for women of childbearing age with these conditions should ensure that the women are given advice about these risks and about the benefits of planning pregnancy. A multidisciplinary team, expert in the care of the autoimmune disease as well as the obstetric and renal features that will impact on maternal and fetal outcome, should be available for prepregnancy advice and counselling.

Table 9.1. Reported outcomes of pregnancy in women with systemic vasculitis[11,35,36]

Systemic vasculitis	Pre-eclampsia	In remission at conception	Active at conception/intrapartum	Presenting in pregnancy
Wegener's granulomatosis		87% live birth 27% relapse	Poor outcome/62% live birth 10% maternal death	70% live birth 10% maternal death
Henoch–Schönlein purpura	Risk with renal/ blood pressure involvement	83% live birth 'usually benign course'	Systemic disease: < 20% renal decline	50% live birth
Churg–Strauss syndrome		> 85% live birth > 50% flare rate	Asthma may need close monitoring	66% live birth 33% maternal death
Polyarteritis nodosa	Risk with renal/ blood pressure involvement	> 80% live birth 12% flare		66% live birth 100% maternal death
Takayasu's arteritis	A particular concern	70–80% live birth 50% fetal growth restriction 15% cardiac failure, renal impairment	Hypertension is a major problem	

24. Hochberg MC. Updating the American College of Rheumatology revised criteria for the classification of systemic lupus erythematosus. *Arthritis Rheum* 1997;40:1725.
25. Pusey CD, Venning MC, Peters DK. Immunopathology of glomerular and interstitial disease. In: Schrier RW, Gottschalk CW, editors. *Diseases of the Kidney*. Boston/Toronto: Little Brown; 1988. p. 1827–83.
26. Clowse ME. Lupus activity in pregnancy. *Rheum Dis Clin North Am* 2007;33:237–52.
27. Ruiz-Irastorza G, Lima F, Alves J, Khamashta MA, Simpson J, Hughes GR. Increased rate of lupus flare during pregnancy and the puerperium: a prospective study of 78 pregnancies. *Br J Rheumatol* 1996;35:133–8.
28. Dixon FJ. The pathogenesis of glomerulonephritis. *Am J Med* 1968;44:493.
29. Austin HA, Klippel JH, Balow JE, le Riche NG, Steinberg AD, Plotz PH, *et al.* Therapy of lupus nephritis: controlled trial of prednisolone and cytotoxic drugs. *N Engl J Med* 1986;314;614–19.
30. Park MC, Park YB, Jung SY, Chung IH, Choi KH, Lee SK. Risk of ovarian failure and pregnancy outcome in patients with lupus nephritis treated with intravenous cyclophosphamide pulse therapy. *Lupus* 2004;13:569–74.
31. Boumpas DT, Austin HA III, Vaughan EM, Yarboro CH, Klippel JH, Balow JE. Risk for sustained amenorrhea in patients with systemic lupus erythematosus receiving intermittent pulse cyclophosphamide therapy. *Ann Intern Med* 1993;119:366–9.
32. Witter FR. Management of the high-risk lupus pregnant patient. *Rheum Dis Clin North Am* 2007;33:253–65.
33. Petri M. The Hopkins Lupus Pregnancy Center: ten key issues in management. *Rheum Dis Clin North Am* 2007;33:227–35.
34. Imbasciati E, Surian M, Bottino S, Cosci P, Colussi G, Ambrososo GC. Lupus nephropathy and pregnancy. *Nephron* 1984;36:46–51.
35. Seo P. Pregnancy and vasculitis. *Rheum Dis Clin North Am* 2007;33:299–317.
36. Langford CA, Kerr GS. Pregnancy in vasculitis. *Curr Opin Rheumatol* 2002;14:36–41.
37. Skorecki KL, Nadler SP, Badr KF, Brenner BM. Renal and systemic manifestations of glomerular disease. In: Brenner BM, Rector FC, editors. *The Kidney*. Philadelphia: WB Saunders; 1986. p. 891–928.
38. McKay DB, Josephson MA. Pregnancy in recipients of solid organs – effects on mother and child. *New Engl J Med* 2006;354:1281–93.
39. Micheloud D, Nuno L, Rodriguez-Mahou M, Sanchez-Ramon S, Ortega MC, Aguaron A, *et al.* Efficacy and safety of Etanercept, high-dose intravenous gammaglobulin and plasmapheresis combined therapy for lupus diffuse proliferative nephritis complicating pregnancy. *Lupus* 2006;15:881–5.

Chapter 10

Diabetic nephropathy in pregnancy

Andrew McCarthy

In contemplating a pregnancy, women with diabetic nephropathy have to consider the dual risks of diabetes and their impaired renal function to a pregnancy. Furthermore, they need advice on the potential for such a pregnancy to further compromise their renal function. They will need to make a considered long-term judgement of the risks involved, which requires that they are well informed about their prognosis even in the absence of pregnancy. It is most appropriate if this information is presented to them in a context that is remote from pregnancy, rather than when they are pregnant, and therefore requires that a system exists to ensure that all women in this situation of childbearing age receive prepregnancy counselling.

Introduction

With the increasing prevalence of type 2 diabetes and increased longevity, diabetes has become the most common cause of end-stage renal disease (reviewed by American Diabetes Association[1] and How and Sibai[2]). Approximately 20–30% of all patients with diabetes progress to nephropathy. A smaller proportion of those with type 2 diabetes progress to end-stage renal disease and death from cardiovascular causes prevents progression to end stage renal disease. It is thought that approximately 8% of renal failure in the diabetic population is due to causes other than diabetic nephropathy and hence wider investigation may be required. Biopsy must be considered if disease progression is atypical, especially in the absence of retinopathy.

Diabetic nephropathy is manifest as scattered sclerosis of glomeruli developing within years of the diagnosis. This initially results in microalbuminuria (30–300 mg in 24 hours) and is then followed by overt nephropathy with increasing proteinuria. Microalbuminuria is a marker for increased cardiovascular risk in future years. As a group, compared with a more general renal population, they will often be younger and more likely to be nulliparous, although this depends on local populations and the risks of type 2 diabetes.

For a historical picture of risk of complications, it is chastening to review the original publications of White[3,4] which led to the clinical classification of women with diabetes in pregnancy. In the paper published in 1945,[3] White refers to fetal mortality rates of 30–60%, the range depending on inclusion of early pregnancy loss. She describes a series of 181 consecutive women with diabetes managed personally between 1936 and 1944, resulting in one maternal death and 29 fetal deaths. It is clear from the discussion that these loss rates are vastly better than those of her peers at the time. A subsequent publication in 1949[4] revealed an 18% fetal mortality among 439 women with diabetes, excluding first-trimester loss.

Epidemiology and progress

Nephropathy is defined in different ways in recent publications, some using 300 mg of protein excretion in 24 hours, others a 500 mg cut-off, assessed in the first half of pregnancy. Urinary albumin excretion before pregnancy and early in gestation has been studied by Ekbom *et al.*[5] and shown to be comparable.

Microalbuminuria is referred to as incipient nephropathy. Hypertension often manifests at the time of development of microalbuminuria in patients with type 1 diabetes. Optimal management includes strict glycaemic control, management of hypertension (the goal of therapy is a blood pressure of less than 130/80 mmHg),[1] use of angiotensin-converting enzyme (ACE) inhibitors and angiotensin II receptor blockers (ARBs), and protein restriction dependent on the stage of nephropathy.

Progression from micro- to macroalbuminuria has varied widely in the many studies performed, with estimates of 2.8 to 13 per 100 person-years in more recent studies. The EURODIAB study[6] suggests that 14% (2 per 100 person-years) of 352 patients with type 1 diabetes with microalbuminuria will progress to macroalbuminuria over 7 years and 51% will regress to normoalbuminuria. HbA_{1c}, albumin excretion rate and body weight at baseline were associated with progression. End-stage renal disease develops in 50% of patients with type 1 diabetes with overt nephropathy within 10 years and in more than 75% in 20 years. The clinical and pathological correlations are outlined in the review of Kitzmiller and Combs.[7]

The Confidential Enquiry into Maternal and Child Health (CEMACH)[8] study in the UK gives a picture of how pregnancy is affected by diabetes. Seventy-three percent had type 1 diabetes, and 27% had type 2. The latter group were more likely to be socially disadvantaged, older, multiparous and belong to ethnic minority communities. In general, this population is at high risk of pregnancy-related complications, with increased risks of preterm delivery (36%), caesarean section (67%), stillbirth (relative risk (RR) of 5) and perinatal mortality (RR 3), and have a two-fold increased risk of congenital abnormality. This chapter will focus on the risks attributable to diabetic nephropathy specifically.

Nephropathy is said to complicate between 5% and 10% of pregnancies of women with diabetes. It has traditionally been associated with increased risks of preterm delivery, pre-eclampsia and general maternal morbidity. The risk of nephropathy may depend on which form of diabetes a woman has. In a separate subset of the CEMACH enquiry,[8] 8% of women with type 1 diabetes had nephropathy and 5% of women with type 2.

It has always been a matter of great concern that pregnancy might exacerbate underlying nephropathy. There is general agreement that glomerular hyperfiltration is the primary problem and that if it is due to increased glomerular capillary pressure and not just increased renal blood flow, then there could be a subsequent loss of function. Glomerular filtration rate (GFR) increases by 50% in pregnancy and theoretically this could therefore increase the rate of progression of underlying nephropathy if accompanied by elevated intraglomerular pressure. The development of hypertension during pregnancy could also have a deleterious effect, as could increased protein intake and any acute complication associated with a pre-renal insult. The degree of glycaemic control can also affect GFR and proteinuria.

ACE inhibitors

Medication exposure is covered in Chapter 11, but there are specific issues relating to ACE inhibition in diabetic nephropathy. It has been demonstrated that ACE inhibition is associated with a 50% reduction in risk of death, dialysis and transplantation in patients with diabetic nephropathy[9] and confers significant benefit in the absence of hypertension. These benefits are clearly very substantial and strategies of care around the time of conception must minimise the loss of such benefits.

Hod *et al.*[10] studied eight women with normotensive insulin-dependent diabetes with confirmed nephropathy (proteinuria more than 500 mg/day). The women took captopril and vigorously pursued optimal blood sugar control, until a missed period followed by positive pregnancy test. All women had significantly lower protein leakage at conception following their captopril treatment (reduced from 1633 ± 666, to 273 ± 146 mg daily), but then experienced increased protein excretion during the pregnancy although not to pre-captopril levels. Postpartum, the level of protein excretion was still below the pretreatment levels. This study may be consistent with a sustained benefit of ACE inhibition prepregnancy or markedly improved glycaemic control. Glycaemic control clearly has the potential to affect the development of nephropathy[11] and will have been an important influence in parallel with ACE inhibition.

Bar *et al.*[12] reported on a series of cases of 24 women with diabetic nephropathy treated with an ACE inhibitor until first positive pregnancy test. In all women in this study, the intensive prepregnancy regimen resulted in a reduction in proteinuria to a range of 10–450 mg/day at conception.

Cooper *et al.*[13] demonstrated in the non-diabetic population a possible two- to three-fold increase in risk of congenital malformation in those exposed to ACE inhibitors in the first trimester. This was in contrast with a prior lack of substantive evidence of teratogenicity in the first trimester (for a review, see How and Sibai[2]). If the concern in the paper of Cooper *et al.* is correct, there must be a possibility of an even greater effect in the diabetic population and hence this warrants a greater degree of caution with prescribing of ACE inhibition to diabetic women of childbearing age. Women with diabetes are at greater risk of congenital abnormality[8] and were specifically excluded from the study of Cooper *et al.* It is not known whether teratogenic risk due to this class of drug may be even greater in this group. However, the potential benefits are substantial and potentially life-saving. Clearly strategies must be employed on an individual basis to maximise the potential benefits and reduce risk. Such strategies may vary depending on background fertility, severity of nephropathy and comorbidities, and may entail cessation of ACE inhibition prior to attempts at conception or a policy of regular pregnancy testing (in the presence of regular menses) with immediate cessation of treatment upon diagnosis of pregnancy.

Levels of comorbidity

There are little data on levels of comorbidity in the pregnant diabetic nephropathic population. Retinopathy is often described and levels of hypertension vary as shown in Table 10.1. Few of the studies make reference to comorbidities such as thromboembolic events or cardiac disease. The data on diabetic nephropathy are weighted towards milder degrees of renal impairment and there will be a clear aversion to pregnancy for those with serious comorbidities. Cardiovascular comorbidity is more frequently mentioned in studies of follow-up following pregnancy. Assessment of risk of coronary artery disease has been studied in this population in other contexts, and Manske *et al.*[14] found that there was a very low level of significant coronary disease where the patient was less than 45 years of age, the duration of diabetes was less than 25 years and no ST–T wave changes were seen on electrocardiogram.

Table 10.1. Characteristics of patient populations with diabetic nephropathy

Study	Country	Number of pregnancies	Percentage with nephropathy	Women with nephropathy		
				Percentage with hypertension	Percentage with nephrotic range proteinuria	Percentage with creatinine > 125 µmol/l
CEMACH (2007)[8]	UK	359	12% (5–8% in separate analysis)			
Khoury *et al.* (2002)[16]	USA	72	Unclear	60%		13%
Ekbom *et al.* (2001)[5]	Denmark	11	5%		55%	
Bar *et al.* (2000)[17]	Israel	24	100%	46%	100%	0
Reece *et al.* (1998)[18]	[Review]	315		42%		
Gordon *et al.* (1996)[19]	USA	49	12%	27%	13%	7%
Mackie *et al.* (1996)[20]	UK	24	9%	17%	13%	21%
Miodovnik *et al.* (1996)[21]	USA	46	25%	41%		
Purdy *et al.* (1996)[22]	USA	14		82%	18%	100%

Barak and Miodovnik[15] reviewed the case reports of coronary events in pregnant women with diabetes. They described 20 cases between 1953 and 1998 who suffered a coronary event around the time of pregnancy. Of the 13 women who suffered an event during pregnancy or in the puerperium, seven mothers and seven infants died. These figures are largely historical, but nonetheless serve to define the natural history of such an event. Major changes in the treatment of coronary events have occurred since the majority of these case reports, but thrombolysis would still pose difficult issues in the perinatal period.

It is clear from Table 10.1 that the literature is weakened by some lack of clarity of the patient population, with varying reporting of hypertension, nephrotic range proteinuria and degree of renal failure.[5,8,16–22] There is a clear paucity of data from prospective studies that characterise the above features prepregnancy. Such data should be available in the near future in cohorts coming through of women exposed to ACE inhibition.

Screening for comorbidity

An electrocardiogram should be performed in early pregnancy in this population. Assessment of cardiovascular and thromboembolic risk should be made. Relevant risk factors would include family or personal history of cardiac or thromboembolic disease, hypertension, raised body mass index, a history of smoking and degree of urinary protein leakage.

There are no specific data on thromboembolic risk in this group of pregnant women. Nonetheless, a strategy to prevent thromboembolism needs to be employed. It would seem reasonable to suggest that all women with nephrotic range proteinuria receive low-molecular-weight heparin (LMWH) prophylaxis throughout pregnancy. Other women with more minor degrees of proteinuria should receive LMWH if other risk factors are present. The dose of LMWH employed will depend on the degree of renal impairment and the woman's weight.

Problems in pregnancy

A number of helpful reviews have been published,[7,15,18,23–26] and results from studies investigating pregnancy complications caused by diabetic nephropathy are summarised in Table 10.2.[5,8,15–22,27–32] The following comments apply to complications from mid-trimester onwards as most studies have excluded first-trimester complications. Reviews of diabetic nephropathy in pregnancy continue to emphasise the problems with this literature, almost invariably retrospective in nature, covering experience in single-site centres of excellence over decades and still with relatively small numbers of women (11–46[23] and 8–62[18]). The situation is further complicated by the fact that level of glycaemic control is a major determinant of outcome in such pregnancies. Furthermore, the diabetic population is continually changing, both in demography (increasing proportions of type 2) and in exposure to treatments such as ACE inhibition. With reference to diabetic nephropathy, it is not possible to subdivide the data available according to prepregnancy treatment with ACE inhibition and the majority of published experience largely predates use of ACE inhibition. Summation of the data in such reviews gives a picture of the relevant population, late twenties in age, with diabetes of 18 years duration and a mean age at onset of 12 years.[18]

Caesarean rates are universally high, reflecting high degrees of intervention in such pregnancies and possibly uncertainty regarding fetal status faced with the dual

Table 10.2. Complications of pregnancy affected by diabetic nephropathy

Study	Country	Number of women	Number of pregnancies	Caesarean section	Mean gestational age (weeks)	Preterm birth	Fetal growth restriction	Perinatal death
CEMACH (2007)[8]		359	359				31%	
Bagg *et al.* (2003)[27]	New Zealand	14	24	83%	36			
Khoury *et al.* (2002)[16]	USA	72	72	68%	35	13% before 32 weeks		3 (4%)
Rossing *et al.* (2002)[28]	Denmark	26	31	39%	37			3 (10%)
Ekbom *et al.* (2001)[5]	Denmark	11	11			45% before 34 weeks		0
Bar *et al.* (2000)[17]	Israel	24	24	62%		17% before 37 weeks	21%	1 (4%)
Biesenbach *et al.* (1999)[29]	Austria	12	14	50%	34		64%	5 (36%)
Dunne *et al.* (1999)[30]	UK	18	21	90%	34		14%	2 (10%)
Reece *et al.* (1998)[18]	[Review; 10 papers]	315	315	74%		22% before 34 weeks	15%	5%
Lauszus *et al.* (1998)[31]	Denmark	11	11					3 (27%)
Gordon *et al.* (1996)[19]	USA	45	49	80%	36	16% before 34 weeks	11%	0
Zhu *et al.* (1997)[32]	Japan	10	10	90%	35			
Mackie *et al.* (1996)[20]	UK	18	24	100%	34	24% before 32 weeks	8%	0
Miodovnik *et al.* (1996)[21]	USA	46	46	76%	35	22% before 34 weeks	9%	9%
Purdy *et al.* (1996)[22]	USA	11	14	29%	34	21% before 32 weeks	7%	0

threats of renal impairment and diabetes, often in the presence of superimposed pre-eclampsia. Gestational age at delivery reflects the same concerns. Definitions of fetal growth restriction are generally centile based, but caution is required with the confounding influences of diabetes and vascular disease. There are strong arguments for regular ultrasound surveillance every 2 weeks, and more frequently in the presence of any acute concern. Perinatal loss rates such as those above are often viewed with optimism, but any perinatal loss in the context of such a high-risk pregnancy is clearly extremely disappointing. It is a double disaster for a woman with diabetic nephropathy to potentially compromise her long-term health and survival and also not achieve a healthy surviving infant.

Hypertension

Carr *et al.*[33] addressed the issue of hypertensive control in pregnancy affected by diabetic nephropathy. This was a retrospective study which identified two groups, one achieving a target blood pressure of mean arterial pressure of less than 100 mmHg and another group failing to meet the target. Approximately 10% of the diabetic population in this study were deemed nephropathic. There was no difference in age or duration of diabetes between the two groups. The group with above-target blood pressure control had greater urinary protein excretion and higher creatinine. Suboptimal control was associated with a significantly increased risk of delivering early, i.e. less than 32 weeks of gestation, even after adjustment for blood glucose control and duration of diabetes.

The study of Carr *et al.*[33] provides some specific data on haemodynamic measurement in pregnancy with diabetic nephropathy. Blood pressure and cardiac output were higher than expected and total peripheral resistance was elevated in the group with above-target blood pressure. The authors concluded that longstanding hypertension is likely to be more severe and to be characterised by vasoconstriction and that treatment regimens should include vasodilators. The issue of target blood pressure is also addressed in the review of Kitzmiller and Combs[7] where they expressed a preference for blood pressure in the range of 120–130/80–85 mmHg.

Sibai *et al.*[34] reported data on a large number of women with type 1 diabetes. The risk of pre-eclampsia increases with increasing White classification of diabetes, attaining a 36% risk in those with retinopathy or nephropathy in comparison with an overall rate of 20%. Proteinuria at baseline, hypertension and nulliparity also predicted pre-eclampsia.

The difficulty in diagnosing pre-eclampsia in a population with diabetic nephropathy is likely to be a significant factor explaining the varying rates of pre-eclampsia in different studies summarised in Table 10.2. Hiilesmaa *et al.*[35] showed a 57% incidence of pre-eclampsia or pregnancy-induced hypertension in mothers with pre-existing nephropathy, Biesenbach *et al.* 57%,[29] Reece *et al.* 41%,[18] Gordon *et al.* 53%,[19] Bar *et al.* 46%,[17] Zhu *et al.* 40% ('severe'),[32] Miodovnik *et al.* 65%[21] and Purdy *et al.* 27%.[22] The incidence of pre-eclampsia has been the subject of a separate review by Sibai.[36] In his review of seven publications there were 333 women with diabetic nephropathy, with an overall incidence of pre-eclampsia of 51% (range 35–66%). The use of low-dose aspirin to prevent pre-eclampsia has not been adequately studied in this population, with the study of Caritis *et al.*[37] failing to show any benefit.

Arguments for advising low-dose aspirin in such pregnancies include the potential to prevent mid-trimester pre-eclampsia, to provide modest protection against thromboembolism in a high-risk group and to prevent coronary events.

Proteinuria

Once pregnant, women with nephropathy do not always adapt to pregnancy with the 50% increase in renal blood flow and glomerular filtration rate that women without nephropathy can achieve. Some will demonstrate the normal physiological rise in GFR, some will remain unchanged and in some a decrement will be noted.[7] It is difficult to tease out the decline in function in pregnancy from the natural history of the condition with falls in GFR of 10–12 ml/minute per year.[7]

Protein leakage is known to generally increase during the course of pregnancy. The study of Hod *et al.*[10] shows the progression of level of proteinuria in a subset of women with diabetes in the different trimesters and postnatally. Proteinuria can be substantial but normally resolves following delivery. Much of the proteinuria must be caused by the hyperfiltration of pregnancy as it resolves reasonably consistently following delivery. Transient deterioration can of course arise as a result of superimposed pre-eclampsia. The greatest clinical concern arises from any subsequent fall in plasma oncotic pressure, with risk of pulmonary oedema. Diuretic treatment may be required in such situations, even though it is conceptually unattractive because of the potential to further reduce intravascular volume in compromised pregnancies. Patterns of weight gain in these pregnancies have not been described.

Urinary protein excretion was summarised in the review of Star and Carpenter[25] which looked at nine studies. Mean protein excretion was typically between 1 and 3 g/day at baseline, but increased to between 4 and 8 g/day in the third trimester. This frequently fell postpartum but not always to baseline values. It is unclear whether persistently high levels postpartum were a reflection of a short follow-up period, disease progression or deterioration secondary to pregnancy.

Preterm delivery

Rates of preterm delivery for this group must be compared with the diabetic population as a whole. These data are available from Sibai *et al.*[38] and from CEMACH.[8] Sibai *et al.* break down rates of delivery as a result of spontaneous labour (16% at less than 37 weeks, 9% at less than 35 weeks) and from indicated delivery such as pre-eclampsia or fetal growth restriction (22% at less than 37 weeks, 7% at less than 35 weeks). Steroids should generally be prescribed prior to 34 weeks albeit with caution, i.e. with monitoring of the blood glucose response, urinary ketones and a temporary increase in insulin treatment as required. There is currently no consensus on use of steroids between 34 and 37 weeks, so any potential benefit has to be balanced against the disadvantage of loss of metabolic control. The greatest argument for steroids in this situation can be made when elective caesarean delivery is considered.

It is clear from many of the studies[19,20] that those women who enter pregnancy with the greatest impairment of renal function are most at risk of very preterm delivery, although mean gestational ages in all studies suggest most babies would be expected to do well, especially with current advances in management of neonatal lung disease. Many of the studies in this area are performed over a substantial time span and many of the papers mentioned in this review include babies born preterm in the 1980s. Neonatal management has improved hugely since then. While this may reassure us that the outcome should be substantially improved, it is also possible that thresholds for delivery have been moved forward to 'protect renal function' or improve overall perinatal survival. Influences likely to result in elective preterm delivery include concern about loss of renal function, presence of pre-eclampsia or concern about risk of stillbirth. Amniocentesis may help provide reassurance about fetal lung maturity while simultaneously assessing fetal status.[39] The latter method of assessment has yet to achieve widespread acceptance.

Factors relating to perinatal outcome

Pregnancies complicated by diabetic nephropathy carry the added burdens of increased risk of congenital malformation, stillbirth and metabolic disturbance in comparison with other forms of renal disease in pregnancy. The literature in this area is more focused on those risks that arise as a result of the impaired renal function as it is this that sets these women apart from the main diabetic population.

Khoury *et al.*[16] describe the problems inherent in calculating risks of complications in pregnancy with diabetic nephropathy, chiefly the small size of many of the studies, reflecting single-site experience. They estimate that to assess an association between severity of diabetic nephropathy and perinatal death, a study of 850 pregnancies would be required. Ekbom *et al.*[5] have examined diabetic pregnancy with a range of urinary albumin excretion. Although the number of patients with nephropathy was low (n = 11), there was a clear association between increasing severity of urinary albumin excretion at baseline and preterm delivery due to pre-eclampsia (but not preterm delivery due to other causes). Lauenborg *et al.*[40] examined the characteristics of women with diabetes that increased risk of stillbirth across three tertiary centres in Denmark over a 10 year period; 27% of women with stillbirths had diabetic nephropathy, as opposed to 5% overall in the reference group. Bar *et al.*[17] described pre-existing hypertension as the only parameter to predict poor outcome.

The CEMACH study[8] used a composite of poor clinical outcome (major anomaly at any gestation, intrauterine death from 20 weeks and any death up to 28 days after delivery). The odds ratio for such an outcome was 2.0 in the nephropathy group (95% CI 1.0–4.2). Excluding congenital anomalies, the adjusted odds ratio for such a poor outcome was 2.6 (95% CI 1.1–6.1).

Salvesen *et al.*[41] examined fetal wellbeing in a group of six fetuses where the mother suffered diabetic nephropathy. Cordocentesis demonstrated that these fetuses were hypoxaemic and acidaemic in the absence of abnormal blood flow studies. This implies the lack of a placental cause and may reflect wider metabolic disturbance. It emphasises the difficulty in being confident regarding fetal outcome even in the presence of normal ultrasound assessment. This difficulty is compounded by the lack of data regarding background risks of placental abruption. It is likely that management of pregnancy in women with diabetic nephropathy will always involve some conflict between stillbirth risk and neonatal morbidity as obstetricians struggle to decide on timing of delivery.

Long-term prognosis

Maternal outcomes

A major issue for women with diabetic nephropathy is the potential risk of a permanent deterioration in renal function attributable to pregnancy, bringing forward the need for renal replacement therapy. A number of studies have attempted to address this issue. There are good reasons why pregnancy may increase the risk of progression of nephropathy, including increasing glomerular hyperfiltration and the risk of development of hypertension. Studies in this area have suffered from small numbers, changing outcome for progression of renal disease due to advances in management, and lack of appropriate control groups. Most studies have found no effect of pregnancy on rate of decline in renal function. The studies are summarised in Table 10.3. There is very wide variation in the follow-up periods reported in such studies, making the data on progression to end-stage renal failure extremely difficult to interpret. These studies focus exclusively on renal outcome and there is no formal assessment of the effect of pregnancy or pre-eclampsia on long-term risk of a cardiovascular event in this high-risk group. The study of Gordin *et al.*[42] adds weight to the general concern that women who suffer from pre-eclampsia are at greater risk of long-term cardiovascular morbidity. In this study women with type 1 diabetes and a history of pre-eclampsia had a higher frequency of diabetic nephropathy at follow-up (41.9% versus 8.9%), were more likely to be on an antihypertensive treatment (50.0% versus 9.8%) and were more likely to have coronary artery disease (12.2% versus 2.2%).

The studies specifically in diabetic nephropathy tend to be retrospective cohort studies, although there are two major prospective cohort studies in diabetic pregnancy in general which provide complementary information.

Retrospective cohort studies

The data on end-stage renal disease and maternal death in the review of Reece *et al.*[18] reflect approximately 3 years of follow-up. The duration of follow-up in the different studies varies and appears to be largely opportunistic.

Studies demonstrating bad progression

Biesenbach *et al.*[29] studied 14 pregnancies in 12 women, all of whom had pre-existing hypertension. They subdivided pregnancies into those that had a physiological increase in creatinine clearance in early pregnancy and those in whom it declined. This resulted in small numbers, in which the latter group was associated with longer duration of diabetes, greater proteinuria and poorer renal function prior to conception. In six

Table 10.3. Studies examining the effect of pregnancy on progression of renal disease

Study	Country	Number of women	Decline in function	Mortality	End-stage renal failure
Bagg *et al.* (2003)[27]	New Zealand	14	NS		36%
Rossing *et al.* (2002)[28]	Denmark	26	NS	35%, mean follow-up 16 years	19%
Bar *et al.* (2000)[17]	Israel	24	None		
Biesenbach *et al.* (1999)[29]	Austria	12	Yes	0	
Dunne *et al.* (1999)[30]	UK	18	No	0	1
Reece *et al.* (1998)[18]	[Review]	315	No	5% (mean follow-up 35 months)	17% (mean follow-up 33 months)
Gordon *et al.* (1996)[19]	USA	45	Yes		3 (6%)
Mackie *et al.* (1996)[20]	UK	24	No	0	4 (17%)
Miodovnik *et al.* (1996)[21]	USA	56	No	1 or 5[a]	26% at 6 years
Purdy *et al.* (1996)[22]	USA	11	Yes		63% at 2–3 years

NS = no significant difference

[a] depending on duration of follow-up

pregnancies there was an improvement in creatinine clearance of 36% up to 24 weeks. In another eight pregnancies it decreased by 16 % over the same early period. In the latter group the deterioration in function persisted postpartum. In the poor prognosis group there was a greater increase in proteinuria during pregnancy and more marked hypertension. In this study, seven out of eight women in the poor prognosis group had a prepregnancy creatinine clearance of less than 70 ml/minute, while all the women with a physiological increase in creatinine clearance had a clearance of more than 70 ml/minute. The groups in this study did not differ in metabolic control as demonstrated by HbA_{1c}.

Gordon *et al.*[19] also found cause for concern. Women were categorised according to degree of renal impairment and no difference in degree of change in the three groups was noted. It is noteworthy that the three with the worst renal impairment progressed to transplantation after the pregnancy, i.e. at intervals of 8, 15 and 41 months after delivery (no control data). Most of their population demonstrated nephrotic range proteinuria by the third trimester. At postnatal follow-up, mean creatinine clearance had decreased but proteinuria was unchanged from early pregnancy measurement. The fall in creatinine clearance in ml/minute per year and the percentage decline in creatinine clearance per year were assessed. Individuals entering pregnancy with proteinuria in excess of 1 g/day and a creatinine clearance of less than 90 ml/minute fared worse by both criteria. The difference was not explained by mean HbA_{1c}, mean arterial blood pressure or use of ACE inhibitor.

Purdy *et al.*[22] examined a group with poor renal function, all with a creatinine of 124 μmol/l or more. They examined reciprocal of creatinine plots over time but there is a clear paucity of data prior to the index pregnancies. Furthermore, there is a lack of clarity about inclusion criteria for the study. Nonetheless, the rate of progression of disease in this group with poor function is of concern.

Rossing *et al.*[28] evaluated the effect of pregnancy on renal function in women with diabetic nephropathy. They found no adverse effect compared with a control group of women with nephropathy but no pregnancies. There were no further details given regarding the control group, raising the possibility that other comorbidities may have been present and sufficient to deter women from pregnancy. The study group did have a shorter duration of diabetes but earlier onset of nephropathy. The pregnancy rate prior to the onset of nephropathy (similar in both groups) argues against any bias due to possible comorbidities.

Data in this study give a sense of the proportion of women that proceed to die prematurely, with nine out of 26 women dead at the end of the follow-up period. Half of these deaths were from cardiovascular disease and between 50% and 60% were smoking at the time of diagnosis of nephropathy. At the end of the follow-up period, 65% of the pregnant group and 53% of the nonpregnant group were still alive and without end-stage renal disease.

Bagg *et al.*[27] provide similar data from women managed from 1985 to 2000. Their study of 24 pregnancies in 14 women found that, at a median follow-up of 6 years postpartum, five (36%) had begun dialysis, four had proliferative retinopathy (one blind), three had ischaemic heart disease, three had stroke and two had peripheral vascular disease. Bar *et al.*[17] found no deterioration in serum creatinine or creatinine clearance in their group of 24 women with diabetic nephropathy. Mackie *et al.*[20] plotted inverse creatinine over the long term in subjects with renal impairment and demonstrated a lack of any effect of pregnancy on long-term decline in renal function.

Studies on parity

Miodovnik *et al.*[21] stratified the risk of developing nephropathy by parity using life-table analysis and showed no significant differences. They also examined the rate of decline in creatinine clearance and found no effect of pregnancy (decreasing at an annual rate of 8–10 ml/minute). No effect of parity on risk of end-stage renal disease was seen. Interestingly, the only factor that made progression to end-stage disease among the group with nephropathy more likely was black ethnicity. Retinopathy, development of hypertension in the pregnancy, development of nephrotic range proteinuria during the pregnancy or glycohaemoglobin did not predict this, although the study was not necessarily powered to address these issues specifically. While this study is reassuring there was no nulliparous control group.

Prospective cohort studies

The Diabetes Control and Complications Trial (DCCT) group[43] allowed intensification of blood glucose control for pregnancy and included 86 women (135 pregnancies) in the conventional treatment group and 94 (135 pregnancies) in the intensive treatment group. There was no difference in the rate of development of microalbuminuria as a result of pregnancy, although some increases in albumin excretion rate were noted in relation to pregnancy.

The EURODIAB prospective complications study[44] examined risk factors for progression to nephropathy in a group of 425 childless women with diabetes and found that, while HbA_{1c} was a significant predictor of progression to microalbuminuria, pregnancy was not (102 gave birth in the study period). This applied to both the nulliparous and multiparous populations. In the same study, while duration of diabetes and HbA_{1c} were predictive of retinopathy, pregnancy again was not. The study examined risk of neuropathy in addition to nephropathy and retinopathy and found that pregnancy was not a risk factor for the development or progression of any diabetic complication.

Neonatal/fetal outcomes

In the study of Bar *et al.*[12] there were two severely disabled infants, both seemingly as a result of shoulder dystocia despite a caesarean rate of 62%. All other survivors to 2 years of age were free of disability.

Reece *et al.*[18] in an earlier review provided data from three previous studies where the incidence of psychomotor impairment was 5.5%, 3.7% and 9%, i.e. an overall incidence of 6%. The studies in question were published in 1981, 1988 and 1995, and one may therefore question their relevance today. However, it is the later study in 1995 that quotes the highest incidence.

Mackie *et al.*[20] reported that one baby delivered at 27 weeks went on to have cerebral palsy. As with the other studies there was no formal neurodevelopmental follow-up of the infants involved.

Omissions in the literature

There are clearly areas of clinical practice that are not addressed by the current literature. The world literature may be from very varied healthcare systems, with varying incidences of type 2 diabetes, access to health care and altered rate of progression of long-term complications, possibly with racial differences. There are few data on first-trimester complications, comorbidities and the potential impact of ACE inhibition prepregnancy, and the literature may not reflect the increasing incidence of type 2 diabetes.

Some guidance needs to be given about the potential reasons to advise against pregnancy. These would include evidence of untreated coronary artery disease, end-stage renal disease (Kitzmiller and Combs[7] suggest creatinine clearance less than 30 ml/minute), uncontrolled hypertension and proliferative retinopathy not in remission. Women with end-stage disease may be better served by assessment for transplantation and consideration of pregnancy afterwards, age permitting.

Conclusion

The above literature spans a number of decades of experience. During this time there have been notable advances in diabetes and renal care, although it cannot be assumed that these have benefited men and women equally.[45] It is likely that, with appropriate care, the vast majority of women with diabetic nephropathy can consider a pregnancy without any threat to their long-term disease progression (see Box 10.1). There is a risk that those with the most severe disease may experience a significant deterioration in renal function and, ultimately, end-stage renal failure. The same women will be most at risk of an adverse outcome to the pregnancy, although most pregnancies will be successful. The demography of this population is changing continually and current cohorts of women may well have an improved outcome largely due to ACE inhibition and statins.

Box 10.1. Management of diabetic nephropathy in pregnancy

- Ensure informed decision about pregnancy (maternal prognosis during and after pregnancy).
- Advise on when to stop angiotensin-converting enzyme (ACE) inhibitors/angiotensin II receptor blockers (ARBs).
- Control glucose.
- Control blood pressure.
- Check for retinopathy and treat.
- Check for other comorbidities such as cardiac or thromboembolic risk.
- Administer 5 mg folic acid.
- Administer 75 mg aspirin.
- Consider low-molecular-weight heparin and monitor dose.
- Review need for thromboprophylaxis regularly (hospitalisation, increasing proteinuria, pre-eclampsia).
- Check maternal weight regularly.
- Arrange regular visits to a multidisciplinary team.
- Perform regular scans to monitor for fetal growth restriction and be aware of confounding influences.
- Deliver for pre-eclampsia only if specific signs of pre-eclampsia are present.
- Restart ACE inhibition postnatally (and consider a statin after breastfeeding).

References

1. American Diabetes Association. Diabetic nephropathy. *Diabetes Care* 2003;26:S94–8.
2. How HY, Sibai BM. Use of angiotensin-converting enzyme inhibitors in patients with diabetic nephropathy. *J Matern Fetal Neonatal Med* 2002;12:402–7.
3. White P. Pregnancy complicating diabetes. *JAMA* 1945;128:181–2.
4. White P. Pregnancy complicating diabetes. *Am J Med* 1949;November:609–16.
5. Ekbom P, Damm P, Feldt-Rasmussen B, Feldt-Rasmussen U, Molvig J, Mathiesen ER. Pregnancy outcome in Type I diabetic women with microalbuminuria. *Diabetes Care* 2001;24:1739–44.
6. Giorgino F, Laviola L, Cavallo Perin P, Solnica B, Fuller J, Chaturvedi N. Factors associated with progression to macroalbuminuria in microalbuminuric Type I diabetic patients: the EURODIAB Prospective Complications Study. *Diabetologia* 2004;47:1020–8.
7. Kitzmiller JL, Combs A. Diabetic nephropathy and pregnancy. *Obstet Gynecol Clini North Am* 1996;23:173–203.
8. Confidential Enquiry into Maternal and Child Health. *Diabetes in Pregnancy: Are We Providing the Best Care? Findings of a National Enquiry: England, Wales and Northern Ireland*. London: CEMACH; 2007.
9. Lewis EJ, Hunsicker LG, Bain RP, Rohde RD, The Collaborative Study Group. The effect of angiotensin-converting enzyme inhibition on diabetic nephropathy. The Collaborative Study Group. *N Engl J Med* 1993;329:1456–62.
10. Hod M, van Dijk DJ, Karp M, Weintraub N, Rabinerson D, Bar J, et *al*. Diabetic nephropathy and pregnancy: the effect of ACE inhibitors prior to pregnancy on fetomaternal outcome. *Nephrol Dial Transplant* 1995;10:2328–83.
11. The Diabetes Control and Complications Trial Research Group. The effect of intensive treatment of diabetes on the development and progression of long-term complications in insulin-dependent diabetes mellitus. *N Engl J Med* 1993;329:977–86.
12. Bar J, Chen R, Schoenfeld A, Orvieto R, Yahav J, Ben-Rafael Z, et *al*. Pregnancy outcome in patients with insulin dependent diabetes mellitus and diabetic nephropathy treated with ACE inhibitors before pregnancy. *J Pediatr Endocrinol Metab* 1999;12:659–65.
13. Cooper WO, Hernandez-Diaz S, Abrogast PG, Dudley JA, Dyer S, Gideon PS, *et al*. Major congenital malformations after first-trimester exposure to ACE inhibitors. *N Engl J Med* 2006;354:2443–51.
14. Manske CL, Thomas W, Wang Y, Wilson RF. Screening diabetic transplant candidates for coronary artery disease: Identification of a low risk subgroup. *Kidney Int* 1993;44:617–21.
15. Barak R, Miodovnic M. Medical complications of diabetes mellitus in pregnancy. *Clin Obstet* 2000;43:17–31.
16. Khoury JC, Miodovnik M, LeMasters G, Sibai B. Pregnancy outcome and progression of diabetic nephropathy. What's next? *J Matern Fetal Med* 2002;11:238–44.
17. Bar J, Ben-Rafael Z, Padoa A, Orvieto R, Boner G, Hod M. Prediction of pregnancy outcome in subgroups of women with renal disease. *Clin Nephrol* 2000;53:437–44.
18. Reece EA, Leguizamon G, Homko C. Pregnancy performance and outcomes associated with diabetic nephropathy. *Am J Perinatol* 1998;15:413–21.
19. Gordon M, Landon MB, Samuels P, Hissrich S, Gabbe SG. Perinatal outcome and long-term follow-up associated with modern management of diabetic nephropathy. *Obstet Gynecol* 1996;87:401–9.
20. Mackie AD, Doddridge MC, Gamsu HR, Brudenell JM, Nicolaides KH, Drury PL. Outcome of pregnancy in patients with insulin-dependent diabetes mellitus and nephropathy with moderate renal impairment. *Diabetic Medicine* 1996;13:90–6.
21. Miodovnik M, Roseen BM, Khoury JC, Grigsby JL, Siddiqi TA. Does pregnancy increase the risk of development and progression of diabetic nephropathy? *Am J Obstet Gynecol* 1996;174:1180–9.
22. Purdy LP, Hantsch CE, Molitch ME, Metzger BE, Phelps RL, Dooley SL, *et al*. Effect of pregnancy on renal function in patients with moderate-to-severe diabetic renal insufficiency. *Diabetes Care* 1996;19:1067–74.
23. Landon MB. Diabetic nephropathy and pregnancy. *Clin Obstet Gynecol* 2007;50:998–1006.
24. Fischer MJ. Chronic kidney disease and pregnancy: maternal and fetal outcomes. *Adv Chronic Kidney Dis* 2007;14:132–45.

25. Star J, Carpenter MW. The effect of pregnancy on the natural history of diabetic retinopathy and nephropathy. *Clin Perinatol* 1998;25:887–916.
26. Imbasciati E, Ponticelli C. Pregnancy and renal disease: predictors for fetal and maternal outcome. *Am J Nephrol* 1991;11:353–62.
27. Bagg W, Neale L, Henley P, MacPherson P, Cundy T. Long-term maternal outcome after pregnancy in women with diabetic nephropathy. *N Z Med J* 2003;116:1180.
28. Rossing K, Jacobsen P, Hommel E, Mathiesen E, Svenningsen A, Rossing P, *et al.* Pregnancy and progression of diabetic nephropathy. *Diabetologia* 2002;45:36–41.
29. Biesenbach G, Grafinger P, Stoger H, Zarzgornik J. How pregnancy influences renal function in nephropathic type I diabetic women depends on their pre-conceptual creatinine clearance. *J Nephrol* 1999;12:41–6.
30. Dunne FP, Chowdhury TA, Hartland A, Smith T, Brydon PA, McConkey C, et *al.* Pregnancy outcome in women with insulin-dependent diabetes mellitus complicated by nephropathy. *Q J Med* 1999;92:451–4.
31. Lauszus FF, Gron PL, Klebe JG. Pregnancies complicated by diabetic proliferative reinopathy. *Acta Obstet Gynecol* 1998;77:814–18.
32. Zhu L, Nakabayashi M, Takeda Y. Statistical analysis of perinatal outcomes in pregnancy complicated with diabetes mellitus. *J Obstet Gynaecol Res* 1997;23:555–63.
33. Carr DB, Koontz GL, Gardella C, Holing EV, Brateng DA, Brown ZA, *et al.* Diabetic nephropathy in pregnancy: suboptimal hypertensive control associated with preterm delivery. *Am J Hypertens* 2006;19:513–19.
34. Sibai BM, Caritis SN, Hauth JC, Lindheimer M, VanDorsten JP, MacPherson C, *et al.* for the National Institute of Child Health and Human Development Maternal-Fetal Medicine Units Network. Risks of preeclampsia and adverse neonatal outcomes among women with pregestational diabetes mellitus. *Am J Obstet Gynecol* 2000;182:364–9.
35. Hiilesmaa V, Suhonen L, Teramo K. Glycaemic control is associated with pre-eclampsia but not with pregnancy-induced hypertension in women with Type I diabetes mellitus. *Diabetologia* 2000;43:1534–9.
36. Sibai BM. Risk factors, pregnancy complications, and prevention of hypertensive disorders in women with pregravid diabetes mellitus. *J Matern Fetal Med* 2000;9:62–5.
37. Caritis S, Sibai B, Hauth J, Lindheimer MD, Klebanoff M, Thom E, *et al.* Low-dose aspirin to prevent pre-eclampsia in women at high risk. *N Engl J Med* 1998;338:701–5.
38. Sibai BM, Caritis SN, Hauth JC, MacPherson C, VanDorsten JP, Klebanoff M, *et al.* Preterm delivery in women with pregestational diabetes mellitus or chronic hypertension relative to women with uncomplicated pregnancies. The National Institute of Child Health and Human Development Maternal–Fetal Medicine Units Network. *Am J Obstet Gynecol* 2000;183:1520–4.
39. Teramo K, Kari MA, Eronen M, Markkanen H, Hiilesmaa V. High amniotic erythropoietin levels are associated with an increased frequency of fetal and neonatal morbidity in type I diabetic pregnancies. *Diabetologia* 2004;47:1695–1703.
40. Lauenborg J, Mathiesen E, Ovesen P, Westergard JG, Ekbom P, Molsted-Pedersen L, *et al.* Audit of stillbirths in women with pregestational type I diabetes. *Diabetes Care* 2003;26:1385–9.
41. Salvesen DR, Higueras MT, Brudenell JM, Drury PL, Nicolaides KH. Doppler velocimetry and fetal heart rate studies in nephropathic diabetics. *Am J Obstet Gynecol* 1992;167:1297–1303.
42. Gordin D, Hiilesmaa V, Fagerudd J, Ronnback C, Kaaja R, Teramo K. Pre-eclampsia but not pregnancy-induced hypertension is a risk factor for diabetic nephropathy in type I diabetic women. *Diabetologia* 2007;50:516–22.
43. The Diabetes Control and Complications Trial Research Group. Effect of pregnancy on microvascular complications in the diabetes control and complications trial. *Diabetes Care* 2000;23:1084–91.
44. Verier-Mine O, Chaturvedi N, Webb D, Fuller JH, the EURODIAB Prospective Complications Study Group. Is pregnancy a risk factor for microvascular complications? The EURODIAB Prospective Complications Study. *Diabet Med* 2005;22:1503–9.
45. Gregg, EW, Gu Q, Cheng YJ, Narayan V, Cowie CC. Mortality trends in men and women with diabetes, 1971–2000. *Ann Intern Med* 2007;147:1–8.

Section 4

Drugs used in renal disease in pregnancy

Chapter 11
Drugs in women with renal disease and transplant recipients in pregnancy

Graham W Lipkin, Mark Kilby and Asif Sarwar

Introduction

An international survey reported that over 80% of unselected pregnant women use over-the-counter or prescribed medicines during pregnancy. Almost all women known to suffer from renal disease require antenatal drug treatment. Most drugs are started prepregnancy for the underlying condition or comorbidity.

This chapter focuses on immunosuppressive agents used by women in the treatment of renal disease as well as erythropoietic-stimulating agents (ESAs) and diuretic agents. Antihypertensive agents are frequently required by people with chronic kidney disease (CKD) and are covered in Chapter 12 on treatment of hypertension in renal disease. For discussion on use of antibiotics in this setting, see Chapter 17.

Prepregnancy counselling is critical to safe and effective drug use in pregnancy by women with known renal disease. Consideration of the risk–benefit balance to both mother and fetus surrounding the initiation or stopping of drug treatment prepregnancy or during pregnancy is a key challenge for the multidisciplinary team caring for these women.

Search strategy

The evidence base available to guide women in this area is limited and relies on case reports, incomplete registry data, case–control series and non-controlled meta-analysis. These were identified from a PubMed search, relevant review articles, TOXbase, the National Teratology Information Service (NTIS), Micromedex, the British National Formulary (BNF 55 (March 2008); Appendix 4), reference guides,[1] expert opinion and relevant pharmaceutical company pregnancy databases.

General principles of teratogenicity

An agent is a teratogen if its administration to the pregnant mother directly or indirectly causes structural or functional abnormalities in the fetus or in the child after birth, which may not be apparent until later life.[2] The belief that the developing fetus was protected by an effective placental barrier from adverse effects of drugs in the maternal circulation was shattered by the experience with thalidomide over 40 years ago. Almost all drugs present in the maternal circulation reach the fetus to a greater or lesser extent. Detection of teratogenicity is problematic for various reasons, as discussed below.

Preclinical/animal studies

All licensed products have undergone extensive prior teratogenicity testing in animals. Extrapolation from preclinical or *in vitro* tests to the clinical situation can be problematic.[3] There is no question that whole-animal teratology studies are helpful in raising concerns about the reproductive effects of drugs but negative animal studies do not guarantee safety in human reproduction.[3] The classic example is thalidomide, which was not shown to be teratogenic in rats and rabbits. Interspecies variability in drug metabolism, clearance and susceptibility, as well as testing methodology, are some confounding factors.

Epidemiological, case series or case–control studies

Birth defects occur in 2–3% of pregnancies in northern Europe. This low incidence makes detecting a drug-induced defect difficult unless the teratogenic effect of a drug results in an extremely unusual fetal abnormality. For example, to be confident that a given drug doubles the incidence of cleft palate (expected incidence less than 1 in 1000 births) with a power of greater than 80%, a study of 23 000 pregnancies would be needed.[1]

Latent period

The challenges of determining adverse consequences of antenatal drug treatment is also highlighted by the experience of the use of maternal diethylstilbestrol, which was given to prevent reproductive problems such as miscarriage. This was associated with an increased risk of vaginal adenocarcinoma developing in the female offspring up to two decades later.[4] More subtle developmental delay would be easily missed and this highlights the need for long-term follow-up of children.

Factors affecting exposure and impact of maternal drugs on the fetus

The interface comprises the uteroplacental circulation, umbilical vein and the uniquely positioned fetal liver through which all drugs must pass to reach the fetal circulation (Figure 11.1). Fetal drug exposure and its impact are determined by a complex interplay of pharmacokinetic and pharmacodynamic factors and many aspects are incompletely understood.

Timing of drug exposure in relationship to fetal development

During the pre-embryonic stage (conception to 17 days), the 'all or nothing' effect is thought to apply. Toxic damage to the dividing blastocyst will either result in its destruction leading to miscarriage or, if damage is incomplete and the toxin short lived, the damaged cells may be replaced allowing continued fetal development. Organogenesis occurs mainly during the embryonic stage, which is largely complete by the 10th week. Thus drug exposure in the first trimester is more likely to increase the rate miscarriage or structural abnormalities (e.g. spina bifida), whereas subsequent exposure is more likely to result in growth restriction.

Factors affecting transplacental drug passage

Placental drug transfer occurs largely by diffusion across a concentration gradient.[4] However, agents of high molecular weight such as epoietin, heparins or insulin are excluded by their size. Non-ionic and lipophilic drugs cross more easily than polar drugs. Metabolism of drugs by the placenta or fetal liver prior to reaching the fetal vena cava can significantly impact on exposure to drugs administered to the mother. Prednisolone is extensively metabolised to inactive products by the placenta with only 10% reaching the fetus. Azathioprine is converted to the active metabolite 6-mercaptopurine (6-MP) by the liver. While azathioprine crosses the placenta, the fetal liver has relatively low levels of the activating enzyme, inosinate pyrophosphorylase, leading to low cord levels of 6-MP possibly protecting the fetus from toxicity.[5]

Differences in susceptibility

It is not clear why exposure to a known teratogen at the same stage in pregnancy at the same dose will give rise to fetal malformation in some but not all pregnancies. Only 20–30% of exposures to thalidomide during the first trimester led to fetal abnormalities.[1] Pharmacogenetic issues may be relevant.

Dose–response relationships

Although idiosyncratic effects are described, most teratogenic effects appear to be dose related. Estimates of the cumulative exposure to the drug may be more important in relation to teratogenic effects than short-term transplacental transfer.[4]

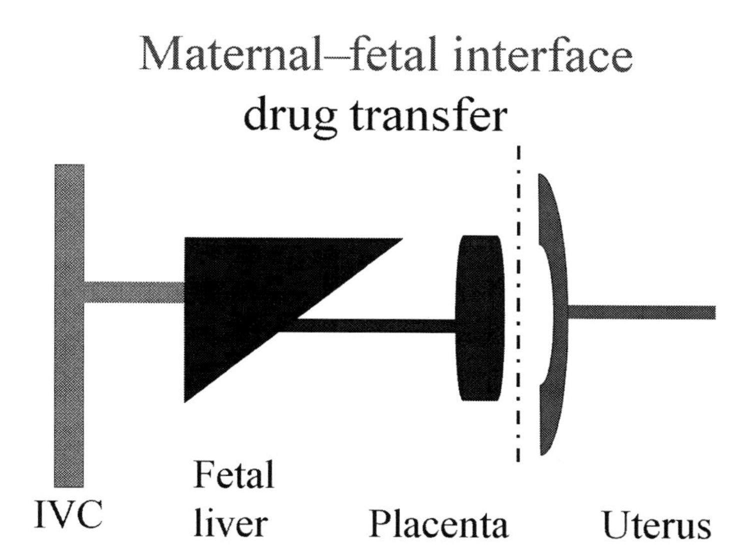

Figure 11.1. Maternal–fetal circulation and drug transfer; IVC = inferior vena cava

Guidance on drug use in pregnancy

Appendix 4 of the British National Formulary (BNF 55) advises on safer drug prescribing in pregnancy (www.bnf.org).

Principles of drug prescription in pregnancy (BNF 55)

- Prepregnancy counselling wherever possible is of particular importance to women with renal disease who are considering pregnancy. Drugs can have harmful effects on the fetus at any time during pregnancy. It is important to bear this in mind when prescribing for a woman of childbearing age. Prepregnancy counselling allows discussion of relevant risks and appropriate modification of drugs in advance of conception.
- During the first trimester, drugs can produce congenital malformations (teratogenesis) and the period of greatest risk is from the third to the eleventh week of pregnancy.
- During the second and third trimesters, drugs can affect the growth and functional development of the fetus or have toxic effects on fetal tissues. Drugs given shortly before term or during labour can have adverse effects on labour or on the neonate after delivery.

The BNF lists drugs that:

- may have harmful effects in pregnancy and indicates the trimester of risk
- are not known to be harmful in pregnancy.

The advice is based upon human data but takes into account information on animal studies.

The following general principles apply to drug prescribing in pregnancy:

- prescribe only if expected benefit is thought to be greater than the risk to the fetus (e.g. immunosuppression in transplantation)
- avoid all non-essential drugs in the first trimester if possible
- use the smallest effective dose and drug-level monitoring wherever possible or relevant
- use drugs that have been extensively used in pregnancy and appear to be usually safe in preference to new or untried drugs
- contribute to the registry evidence base wherever possible.

Alternative sources of information

Information on drugs and pregnancy is also available from the UK National Teratology Information Service (www.nyrdtc.nhs.uk/Services/teratology/teratology.html).

The US Food and Drug Administration has adopted a classification that codes the safety categories of drugs when used in pregnancy (Table 11.1). These categories have limitations when applied to women with renal disease in pregnancy. Many of the data are not derived from pregnant women.

Issues specific to patients with renal disease

In women with CKD, as in all pregnant women, glomerular filtration increases substantially above baseline early in pregnancy.[6] For agents excreted by the kidney,

Table 11.1. US Food and Drug Administration categorisation of drugs in pregnancy

Category	Interpretation
A	Controlled studies show no risk. Adequate, well-controlled studies in pregnant women have failed to demonstrate risk to the fetus
B	No evidence of risk in humans. Either animal findings show risk (but human findings do not) or, if no adequate human studies have been done, animal findings are negative.
C	Risk cannot be ruled out. Human studies are lacking and animal studies are either positive for fetal risk or lacking as well. However, potential benefits may justify the potential risk.
D	Positive evidence of risk. Investigational or post marketing data show risk to fetus. Nevertheless, potential benefits may outweigh the risk.
X	Contraindicated in pregnancy. Studies in animals or humans, or investigational or post marketing reports, have shown fetal risk which clearly outweighs any possible benefit to the patient.

drug clearance also increases and may require dose increase to maintain therapeutic plasma levels. Women with CKD may experience a marked increase in proteinuria to nephrotic levels and exhibit an exaggerated fall in serum albumin during pregnancy which impacts on handling of drugs with extensive protein binding.

For the nonpregnant situation, the US National Kidney Foundation classification of severity of CKD codes 5 stages of CKD based on calculation of estimated glomerular filtration rate (eGFR). This employs the patient's serum creatinine, sex, race and age[7] and helps to overcome the limitations of using serum creatinine alone to assess renal function. Unfortunately, the equation used to calculate eGFR is not valid in pregnancy.[7] This complicates adjustment of drug dosing in pregnancy in women with renal disease.

Breastfeeding

Breastfeeding is beneficial to both mother and child; the immunological and nutritional value of breast milk to the infant is greater than that of formula feeds and breastfeeding enhances bonding.

The BNF concludes: 'although there is concern that drugs taken by the mother might affect the infant, there is very little information on this. In the absence of evidence of an effect, the potential for harm to the infant can be inferred from:

- the amount of drug or active metabolite of the drug delivered to the infant (dependent on the pharmacokinetic characteristics of the drug in the mother);
- the efficiency of absorption, distribution and elimination of the drug by the infant (infant pharmacokinetics);
- the nature of the effect of the drug on the infant (pharmacodynamic properties of the drug in the infant)'.

This chapter presents the view of the authoritative texts such as Briggs *et al.*[1] and those of the current BNF together with existing information from literature review in human studies.

Immunosuppressive agents and pregnancy

Consensus guideline statements and reviews covering the use of transplantation immunosuppression in pregnancy have recently been published.[5,8]

Glucocorticosteroids (FDA pregnancy class B)

Women who have undergone organ transplantation or who suffer immunological renal disease such as systemic lupus erythematosus (SLE) often receive chronic steroid treatment. The risks of stopping immunosuppressive medications in pregnancy are frequently outweighed by the benefits of continuation and the fetus is inevitably exposed to potentially feto-toxic and potentially teratogenic agents throughout its development.

The most commonly used glucocorticoids are the short-acting agents prednisolone and methylprednisolone and the longer acting dexamethasone and betamethasone. They easily traverse the placenta. The maternal–cord blood prednisolone ratio is 1 : 10, suggesting substantial protection of the fetus from maternal prednisolone exposure because of high levels of the inactivating hormone 11-beta-hydroxysteroid dehydrogenase.[5] In comparison, dexamethasone and betamethasone reach higher concentrations in the fetus because they are less efficiently metabolised by the placenta.

Animal studies have suggested an increased risk of cleft palate in neonates exposed to prednisolone in early pregnancy. In a prospective study, 184 women exposed to prednisolone in the first trimester of pregnancy were studied in a Canadian case–control series.[9] The primary outcome was the rate of major birth defects. There was no statistical difference in the rate of major anomalies between the corticosteroid-exposed and control groups. The same group also conducted a meta-analysis of existing epidemiological studies of glucocorticoid exposure in pregnancies. In the meta-analysis there was no increase in the rate of major malformations (3.6% versus 2.0%) and no cluster of malformations suggestive of a common cause. However, the case–control study indicated that the odds ratio for oral clefts was significantly increased (OR 3.35, 95% CI 1.97–5.69). These studies included women treated with steroids in high doses for many different indications, some of which in themselves are associated with an increased risk of malformations.[9]

No increased teratogenic risk has been demonstrated in mothers exposed to lower doses of prednisolone (BNF 55). Cases of fetal adrenal suppression and fetal immunosuppression have been described with maternal use of higher prednisolone doses but not where the maternal prednisolone dose is kept below 15 mg/day.[10]

Maternal risks

Prolonged courses of antenatal glucocorticoids increase the risk of gestational diabetes, especially when combined with other diabetogenic agents such as tacrolimus, exacerbate hypertension, increase the loss of bone mineral density and increase the risk of preterm rupture of membranes.[11–13]

The consensus view is that prednisolone use in pregnancy is not associated with an increased risk of fetal malformations (BNF). However, pregnancies in women receiving steroid therapy necessitate close maternal and fetal monitoring including random blood glucose monitoring. Formal glucose tolerance testing at the beginning of the third trimester is recommended.

Breastfeeding

The BNF states: 'systemic effects in infant unlikely with maternal dose of prednisolone up to 40 mg daily; monitor infant's adrenal function with higher doses'. Following a 10 mg oral dose, trace amounts are found in breast milk. Milk concentrations range from 5–25% of maternal blood levels.[1] A formal pharmacokinetic study on the effects of a 50 mg intravenous dose demonstrated only 0.025% recovery from breast milk, which is unlikely to be of clinical significance to the baby.[14] As such it would appear that prednisolone is compatible with safe breastfeeding.

Azathioprine

Azathioprine is used as a component of prophylaxis from rejection in solid organ transplant recipients and in those patients with native renal disease requiring immunosuppression, such as those with SLE. It is usually combined with other immunosuppressive treatment including glucocorticoids. There is extensive experience of this drug in pregnant women. The US Food and Drug Administration categorises azathioprine as class D on the basis of animal toxicity and of anecdotal reports in pregnant women of fetal immunosuppression.

Teratogenic effects are demonstrated in animals treated with very high doses of azathioprine.[1] In pregnant rats, azathioprine (6 mg/kg) can cause fetal resorption and death, while lower doses result in skeletal and visceral teratogenicity in rats and rabbits. Lower doses comparable with those used in the clinical setting may not interfere with normal implantation and fetal development.[1]

Azathioprine freely crosses the placenta but to be active requires conversion to the active metabolite 6-MP in the liver by the enzyme inosinate pyrophosphorylase, which is deficient in the developing fetal liver. The fetal liver metabolises azathioprine to the inactive metabolite thiouric acid rather than 6-MP. A radioactive-labelling study in human pregnancy reported that 64–93% of azathioprine administered to mothers appears in fetal blood as inactive metabolites.[15] It is thus possible that the fetus is to some extent protected from the teratogenic effects of azathioprine.

Randomised trials to evaluate the safety of azathioprine in pregnancy in this setting are neither ethical nor practical. Research therefore relies on case series and registry data to determine adverse fetal effects in humans. No increased risk for general or specific structural defects in exposed babies has been noted in these studies, although sample size is not sufficient to rule out a small risk.[16] The reported rate of miscarriage appears to be similar to that of the general population. Azathioprine has been associated with dose-related myelosuppression in the fetus.[17] In this study maternal azathioprine dose at 32 weeks and at term correlated with cord blood leucocyte count. Leucopenia is not usually a problem if the maternal dose of azathioprine is less than 2 mg/kg and the maternal white cell count is greater than 7500/l.[10]

The US National Transplantation Pregnancy Registry (NTPR) evaluated 146 kidney transplant recipients who received azathioprine and prednisolone (90.4%), azathioprine alone (2.1%) or prednisolone alone (7.5%).[18] Complications in the azathioprine-treated group included low birthweight and preterm birth. It is likely that these adverse outcomes reflected maternal disease (renal dysfunction, hypertension, diabetes, etc.) rather than the drug itself.[5] There were isolated cases of fetal abnormality that were not in excess of that expected. The UK Transplant Pregnancy Registry reported pregnancy outcomes in 209 cardiothoracic, liver and renal transplant recipients, most of whom received azathioprine. There was no increased risk of first-trimester miscarriage or fetal abnormalities.[19] Likewise, no increased risk of structural abnormality is reported in babies of women treated with azathioprine during pregnancy for lupus.[16]

A Danish Registry study of 900 children born to women with Crohn's disease exposed to various immunosuppressants between 1996 and 2004 suggested a greater incidence of congenital abnormalities in those receiving azathioprine even after adjusting for confounders.[20] However, the frequency of congenital abnormalities described at 2.9% is similar to the expected background risk in the northern European population and the significance of this study remains to be determined.

Azathioprine may interfere with the contraceptive efficacy of copper intrauterine contraceptive devices used in renal transplant recipients who were also treated with steroids, an effect reflecting its immunosuppression action.[21] However, this finding was not confirmed in a study of women immunosuppressed with steroids and azathioprine for SLE. Only one of 54 women who used the copper intrauterine device conceived.[22]

The present consensus is that azathioprine should not be suspended during pregnancy out of concern regarding teratogenicity. Conception while taking azathioprine is not in itself grounds to recommend termination of pregnancy. There is no current evidence of teratogenicity in human pregnancy. Nevertheless, women requiring azathioprine use in pregnancy for renal disease or transplantation should be considered at high risk of complications related to the underlying condition. Their care requires careful overview in a centre experienced in management of these women and their babies require expert neonatal review.

Breastfeeding

The BNF recommends 'discontinuation of breast feeding' in women prescribed azathioprine. In practice, many units have experienced no significant problems related to breastfeeding in babies of mothers who receive this drug. Consensus opinion is that breastfeeding is not absolutely contraindicated.[23] A study of azathioprine-treated lactating women reported low levels of 6-MP in only two of 31 breast milk samples and undetectable levels in ten breastfed babies with no signs of immunosuppression.[24]

Ciclosporin and tacrolimus

Ciclosporin is a novel cyclic undecapeptide that possesses potent immunosuppressive properties and has been widely used in the prevention of acute rejection in solid organ transplantation as well as in treatment of immune-mediated disease. Tacrolimus has a similar mode of action and clinical toxicity profile including nephrotoxicity and hypertension. Both drugs have a narrow therapeutic window and are associated with both functional reversible and structural nephrotoxity in humans. Ciclosporin crosses the human placenta and ciclosporin levels in the placenta are equivalent to those in maternal blood.[25]

Studies in pregnant rats have found no effect of ciclosporin or tacrolimus on organogenesis, although some renal proximal tubular cell damage can occur.[26] Growth delay is reported in rodents treated with high doses of both drugs. Pregnancy data on ciclosporin and tacrolimus use in humans are primarily derived from data in transplant recipients.

High rates of miscarriage may give a clue to possible early drug-induced feto-toxicity. Table 11.2 lists the rates seen in registry series. It is likely that there is underreporting of miscarriage in these series and as such it may be that miscarriage rates are slightly higher than the quoted incidence in the general population of 8–9%, although this requires confirmation.[19]

A meta-analysis of pregnancy outcomes in solid organ transplant recipients taking ciclosporin ($n = 410$) reported a non-significant trend to a greater malformation risk (OR 3.83) when compared with controls who received alternative immunosuppression.[27] However, the absolute rate of congenital abnormalities was 4.1%, which was not substantially different from the general population. In addition, there were methodological problems with this meta-analysis and the finding requires further confirmation. Numerous single-centre and registry reports have shown no evidence of an increase in structural abnormalities in babies born to transplant recipients taking ciclosporin or tacrolimus in pregnancy.[5,18,19] The prevalence of major structural malformations according to the NTPR was approximately 4–5%, similar to the incidence of 3% reported in pregnant women without disease.[13]

There is clear evidence of a greater incidence of low birthweight and preterm birth in ciclosporin- and tacrolimus-treated women as compared with the general population.[5,18,19] Again, the latter finding could well be more related to patient comorbidity than to the drug itself. The NTPR registry explored the issue of whether ciclosporin might be the cause of low birthweight in renal transplant recipients. Compared with those women treated with the combination of prednisolone, azathioprine and ciclosporin (156 pregnancies), women who received steroids and azathioprine alone (249 pregnancies) gave birth to babies with higher birthweight (2.7 kg versus 2.4 kg) and to fewer very low birthweight babies (8% versus 18%).[5,18,19] However, on further inspection the two populations were clearly different. Prepregnancy hypertension and type 2 diabetes mellitus, both factors associated with adverse fetal outcome, were more common in the ciclosporin-treated group. The recent UK Transplant Registry report on pregnancy outcome examines the low birthweight issue and ascribes it to known predisposing factors including drug-treated hypertension and prematurity.[19]

The maternal and fetal outcomes of tacrolimus or ciclosporin-treated transplant recipients in pregnancy are similar[13] although diabetes may be more frequently seen in those treated with tacrolimus (Table 11.3). Babies born to women treated with tacrolimus may have transient renal impairment and hyperkalaemia.

Table 11.2. Comparison of outcome of pregnancy in ciclosporin- and prednisolone-treated renal transplant recipients

Outcome	UK Transplant Registry[5,18,19]	US National Transplantation Pregnancy Registry[5]	
		Ciclosporin-treated	Steroid/azathioprine-treated
Miscarriage (before 24 weeks)	11%	16%	7%

Table 11.3. Pregnancy outcomes in transplant recipients reported to the US National Transplantation Pregnancy Registry[28]

Outcome	Ciclosporin (Neoral)-treated women (146 pregnancies)	Tacrolimus-treated women (70 pregnancies)
Hypertension	72%	58%
Diabetes during pregnancy	3%	10%
Miscarriage	19%	24%
Live births	79%	71%
Low birthweight	50%	50%
Newborn complications	50%	54%

Complex pharmacokinetic changes are seen in ciclosporin- and tacrolimus-treated women in pregnancy. These include increased volume of distribution due to increase in body weight, proportion of adipose tissue, red cell mass and hormone-induced changes in liver metabolism and bile salt handling. As a consequence, dose increases of ciclosporin of around 50% are frequently required to maintain therapeutic ciclosporin levels (see Figure 11.2).[29] Similarly tacrolimus trough blood levels should be monitored monthly, and more frequently if interacting drug therapy is introduced or withdrawn (check BNF for details).

A recent report suggests an increased risk of obstetric cholestasis in ciclosporin-treated (but not tacrolimus-treated) renal transplant recipients, an effect possibly mediated by ciclosporin-induced inhibition of the bile salt excretion pump.[30] Seven of 23 ciclosporin-treated renal transplant recipients suffered this complication against a background incidence of around 1%.

The effects of *in utero* drug exposure may not be apparent at birth and subtle effects on neurocognitive or immunological function or long-term blood pressure or renal function may not be seen for over a decade or more.

There are inconsistent reports of immunological abnormalities in neonates born to transplant recipients.[5] Neurocognitive development was assessed in a follow-up study of children born to ciclosporin-treated female transplant recipients.[31] Twenty-four percent showed some delay but the relationship to drug treatment rather than preterm birth was unclear.

Rabbits exposed to ciclosporin *in utero* exhibit reduced nephron number and develop hypertension and progressive CKD in adult life.[32] Human studies in the general population show an inverse correlation between birthweight and blood pressure in later life. Preliminary data suggest renal function and blood pressure of children born

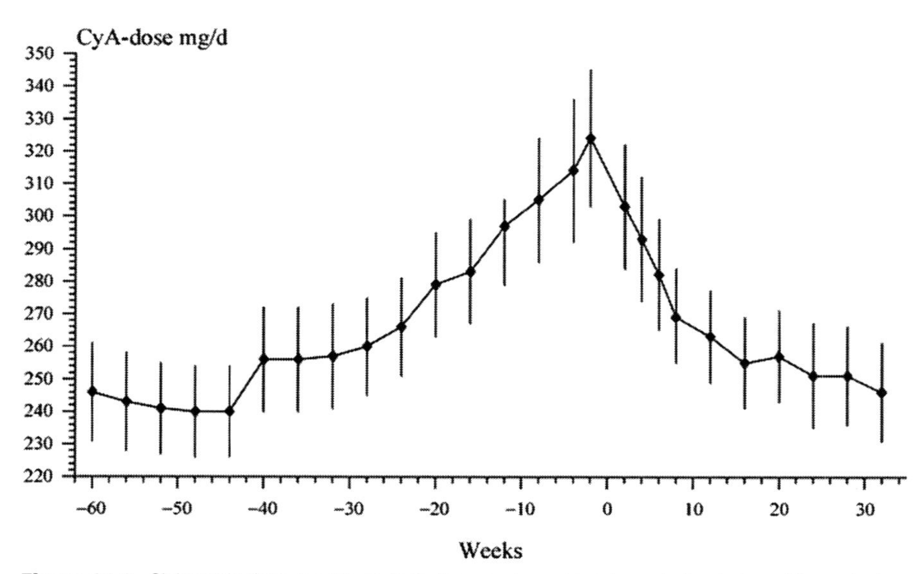

Figure 11.2. Ciclosporin dose requirements during pregnancy in ciclosporin-treated renal transplant recipients; week 0 represents birth; reproduced with permission from Fischer *et al.*[29]

to mothers treated with ciclosporin during pregnancy appear to be normal.[33] However, long-term follow-up studies of children from these mothers are awaited.

Accumulated experience with the use of ciclosporin and tacrolimus during pregnancy supports the use of these agents if immunosuppression is necessary. Currently there is no evidence of teratogenicity. Preterm birth and small-for-gestational-age infants are not uncommon outcomes and pregnancy in women taking these agents should be carefully monitored, including blood pressure and renal function. The drug dose requires review based on trough levels and gestational diabetes may occur with both drugs, although it is more common with tacrolimus treatment. Whether there will be long-term immunomodulatory or renal effects, effects in offspring who have been exposed to ciclosporin *in utero* are unknown.

Breastfeeding

The BNF comments: 'present in breast milk – manufacturer advises avoid'. There are, however, limited data on which to advise. Again, several experienced units, including our own, have allowed breastfeeding in ciclosporin-treated women and have noted no drug-related problems in their babies. Reports of ciclosporin levels in breast milk approach those in maternal blood. However, ciclosporin was detected in only one out of six infants tested and infant development up to 1 year was reported as normal.[34,35]

Two reports identify minimal tacrolimus transfer to the infant by breastfeeding, with calculated dose exposure being between 0.02% and 0.5% of the mother's weight-adjusted dose.[36,37] The consensus opinion is that breastfeeding is not absolutely contraindicated. Clearly, however, babies should be closely monitored and immunosuppressive levels in the infant checked.[23]

Mycophenolate mofetil and enteric-coated mycophenolic acid

Mycophenolate mofetil (MMF) (CellCept) is the ester prodrug of mycophenolic acid (MPA), a reversible inhibitor of inosine monophosphate dehydrogenase that blocks *de novo* purine synthesis in T and B lymphocytes. It is licensed for the prevention of acute rejection following solid organ transplantation and has become the standard of care, usually in combination with steroids and tacrolimus, as first-line immunosuppression in renal transplantation in the USA and mainland Europe and is increasingly used in the UK. MMF is now also employed for treatment of severe renal manifestations of SLE, an autoimmune disorder disproportionately affecting women in the fertile age range.[38]

Teratology studies in rats and rabbits exposed to MMF resulted in fetopathy and malformations such as anophthalmia, agnathia, hydrocephaly, cardiovascular and renal abnormalities even when administered at half the therapeutic dose recommended in clinical practice (Summary of Product Characteristics for Cellcept).[39]

Transplacental transfer of MPA has been demonstrated in pregnant women, achieving fetal plasma levels similar to those found in the mother.[40] Case reports describe fetal abnormalities in women taking MMF during pregnancy. Le Ray *et al.*[41] report a case of major fetal malformation in a renal transplant recipient receiving MMF, tacrolimus and steroids during the first trimester after which MMF was replaced by azathioprine. Multiple malformations were detected at 22 weeks of gestation leading to therapeutic termination. Cleft lip and palate, micrognathia, microtia, ectopic left kidney and corpus callosum agenesis were identified at autopsy.[41] One case of non-immune severe fetal anaemia and hydrops as well as microtia was recently reported in a renal transplant recipient taking MMF throughout pregnancy as well as a number of other medications.[40]

Twenty-six cases of early exposure to MMF during pregnancy in 18 renal transplant recipients had been reported to the US NTPR as of late 2006. Upon discovery of pregnancy, MMF dose was decreased or stopped and some women were converted to azathioprine. An unexpectedly high rate of first-trimester miscarriage was noted (42%) and four out of 15 live births were associated with structural malformations (27%). Abnormalities bore similarity to those described in preclinical studies, including cleft lip and palate, microtia, diaphragmatic hernia, hypoplastic nails, shortened finger and congenital heart defects. There were seven pregnancies reported in six recipients of other transplants (one simultaneous kidney/pancreas, three liver and two heart recipients (three pregnancies)). Four resulted in miscarriage. There were no structural abnormalities recorded in this group.[42]

The manufacturer has 137 pregnancies with exposure to MMF on file as of 2006. Of the 41 reports of live births, ten babies were defined as having birth defects and nine 'another disorder'. Babies conceived by men taking MMF appear to have no higher rate of congenital abnormality than expected (personal communication).

The management of a woman who conceives while taking MMF is unclear. Potential problems appear to relate to the period of organogenesis. Immunosuppression drug change in pregnancy is not without some risk of toxic adverse effects or rejection. Each case should be assessed on its individual merits taking into account stage of pregnancy, past history of rejection and complications.

There are no data on MPA excretion in human breast milk, although animal studies indicate that transfer does take place. At present breastfeeding should be discouraged in women taking MMF.

The manufacturer's Summary of Product Characteristics states that Cellcept is not recommended during pregnancy and should be discontinued at least 6 weeks prior to conception. Secure contraception should be practiced by all fertile women taking MMF. The FDA classifies this drug as pregnancy category C (Table 11.1).

The animal and clinical data, in particular the apparent high frequency of early miscarriage and incidence and similarity of human and animal birth defects, certainly raise concern that MPA may be a teratogen. It is vital that implications for pregnancy are considered and discussed with women of fertile age at the time of choosing initial transplant immunosuppression or using MMF for treatment of SLE or vasculitis.

It is our own practice to avoid the use of MMF as baseline immunosuppression in women in this group unless clearly strongly indicated for other reasons such as high immunological risk of transplant rejection. If this pertains, the implications should be highlighted at the time of consent for transplant. Prepregnancy counselling is particularly important in any woman considering pregnancy who is already taking MMF or enteric-coated MPA. Where clinically appropriate, the risks of prepregnancy cessation or change of MMF to azathioprine should be carefully discussed with the woman and her partner. The appropriate management of a woman who conceives while taking MMF is at present unclear and the options should be discussed on an individual basis with the woman and her partner. It should be remembered that case reports and case series relying on voluntary reporting might overestimate the risks associated with a drug in pregnancy. No causal association between MMF and birth defects or miscarriage has been determined at present but concerns exist.

The long-term impact of exposure of the fetus to MPA remains at present unknown and requires careful follow-up until babies born to women taking such therapy reach reproductive age.

Sirolimus and everolimus

Sirolimus (rapamycin) and everolimus are potent macrolide immunosuppressive agents whose primary mechanism of action is inhibition of intracellular mTOR (metabolic target of Rapamycin). This results in inhibition of cytokine-driven T cell proliferation. They are licensed in the UK for prevention and treatment of acute rejection following solid organ transplantation (Summary of Product Characteristics). The FDA categorises them as pregnancy class C.

Data on the impact on sirolimus on pregnancy outcomes are limited. Studies in animals indicate transplacental drug transfer. Sirolimus resulted in toxicity when administered to pregnant rats (Summary of Product Characteristics), manifested as feto-toxicity and reduced fetal weight, with associated delays in ossification. There was no evidence of teratogenicity. Embryotoxicity was increased when sirolimus was co-administered with ciclosporin, consistent with the well-recognised increased nephrotoxicity in this setting.

Guardia *et al.*[43] reported a 30-year-old renal transplant recipient who delivered a healthy normal baby at term while taking sirolimus throughout pregnancy in combination with ciclosporin. The dose of both ciclosporin and sirolimus needed to be increased in pregnancy to maintain prepregnancy therapeutic target blood levels. In a second case report a 21-year-old liver transplant recipient received sirolimus for the first 6 weeks of pregnancy, after which she was switched to tacrolimus and delivered a normal 3 kg healthy baby at term.[44]

The NTPR as of 2006 reported the outcomes of seven transplant (four kidney, one kidney/pancreas and two liver) recipients exposed to sirolimus during pregnancy. In four cases, sirolimus was discontinued or switched to azathioprine ($n = 2$) on diagnosis of pregnancy (within first 6 weeks). Of these seven cases, three pregnancies ended in miscarriage and four live births at 27, 31, 36 and 38 weeks of gestation. One unrelated structural abnormality was reported in a woman switched to sirolimus at 24 weeks.[42]

Sirolimus and everolimus are associated with impaired wound healing post transplant or during subsequent surgery.[45] In fact these agents are powerful growth inhibitors used extensively to prevent neointimal hyperplasia following transluminal coronary angioplasty. There are currently no reports of delayed caesarean section scar healing or prolonged postpartum recovery in these women. Roos *et al.*[46] demonstrated that the placental mTOR-signalling pathway regulates transport of the amino acid leucine and may be involved in the trafficking of this amino acid in human pregnancies complicated by fetal growth restriction. Whether further observational data suggest a role of sirolimus in small-for-gestational-age babies remains to be determined.

Breastfeeding

There are currently no data on breast milk transfer in lactating women treated with mycophenolate, sirolimus or everolimus. Until this becomes available, we would recommend avoiding breastfeeding.

Erythropoietic-stimulating agents in pregnancy

In normal pregnancy a greater increase in intravascular volume compared with red cell mass results in dilutional or physiological anaemia (haemoglobin less than 10.5 g/dl) (see Figure 11.3). This becomes most apparent at 30–34 weeks of gestation. Increased plasma erythropoietin (EPO) produced by the healthy kidney induces the rise in red cell mass, which partially supports the higher metabolic requirement for oxygen in this setting.[47]

Outside of pregnancy, anaemia is common in women with more advanced CKD (including transplant recipients) and in those with established renal failure treated by dialysis. The principal cause is reduced EPO production by the diseased kidneys, and correction of anaemia by administration of an exogenous erythropoietic-stimulating agent (ESA) is a standard of care of these patients, improving cardiovascular function and quality of life.

Women with CKD including renal transplant recipients experience a greater decrement in haemoglobin than do normal women in pregnancy and often require red cell transfusion with its inherent risks, including human leucocyte antigen (HLA) sensitisation.[10] The diseased kidney fails to adequately achieve the required pregnancy-induced increase in EPO production.[48]

Safety and efficacy of exogenous treatment with EPO in women with renal disease in pregnancy

Pregnant rats that received high-dose exogenous EPO showed no evidence of feto-toxic or teratogenic effects and it appears that ESAs do not cross the placenta into the fetal circulation. There is no correlation between serum EPO in the fetus and in the mother.[49]

There are several small case series or registry data indicating the effective use of ESAs in increasing haemoglobin after correction of haematinic deficiency in women with renal disease (including those with CKD, dialysis dependency and renal transplant recipients) in pregnancy.[50,51] EPO use in nonpregnant women with CKD is often

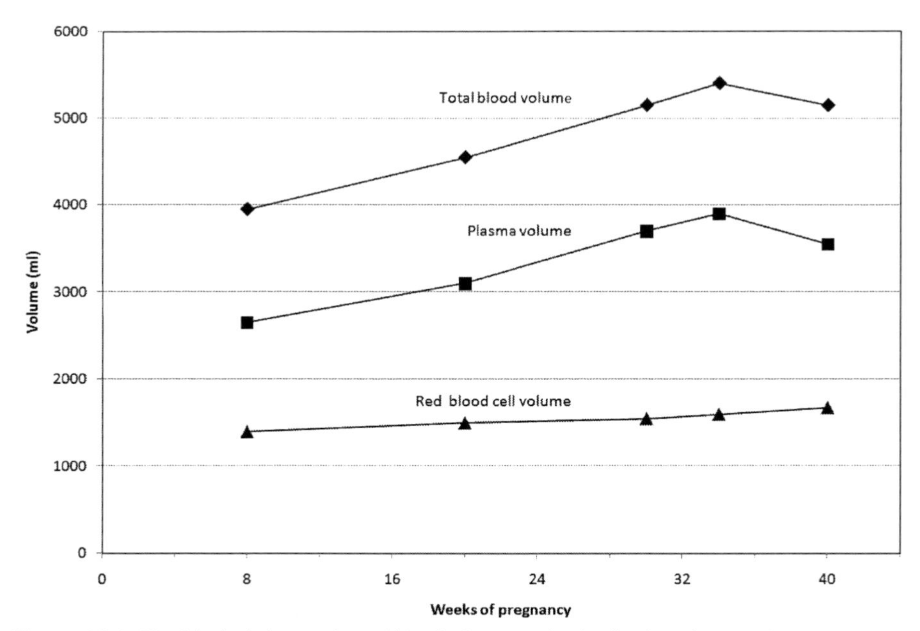

Figure 11.3. Physiological changes in total blood, plasma and red cell volume in normal pregnancy

combined with administration of intravenous iron. This better overcomes functional iron deficiency than does oral iron alone and leads to a greater erythopoietic response. Intravenous iron has also been employed with ESAs in women with anaemia of CKD in pregnancy and appears to be safe, although it is recommended that intravenous iron is given more frequently in low doses to reduce the potential risk of fetal iron toxicity.[52] A recent Cochrane systematic review[53] of intravenous iron for treatment of anaemia in normal pregnancy concluded that the evidence base surrounding its use is limited in the antenatal setting.

The most frequent and serious adverse effect of ESA use outside pregnancy is new-onset or worsening of existing hypertension. This appears to be mediated by reversal of anaemia-induced vasodilation without a corresponding fall in cardiac output. As pregnancy itself is frequently associated with worsening blood pressure control, any additional impact of EPO is difficult to assess.

EPO is effective in correcting the anaemia of CKD in pregnancy. Okundaye *et al.*[54] reported a series of 42 pregnant women on dialysis who received ESA. Transfusion requirement was reduced from 77% to 26% by ESA administration. Three-quarters of women required initiation or increase of ESA dose in the antenatal period. EPO use was reported in a further series of 18 and 34 pregnancies in women who required chronic dialysis. A significant ESA dose increase was required to maintain haematocrit, with one report recommending that the diagnosis of pregnancy be considered for women having dialysis who unexpectedy require sudden dose increases of EPO.[55,56] Reports of hypertension clearly related to EPO in pregnancy are sparse.[57] Hou[10] reported no difference in pregnancy outcome from 19 women on dialysis treated with EPO as compared with 11 contemporary women who were not on dialysis.

Anaemia frequently complicates renal transplant pregnancies in which serum endogenous EPO is inappropriately low and rate of erythropoiesis blunted.[48] Treatment with ESA has been reported as being effective in raising haematocrit in renal transplant recipients. Dose increases have been noted and some of these pregnancies have been complicated by pre-eclampsia. The role, if any, of EPO in the development or worsening of hypertension in pregnancy remains unclear.[58,59]

In summary ESAs do not cross the placenta. A 50% dose increase above prepregnancy is usually required to achieve the haemoglobin target.[52] Intravenous iron appears to be safe but should be administered in frequent low-dose regimens. Target haemoglobin of 10–11 g/dl is recommended and ESA doses should be adjusted to approach the haemoglobin target slowly as in the nonpregnant population. There is no clear impact of ESA treatment on hypertension in pregnancy but close antenatal blood pressure monitoring is mandatory in these women.

Diuretics

Diuretics are widely employed in the nonpregnant state to manage disease states associated with extracellular fluid volume expansion such as cardiac failure and nephrotic syndrome as well as some cases of renal hypertension. Oedematous states, especially dependent peripheral oedema, are common in pregnant women but rarely merit diuretic treatment. The oedema of pre-eclampsia is caused in part by increased capillary permeability while overall extracellular fluid volume in severe cases is often reduced.[60]

No increase in the frequency of malformations was observed among the offspring of rats treated with thiazide or loop diuretics in doses many times higher than used in humans.[1] In a collaborative report of 5000 pregnant women treated with diuretics, no excess embryo or feto-toxicity was shown.[1] Olsen *et al.* recently reported registry data on 35 and 43 women who received thiazide or loop diuretics, respectively, during the first trimester. No increased rate of teratogenicity was noted.[1]

The effect of diuretics on plasma volume in pregnancy was explored in a small randomised prospective trial of 20 women receiving chronic thiazide treatment for mild hypertension. Reduced plasma volume may impair placental perfusion. Diuretics attenuated the expected physiological pregnancy-related plasma volume expansion (8% versus 52%) although ultimate perinatal outcomes were similar.[61] In contrast, the Danish pregnancy registry reports that women who received diuretics in pregnancy delivered more premature and smaller babies than those not taking these drugs.[1] It is likely that at least a component of this is the impact of the primary condition on pregnancy rather than the drugs themselves.

Thiazide, loop and aldosterone antagonist diuretics cross the placenta, enter the fetal circulation and can impact on fetal renal function. Maternal diuretic given just prior to delivery can lead to electrolyte disturbance in human babies. Diuretics used to treat hydrops fetalis have led to isolated case reports of thrombocytopenia and prolonged labour and also reports suggesting that it may promote patent ductus arteriosus in preterm neonates.[62] Furosemide-induced ototoxicity is reported when used in high doses in adults. Based on this, case–control studies were performed, suggesting a possible link between *in utero* furosemide exposure and sensorineural deafness in neonates, especially when combined with antenatal aminoglycoside.[63]

Spironolactone, an aldosterone antagonist, has well-recognised antiandrogenic adverse effects. Despite this, there are no reports of specific birth defects in neonates or of feminisation of male babies born to mothers taking this drug. As yet there are no reports regarding use of the newer agent eplerenone. This class of diuretic should, however, be avoided because of theoretical concerns.

Diuretics should not be considered as first-line treatment of maternal hypertension in pregnancy because of possible impact on physiological volume expansion. They do not appear to have a major teratogenic effect. When use is considered essential, hydrochlorothiazide and furosemide are the agents for which there is greatest experience in pregnancy.

Breastfeeding

Furosemide is excreted in breast milk, although no reports of adverse effects in nursing mothers have been reported. Thiazide diuretics have very low breast milk : plasma ratios. These drugs are likely to be compatible with safe breastfeeding under careful supervision.[1]

References

1. Briggs GG, Freeman RK, Yaffe SJ. *Drugs in Pregnancy and Lactation : a Reference Guide to Fetal and Neonatal Risk.* 7th ed. Philadelphia/London: Lippincott Williams & Wilkins; 2005.
2. Koren G, Pastuszak A, Ito S. Drugs in pregnancy. *N Engl J Med* 1998;338:1128–37.
3. Brent RL. Utilization of animal studies to determine the effects and human risks of environmental toxicants (drugs, chemicals, and physical agents). *Pediatrics* 2004;113(4 Suppl):984–95.
4. Garbis H, Elefant E, Diav-Citrin O, Mastroiacovo P, Schaefer C, Vial T, *et al.* Pregnancy outcome after exposure to ranitidine and other H2-blockers. A collaborative study of the European Network of Teratology Information Services. *Reprod Toxicol* 2005;19:453–8.
5. McKay DB, Josephson MA. Pregnancy in recipients of solid organs – effects on mother and child. *N Engl J Med* 2006;354:1281–93.

6. Fischer MJ. Chronic kidney disease and pregnancy: maternal and fetal outcomes. *Adv Chronic Kidney Dis* 2007;14:132–45.
7. Levey AS, Bosch JP, Lewis JB, Greene T, Rogers N, Roth D. A more accurate method to estimate glomerular filtration rate from serum creatinine: a new prediction equation. Modification of Diet in Renal Disease Study Group. *Ann Intern Med* 1999;130:461–70.
8. European best practice guidelines for renal transplantation. Section IV: Long-term management of the transplant recipient. IV.10. Pregnancy in renal transplant recipients. *Nephrol Dial Transplant* 2002;17 Suppl 4:50–5.
9. Park-Wyllie L, Mazzotta P, Pastuszak A, Moretti ME, Beique L, Hunnisett L, *et al.* Birth defects after maternal exposure to corticosteroids: prospective cohort study and meta-analysis of epidemiological studies. *Teratology* 2000;62:385–92.
10. Hou S. Pregnancy in chronic renal insufficiency and end-stage renal disease. *Am J Kidney Dis* 1999;33:235–52.
11. Empson M, Lassere M, Craig J, Scott J. Prevention of recurrent miscarriage for women with antiphospholipid antibody or lupus anticoagulant. *Cochrane Database Syst Rev* 2005;(2):CD002859.
12. Ostensen M, Khamashta M, Lockshin M, Parke A, Brucato A, Carp H, *et al.* Anti-inflammatory and immunosuppressive drugs and reproduction. *Arthritis Res Ther* 2006;8:209.
13. Armenti VT, Radomski JS, Moritz MJ, Philips LZ, McGrory CH, Coscia LA. Report from the National Transplantation Pregnancy Registry (NTPR): outcomes of pregnancy after transplantation. *Clin Transpl* 2000:123–34.
14. Greenberger PA, Odeh YK, Frederiksen MC, Atkinson AJ Jr. Pharmacokinetics of prednisolone transfer to breast milk. *Clin Pharmacol Ther* 1993;53:324–8.
15. Saarikoski S, Seppala M. Immunosuppression during pregnancy: transmission of azathioprine and its metabolites from the mother to the fetus. *Am J Obstet Gynecol* 1973;115:1100–6.
16. Chambers CD, Tutuncu ZN, Johnson D, Jones KL. Human pregnancy safety for agents used to treat rheumatoid arthritis: adequacy of available information and strategies for developing post-marketing data. *Arthritis Res Ther* 2006;8:215.
17. Davison JM, Dellagrammatikas H, Parkin JM. Maternal azathioprine therapy and depressed haemopoiesis in the babies of renal allograft patients. *Br J Obstet Gynaecol* 1985;92:233–9.
18. Armenti VT, Ahlswede KM, Ahlswede BA, Jarrell BE, Moritz MJ, Burke JF. National transplantation Pregnancy Registry – outcomes of 154 pregnancies in cyclosporine-treated female kidney transplant recipients. *Transplantation* 1994;57:502–6.
19. Sibanda N, Briggs JD, Davison JM, Johnson RJ, Rudge CJ. Pregnancy after organ transplantation: a report from the UK Transplant pregnancy registry. *Transplantation* 2007;83:1301–7.
20. Norgard B, Pedersen L, Christensen LA, Sorensen HT. Therapeutic drug use in women with Crohn's disease and birth outcomes: a Danish nationwide cohort study. *Am J Gastroenterol* 2007;102:1406–13.
21. Davison JM, Lindheimer MD. Pregnancy in renal transplant recipients. *J Reprod Med* 1982;27:613–21.
22. Sanchez-Guerrero J, Uribe AG, Jimenez-Santana L, Mestanza-Peralta M, Lara-Reyes P, Seuc AH, *et al.* A trial of contraceptive methods in women with systemic lupus erythematosus. *N Engl J Med* 2005;353:2539–49.
23. McKay DB, Josephson MA, Armenti VT, August P, Coscia LA, Davis CL, *et al.* Reproduction and transplantation: report on the AST Consensus Conference on Reproductive Issues and Transplantation. *Am J Transplant* 2005;5:1592–9.
24. Sau A, Clarke S, Bass J, Kaiser A, Marinaki A, Nelson-Piercy C. Azathioprine and breastfeeding: is it safe? *BJOG* 2007;114:498–501.
25. Venkataramanan R, Koneru B, Wang CC, Burckart GJ, Caritis SN, Starzl TE. Cyclosporine and its metabolites in mother and baby. *Transplantation* 1988;46:468–9.
26. Schmid BP. Monitoring of organ formation in rat embryos after *in vitro* exposure to azathioprine, mercaptopurine, methotrexate or cyclosporin A. *Toxicology* 1984;31:9–21.
27. Bar Oz B, Hackman R, Einarson T, Koren G. Pregnancy outcome after cyclosporine therapy during pregnancy: a meta-analysis. *Transplantation* 2001;71:1051–5.

28. Armenti VT, Radomski JS, Moritz MJ, Gaughan WJ, Hecker WP, Lavelanet A, *et al.* Report from the National Transplantation Pregnancy Registry (NTPR): outcomes of pregnancy after transplantation. *Clin Transpl* 2004:103–14.
29. Fischer T, Neumayer HH, Fischer R, Barenbrock M, Schobel HP, Lattrell BC, *et al.* Effect of pregnancy on long-term kidney function in renal transplant recipients treated with cyclosporine and with azathioprine. *Am J Transplant* 2005;5:2732–9.
30. Day C, Hewins P, Sheikh L, Kilby M, McPake D, Lipkin G. Cholestasis in pregnancy associated with ciclosporin therapy in renal transplant recipients. *Transpl Int* 2006;19:1026–9.
31. Stanley CW, Gottlieb R, Zager R, Eisenberg J, Richmond R, Moritz MJ, *et al.* Developmental well-being in offspring of women receiving cyclosporine post-renal transplant. *Transplant Proc* 1999;31:241–2.
32. Tendron-Franzin A, Gouyon JB, Guignard JP, Decramer S, Justrabo E, Gilbert T, *et al.* Long-term effects of *in utero* exposure to cyclosporin A on renal function in the rabbit. *J Am Soc Nephrol* 2004;15:2687–93.
33. Giudice PL, Dubourg L, Hadj-Aissa A, Said MH, Claris O, Audra P, *et al.* Renal function of children exposed to cyclosporin *in utero*. *Nephrol Dial Transplant* 2000;15:1575–9.
34. Munoz-Flores-Thiagarajan KD, Easterling T, Davis C, Bond EF. Breast-feeding by a cyclosporine-treated mother. *Obstet Gynecol* 2001;97:816–18.
35. Moretti ME, Sgro M, Johnson DW, Sauve RS, Woolgar MJ, Taddio A, *et al.* Cyclosporine excretion into breast milk. *Transplantation* 2003;75:2144–6.
36. Gardiner SJ, Begg EJ. Breastfeeding during tacrolimus therapy. *Obstet Gynecol* 2006;107:453–5.
37. French AE, Soldin SJ, Soldin OP, Koren G. Milk transfer and neonatal safety of tacrolimus. *Ann Pharmacother* 2003;37:815–18.
38. D'Cruz DP, Khamashta MA, Hughes GR. Systemic lupus erythematosus. *Lancet* 2007;369:587–96.
39. Tendron A, Gouyon JB, Decramer S. *In utero* exposure to immunosuppressive drugs: experimental and clinical studies. *Pediatr Nephrol* 2002;17:121–30.
40. Tjeertes IF, Bastiaans DE, van Ganzewinkel CJ, Zegers SH. Neonatal anemia and hydrops fetalis after maternal mycophenolate mofetil use. *J Perinatol* 2007;27:62–4.
41. Le Ray C, Coulomb A, Elefant E, Frydman R, Audibert F. Mycophenolate mofetil in pregnancy after renal transplantation: a case of major fetal malformations. *Obstet Gynecol* 2004;103:1091–4.
42. Sifontis NM, Coscia LA, Constantinescu S, Lavelanet AF, Moritz MJ, Armenti VT. Pregnancy outcomes in solid organ transplant recipients with exposure to mycophenolate mofetil or sirolimus. *Transplantation* 2006;82:1698–702.
43. Guardia O, Rial Mdel C, Casadei D. Pregnancy under sirolimus-based immunosuppression. *Transplantation* 2006;81:636.
44. Jankowska I, Oldakowska-Jedynak U, Jabiry-Zieniewicz Z, Cyganek A, Pawlowska J, Teisseyre M, *et al.* Absence of teratogenicity of sirolimus used during early pregnancy in a liver transplant recipient. *Transplant Proc* 2004;36:3232–3.
45. Valente JF, Hricik D, Weigel K, Seaman D, Knauss T, Siegel CT, *et al.* Comparison of sirolimus vs. mycophenolate mofetil on surgical complications and wound healing in adult kidney transplantation. *Am J Transplant* 2003;3:1128–34.
46. Roos S, Jansson N, Palmberg I, Saljo K, Powell TL, Jansson T. Mammalian target of rapamycin in the human placenta regulates leucine transport and is down-regulated in restricted fetal growth. *J Physiol* 2007;582:449–59.
47. Milman N, Graudal N, Nielsen OJ, Agger AO. Serum erythropoietin during normal pregnancy: relationship to hemoglobin and iron status markers and impact of iron supplementation in a longitudinal, placebo-controlled study on 118 women. *Int J Hematol* 1997;66:159–68.
48. Magee LA, von Dadelszen P, Darley J, Beguin Y. Erythropoiesis and renal transplant pregnancy. *Clin Transplant* 2000;14:127–35.
49. Schneider H, Malek A. Lack of permeability of the human placenta for erythropoietin. *J Perinat Med* 1995;23:71–6.
50. Hou SH. Frequency and outcome of pregnancy in women on dialysis. *Am J Kidney Dis* 1994;23:60–3.

51. Szurkowski M, Wiecek A, Kokot F, Daniel K. Safety and efficiency of recombinant human erythropoietin treatment in anemic pregnant women with a kidney transplant. *Nephron* 1994;67:242–3.
52. Holley JL, Reddy SS. Pregnancy in dialysis patients: a review of outcomes, complications, and management. *Semin Dial* 2003;16:384–8.
53. Reveiz L, Gyte GM, Cuervo LG. Treatments for iron-deficiency anaemia in pregnancy. *Cochrane Database Syst Rev* 2007;(2):CD003094.
54. Okundaye I, Abrinko P, Hou S. Registry of pregnancy in dialysis patients. *Am J Kidney Dis* 1998;31:766–73.
55. Chao AS, Huang JY, Lien R, Kung FT, Chen PJ, Hsieh PC. Pregnancy in women who undergo long-term hemodialysis. *Am J Obstet Gynecol* 2002;187:152–6.
56. Toma H, Tanabe K, Tokumoto T, Kobayashi C, Yagisawa T. Pregnancy in women receiving renal dialysis or transplantation in Japan: a nationwide survey. *Nephrol Dial Transplant* 1999;14:1511–16.
57. Kashiwagi M, Breymann C, Huch R, Huch A. Hypertension in a pregnancy with renal anemia after recombinant human erythropoietin (rhEPO) therapy. *Arch Gynecol Obstet* 2002;267:54–6.
58. Thorp M, Pulliam J. Use of recombinant erythropoietin in a pregnant renal transplant recipient. *Am J Nephrol* 1998;18:448–51.
59. Goshorn J, Youell TD. Darbepoetin alfa treatment for post-renal transplantation anemia during pregnancy. *Am J Kidney Dis* 2005;46:e81–6.
60. Hladunewich M, Karumanchi SA, Lafayette R. Pathophysiology of the clinical manifestations of preeclampsia. *Clin J Am Soc Nephrol* 2007;2:543–9.
61. Sibai BM, Grossman RA, Grossman HG. Effects of diuretics on plasma volume in pregnancies with long-term hypertension. *Am J Obstet Gynecol* 1984;150:831–5.
62. Green TP, Thompson TR, Johnson DE, Lock JE. Furosemide promotes patent ductus arteriosus in premature infants with the respiratory-distress syndrome. *N Engl J Med* 1983;308:743–8.
63. Rybak LP. Furosemide ototoxicity: clinical and experimental aspects. *Laryngoscope* 1985;95(9 Pt 2 Suppl 38):1–14.

Chapter 12
Management of hypertension in renal disease in pregnancy

Mark Kilby and Graham W Lipkin

Introduction

Chronic kidney disease (CKD) is relatively common and therefore, in women of childbearing age, is likely to be a common cause of secondary hypertension. In the nonpregnant state, CKD is defined either as kidney damage (which is confirmed by renal biopsy or secondary markers of damage) or the presence of a glomerular filtration rate (GFR) of less than 60 ml/minute/1.73 m^2 for a period of greater than 3 months.[1] It is likely that the prevalence of CKD will increase in general terms within the UK, with the introduction of the estimated GFR (eGFR)[2] and that, with the ageing population of women embarking on pregnancy, this increase will be disproportionate amongst women pregnant for the first time.[3] Recent data collected from the USA indicate that approximately 5% of the overall population suffers from reduced GFR (less than 60 ml/minute/1.73 m^2).[4] Chronic kidney disease is strongly associated with hypertension and the greater the severity of renal impairment the higher the risk. In end-stage renal disease, 80% of patients have associated hypertension.

The prevalence of hypertension varies somewhat with the aetiology of the underlying disease, with approximately 40% prevalence in chronic interstitial nephritis, immunoglobulin A (IgA) nephropathy and minimal change disease in the nonpregnant population, whereas rates of above 60% are associated with diabetic nephropathy, adult-type polycystic renal disease and focal segmental glomerulosclerosis.[5] Interestingly, in the end-stage renal disease patient, systolic hypertension is more common than combined systolic and diastolic hypertension.

In general, in the nonpregnant and probably the prepregnant population, the control of hypertension is relatively poor. Estimates indicate that only a quarter of patients with recognised hypertension are adequately treated. Studies investigating this phenomenon within the cohorts of patients with CKD indicate that hypertensive treatment is no better and may even be worse.[6] This is important, as substandard treatment will drive worsening kidney function owing to continuing nephron attrition mitigated by antihypertensive therapy and also increases overall cardiovascular morbidity and mortality. Large epidemiological studies of nonpregnant people with CKD have demonstrated increased cardiovascular mortality even in moderate renal failure.[7,8] A recent meta-analysis of 85 publications demonstrates that the threshold for an increase in cardiovascular risk is when the GFR falls below 75 ml/minute/1.73 m^2, with the risk increasing steeply with reducing GFR.[9] When people with CKD start dialysis, the cardiovascular mortality rate increases five- to ten-fold and those with end-stage renal disease and dialysis have a risk that is 100-fold increased.[10] However, hypertension is just one factor in people with chronic renal impairment, and dyslipidaemia, insulin resistance, anaemia, hyperhomocysteinaemia, reduced nitric oxide availability and chronic inflammation also add to the cardiovascular risk in such patients.

In the Multiple Risk Factor Intervention Trial (MRFIT), blood pressure was noted to be a strong predictor of worsening renal disease, with primary hypertensive nephrosclerosis (with associated hyalinisation and sclerosis of afferent renal arterioles) being a significant cause of chronic renal impairment.[11] Many factors may exist in an individual (of reproductive age or not) that may be responsible for blood pressure elevation (Box 12.1). The added mortality and cardiovascular risk induced by hypertension are significant and the effects of blood pressure control through dialysis technology and antihypertensive medication important.

In addition, hypertension is a common medical disorder of pregnancy, affecting 10–15% of all pregnancies. It is also a significant cause of maternal morbidity and mortality both worldwide and within the UK.[12] The condition also increases perinatal mortality and morbidity, by increasing the risk of preterm birth, fetal growth restriction and placental abruption. Pre-existing or chronic hypertension is one of the most rapidly growing causes of hypertension in pregnancy. A combination of factors appears to be important in this rise in prevalence, including the postponement of childbearing to a more advanced age and the increased 'essential' hypertension, often coupled with obesity and insulin resistance. Although less common than essential hypertension, in women of reproductive age, three forms of secondary hypertension require exclusion. These include endocrine causes, such as pheochromocytoma and primary hyperaldosteronism, and cardiac causes such as aortic coarctation and renovascular hypertension. Additionally, many apparently healthy young women may not have had any blood pressure assessment prior to pregnancy. As has been indicated, the physiological mechanisms of gestational blood pressure alteration and increased vasodilation in the second trimester may mask chronic hypertension. This will then only be revealed in the second half of pregnancy and may be difficult to differentiate

Box 12.1. Possible mechanisms for hypertension in people with chronic kidney disease

- pre-existing essential hypertension
- extracellular fluid volume expansion
- renin–angiotensin–aldosterone system stimulation
- increased activity of the sympathetic nervous system
- increased body mass index (BMI)
- erythropoietin (EPO) administration
- parathyroid hormone (PTH) secretion and increased intracellular calcium concentrations
- calcification of the arterial tree
- renal artery disease
- alterations in endothelial-derived factors (e.g. nitric oxide, endothelin and prostaglandins)
- chronic allograft dysfunction
- cadaveric allografts (especially if donor has family history of hypertension)
- chronic pharmacotherapy for immunosuppression (e.g. ciclosporin, tacrolimus and corticosteroids)

from gestational hypertension or pre-eclampsia. Indeed, a recent review of renal biopsy data in women close to pregnancy has again reiterated the fact that a small but significant number of women with pre-eclampsia have underlying pre-existing renal disease with hypertension mistaken as severe pre-eclampsia.[13]

Superimposed pre-eclampsia

A full discussion of pre-eclampsia and gestational hypertension is outside the remit of this chapter (see Chapter 15). However, because pre-eclampsia is such a common and important complication in pregnant women with pre-existing hypertension and CKD, 'superimposed pre-eclampsia' is discussed at this point. 'Pure' pre-eclampsia complicates 5–6% of (usually nulliparous) pregnancies. In addition, it may be superimposed on 20–40% of pregnant women who have underlying chronic hypertension or a predisposing medical disorder, including even minor renal disease of any aetiology, including early diabetic nephropathy, autoimmune disease or even microscopic haematuria. It must thus be (re-)emphasised that prepregnancy care and advice (whether it be in the primary or secondary medical setting) is important in limiting this complication of pregnancy (see Chapter 2). Superimposed pre-eclampsia tends to be more severe and to reveal itself at an earlier gestational age than pre-eclampsia without an underlying medical cause. It is therefore not surprising that it tends to recur in subsequent pregnancies.[14] Likewise, given the persistence (and lack of treatment) of the underlying risk factor, its presence may lead to 'pre-eclampsia' (with associated placental failure) and more severe hypertension, which represent the two major risks of chronic hypertension in pregnancy. It may be clinically difficult to differentiate between superimposed pre-eclampsia and worsening hypertension and proteinuria. Indeed, a now classic study[15] indicated that in only 58% of cases could a nephrologist and obstetrician distinguish true/primary pre-eclampsia from that of superimposed disease. However, more recently, the use of serum or plasma soluble fms-like tyrosine kinase 1 (sFlt1) noting an association between the typical renal lesion of 'glomerular endotheliosis' and elevated maternal levels will mean the sensitivity and specificity of diagnosis may increase.[16] However, the key to management appears to be the identification and treatment of underlying hypertension and/or renal disease.

Goals of antihypertensive treatment in kidney disease: nonpregnant patients

In people with CKD it is important to manage both components of hypertension – hypervolaemia and vasoconstriction. According to the 7th Report of the Joint National Committee in the USA (JNC7), the blood pressure goal for nonpregnant patients with CKD and hypertension is less than 130/80 mmHg.[17] Two multicentre outcome studies (one from the USA and one from the UK) that randomised to different levels of blood pressure have demonstrated a significant reduction in cardiovascular mortality in the groups of patients with microvascular disease (mainly of diabetic aetiology) and renal disease that achieved lower levels of blood pressure and were the main reason for JNC7 to choose the less than 130/80 mmHg threshold.[18,19] An analysis of long-term clinical trials in patients with diabetic and non-diabetic kidney disease clearly demonstrates that lowering blood pressure also leads to greater preservation of kidney function. It is not just the JNC7 proceedings that advocate the reduction of blood pressure to less than 130/80 mmHg. The evidence in favour of such tight blood pressure control to reduce the rates of both progressive renal impairment and cardiovascular events is so strong that it is recommended by the European Society of Hypertension, the European Society of Cardiology and the NKF-KDOQI working group. All recommend a goal of blood pressure to below 130/80 mmHg for patients with CKD with or without diabetes and an even lower threshold of 125/75 mmHg or less if concomitant proteinuria of more than 1 g/day exists.[20]

In nonpregnant patients with end-stage renal disease undergoing dialysis, determining the target blood pressure is more complicated. In contrast to the other studies of chronic renal impairment and hypertensive control, several studies have failed to demonstrate that blood pressure above 130/80 mmHg is associated with increased long-term cardiovascular mortality. This has led to concerns that in this cohort of subjects there is a J-shaped relationship between mean arterial blood pressure (MAP) and mortality, with increased mortality in patients with both low or high pre-dialysis blood pressure.[21,22]

In people with CKD who are not on dialysis, it is commonplace in the nonpregnant patient to initiate antihypertensive therapy with a renin–angiotensin–aldosterone blocker, which eliminates vasoconstriction (except some structural vascular changes) and some of the sympathetic hyperactivity.[23] Residual hypertension often indicates the hypervolaemic component and this can often be treated using diuretics and any residual sympathetic effects treated by β-blockade. Long-term outcome studies utilising angiotensin-converting enzyme (ACE) inhibitors or angiotensin II receptor blockers (ARBs) demonstrate long-term improvement of renal function with treatment in CKD. Such effects appear to be most effective if protein excretion is less than 1 g/day but demonstrates improved renal outcome even when significant protein excretion (more than 1 g/day) is present (Figure 12.1).[24]

In people with end-stage renal failure, volume has to be controlled by ultrafiltration. Inadequate blood pressure control is present when there is volume excess as exhibited

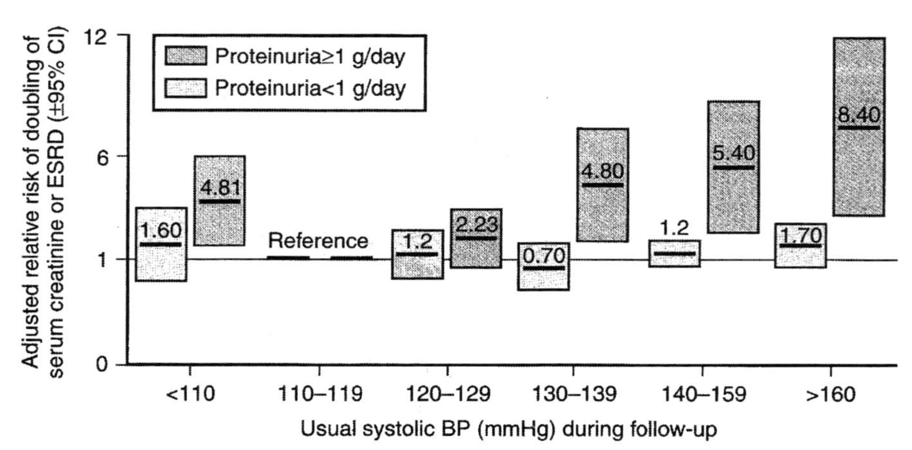

Figure 12.1. Relative risk of kidney disease progression based upon current level of systolic blood pressure and urine protein excretion, based on a meta-analysis of 11 randomised controlled trials (the reference group for each was a systolic blood pressure of 110–119 mmHg); reproduced with permission from Sarafidis and Bakris[57]

by a large interdialytic weight increase. In such patients, the problem of blood pressure control is often exacerbated as antihypertensive medication is often withheld on the day of dialysis and dietary sodium restriction is not instituted. In nonpregnant patients with end-stage renal disease, however, 'double blockade' with an ARB and an ACE inhibitor appears to confer benefit (in both diabetic and non-diabetic patients) reducing proteinuria, protecting renal function and improving cardiac function.

Such data are interesting and women of reproductive age will often be placed on such therapeutic regimens. As the use of many of these pharmacological agents are contraindicated in pregnancy, the management of hypertension associated with renal disease in prepregnancy and in the antenatal period is of utmost importance and has significant effects on outcomes for both mother and baby.[25]

Hypertension, renal disease and pregnancy

Chronic hypertension increases the risks of several morbid pregnancy outcomes.[26–28] A review that evaluated the magnitude of maternal and fetal risks[27] during pregnancy in these women found a three-fold increase in perinatal mortality (OR 3.4, 95% CI 3.0–3.7), a two-fold increase in placental abruption (OR 2.1, 95% CI 1.1–3.9) and an increased frequency of impaired fetal growth compared to normotensive women (even in the absence of pre-eclampsia). The absolute ranges of risk for adverse pregnancy outcome reported in observational studies of women with mild chronic hypertension were:[28]

- superimposed pre-eclampsia 10–25%
- placental abruption 0.7–1.5%
- preterm birth before 37 weeks 12–34%
- fetal growth restriction 8–16%.

These risks are even higher in women with severe chronic hypertension in the first trimester (pre-eclampsia 50%, abruption 5–10%, preterm birth 62–70%, growth restriction 31–40%), and were highest in those with severe hypertension and superimposed pre-eclampsia.

A recent retrospective study of an obstetric renal cohort of 358 women (400 pregnancies) from the maternity hospitals in Birmingham, Leicester and Hammersmith in London compared pregnancy outcomes with a control cohort of 113 782 women without renal disease (the CORD study; published as abstract at the British Maternal & Fetal Medicine Society 2005 annual conference).[29]

Chronic hypertension (with diastolic blood pressures of 90 mmHg or higher (in those treated or untreated)) was independently associated with neonatal death, and both chronic hypertension and renal impairment with preterm birth in multivariate analysis (Table 12.1). The Kaplan–Meier perinatal survival data indicate that hypertension reduces duration of pregnancy, whatever the severity of chronic renal impairment (i.e. serum creatinine) (Figure 12.2). This perinatal risk increased in parallel with greater degrees of baseline maternal renal dysfunction. In the presence of both risk factors, the duration of pregnancy was greatly reduced. In those with severe hypertension and creatinine above 1.4 mg/dl in early pregnancy, median gestational age at delivery was 31.6 weeks. A significantly increased risk of caesarean section accompanied both increasing maternal age and renal impairment.

Other potential problems stem from the known risks of hypertensive disease, such as heart failure, hypertensive encephalopathy, retinopathy, cerebral haemorrhage and

Table 12.1. Maternal variables associated with adverse obstetric outcomes in multivariate analysis

Adverse outcome	Associated variable	Odds ratio	95% confidence interval	Significance
Risk of neonatal death ($n = 244$)	Diastolic blood pressure (mmHg):			
	< 70	1		
	70–80	4.5	0.4–50	0.23
	80–90	4.3	0.3–71	0.31
	> 90 or treated	17	2.0–140	0.009
Preterm birth before 37 weeks ($n = 224$) (hazard ratio)	Creatinine (mg/dl):			
	< 0.8	1		
	0.8–1.4	1.7	0.9–3.0	0.08
	1.4–2	2.9	1.1–7.8	0.03
	> 2	5.7	1.8–18	0.002
	Diastolic blood pressure (mmHg):			
	< 70	1		
	70–80	1.2	0.5–2.9	0.66
	80–90	1.5	0.6–4.2	0.40
	> 90 or treated	3.6	1.8–7.5	< 0.001
Caesarean section ($n = 220$)	Maternal age (years):			
	< 28	1		
	28–32½	3.3	1.5–7.2	0.003
	> 32½	4.5	2.1–9.9	< 0.001
	Creatinine (mg/dl):			
	< 0.8	1		
	0.8–1.4	3.1	1.6–6.1	0.001
	1.4–2.0	9.6	1.8–52	0.009
	> 2.0	19	2.1–160	0.008
Small for gestational age ($n = 334$)	Ethnicity			
	Caucasian	1		
	Asian	3.0	1.7–5.2	< 0.001
	African-Caribbean	1.8	0.7–4.5	0.24

acute renal failure. Despite these risks, the treatment of chronic hypertension during pregnancy is controversial. Beneficial effects of treatment appear to be limited to prevention of maternal morbidity and depend upon the severity of the disease.

Maternal evaluation

Baseline laboratory tests that have been recommended in pregnancy include urinalysis, urine culture, serum creatinine, blood urea nitrogen, glucose, and electrolytes.[28] These tests will effectively exclude many causes of previously unrecognised secondary hypertension, such as renal disease, and will also identify important comorbidities, such as diabetes. If qualitative testing for urine protein is negative, quantitative testing is not necessary. Women who develop evidence of proteinuria on a urine dipstick should have a quantitative test for urine protein. An electrocardiogram should be obtained in women with longstanding hypertension.

Management of hypertension in pregnancy

Prophylaxis

A detailed discussion of prophylaxis in preventing 'superimposed pre-eclampsia' is outside the remit of this chapter. However, antihypertensive therapy and lowering blood pressure alone *per se* fail to prevent pre-eclampsia. Similarly, neither salt restriction nor

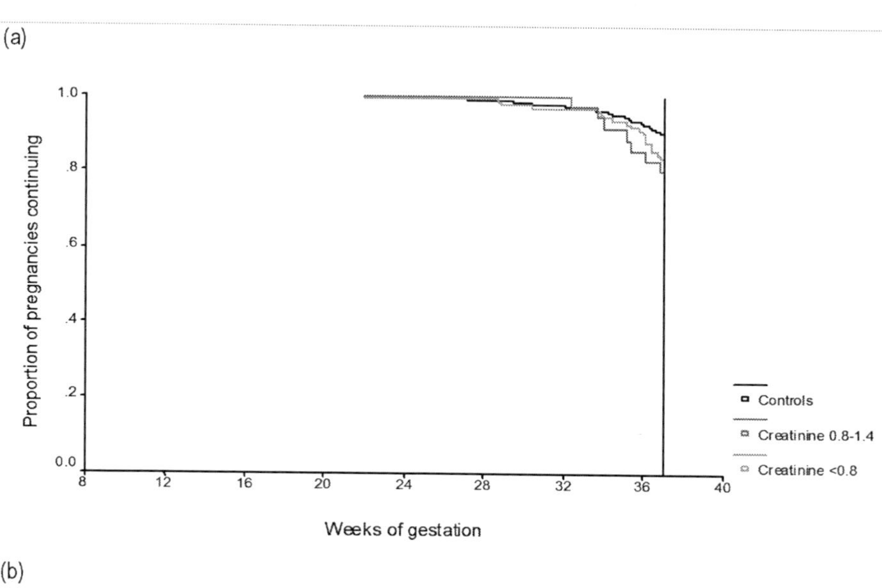

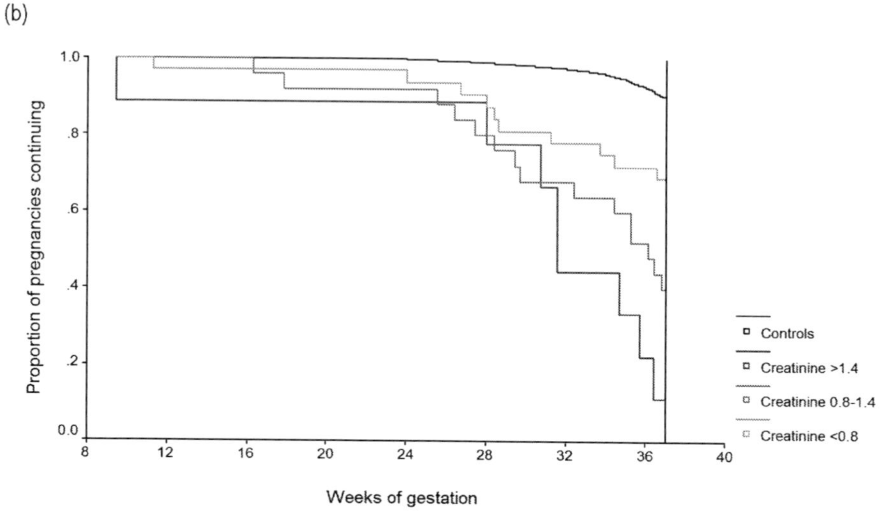

Figure 12.2. (a) Duration of pregnancy in those women without hypertension (untreated diastolic blood pressure < 90 mmHg) according to maternal serum creatinine (mg/dl); (b) Duration of pregnancy in those women with hypertension (treated, or diastolic blood pressure > 90 mmHg) according to maternal serum creatinine (mg/dl)

prophylactic diuretic therapy prevent pre-eclampsia. It is thus important to consider the evidence for therapeutic strategies that may be adjuvant to antihypertensive treatment in the pregnant women with pre-existing hypertension and renal disease.

Physiological observations of an imbalance in arachidonic acid metabolism in pre-eclampsia, favouring autocrine imbalance between thromboxane A2 over prostacyclin has led to the rationale for primary prevention studies using low-dose aspirin (60–100 mg/day). Many relatively small, uncontrolled studies demonstrated benefit in prophylaxis but unfortunately the promise of these studies was not upheld with larger randomised controlled trials.[30,31] Indeed, although some group analysis indicated that there may be some benefit in 'high-risk cohorts', such as women with pre-existing renal disease, the results have been mixed. However, a recent systematic review from the PARIS group[32] has indicated that aspirin has few morbid associations and in general terms the number needed to treat is 50 to prevent one acquiring pre-eclampsia.

Observational data that pre-eclampsia is associated with hypocalciuria has led to studies investigating the supplementation of women with calcium. A recent and relatively large randomised controlled trial failed to demonstrate any beneficial effect of calcium supplementation on the incidence of pre-eclampsia but those developing the disease did so at a later gestational age, had a lower incidence of eclampsia and severe hypertensive complications and had lower perinatal morbidity.[33] This has led to a call for the use of calcium prophylaxis in women at high risk of developing pre-eclampsia.

In vitro evidence of uteroplacental and systematic oxidative stress in pre-eclampsia led to the hypothesis that prophylaxis with the antioxidants vitamins C and E may reduce severe complications of hypertension. However, a randomised study, the Vitamin in Pregnancy (VIP) trial,[34] demonstrated that the cohort of women receiving vitamins C and E had a non-significant increased incidence of pre-eclampsia, more severe hypertension, lower birthweight babies and increased perinatal morbidity. A further study from Australasia[35] demonstrated no worsening of outcome but no significant benefit in the group receiving antioxidants.

Evaluation and management of hypertension in pregnancy

Women with uncomplicated chronic hypertension who are normotensive or mildly hypertensive on medication may continue their therapy or have their antihypertensive agents tapered and/or stopped during pregnancy, with close monitoring of the maternal blood pressure response.[36] Acceptable blood pressures (systolic less than 140–159 mmHg or diastolic less than 90–99 mmHg) in the absence of their usual antihypertensive therapy is not uncommon in the second trimester owing to the normal decrease in blood pressure at this time. There is no consensus on the best approach.

Mild essential hypertension

The indications for instituting antihypertensive drugs in uncomplicated patients with mild essential hypertension (systolic 140–159 mmHg or diastolic 90–99 mmHg) who have not previously been treated or who have discontinued therapy are not clear. Neither the woman nor the fetus appears to be at risk from mild hypertension during pregnancy. Furthermore, controlled studies have not demonstrated that lowering the blood pressure with antihypertensive medications reduces the risk of pre-eclampsia or abruption, or improves fetal or maternal outcome.[37–41] However, two systematic reviews concluded that therapy does reduce the incidence of severe hypertension.[36,41]

Despite a large number of trials on treatment of hypertension in pregnancy, these trials lack sufficient power, even with meta-analysis, to detect modest (20–30%) treatment effects and usually do not differentiate among degrees of severity of mild hypertension.

Based on the available data, the conclusion would be not to initiate treatment of pregnant women with uncomplicated mild essential hypertension, especially in the first trimester, since blood pressure may decrease as pregnancy progresses. In women already taking antihypertensive therapy who have early pregnancy blood pressures less than 120/80 mmHg, again the data suggest tapering/discontinuing antihypertensive drugs and closely monitoring the blood pressure response.

The indications for initiating or re-instituting antihypertensive therapy are persistent diastolic pressures of 95–99 mmHg, systolic pressures greater than 150 mmHg, or signs of hypertensive end-organ damage. These thresholds, although not in the severe range, allow non-emergent intervention with oral drugs while hypertension is only moderately elevated.

The recently published CHIP randomised controlled trial[42] was a 'pilot' study designed to determine whether 'less tight' (versus 'tight') control of non-severe hypertension results in a difference in diastolic blood pressure (dBP) between groups at seventeen obstetric centres in Canada, Australia, New Zealand and the UK. Pregnant women with dBP 90–109 mmHg, pre-existing/gestational hypertension, live fetus(es) and duration of pregnancy of 20 weeks to 33 weeks and 6 days were included. Randomisation of subjects to less tight (target dBP of 100 mmHg) or tight (target dBP of 85 mmHg) blood pressure control was performed. A total of 132 women were randomised to less tight ($n = 66$; seven had no study visit) or tight control ($n = 66$; one was lost to follow-up; seven had no study visit). The mean dBP was significantly lower with tight control, at a difference of −3.5 mmHg (95% CI −6.4 to −0.6). Clinician compliance was 79% in both groups. Women were satisfied with their care. With less tight (versus tight) control, the rates of other treatments and outcomes were as follows:

- post-randomisation antenatal antihypertensive medication use 46 (69.7%) versus 58 (89.2%)
- severe hypertension 38 (57.6%) versus 26 (40.0%)
- proteinuria 16 (24.2%) versus 20 (30.8%)
- serious maternal complications 3 (4.6%) versus 2 (3.1%)
- preterm birth 24 (36.4%) versus 26 (40.0%)
- birthweight 2675 ± 858 versus 2501 ± 855 g
- neonatal intensive care unit (NICU) admission 15 (22.7%) versus 22 (34.4%)
- serious perinatal complications 9 (13.6%) versus 14 (21.5%).

Although this was a relatively small pilot study, it has provided a rationale to increase the numbers in the study to power for outcomes such as perinatal loss and to study 'at risk' subgroups, such as those women with pre-existing renal disease and hypertension.[42]

Complicated and secondary hypertension

Subgroups of women with mild hypertension appear to be at greater risk of maternal or fetal complications and may benefit from antihypertensive therapy. Therapy has been suggested for women with:[28,40]

- secondary, rather than essential, hypertension (e.g. renal disease, collagen vascular disease, coarctation of the aorta)

- end-organ damage (e.g. ventricular dysfunction, retinopathy)
- dyslipidaemia
- maternal age over 40 years
- microvascular disease
- history of stroke
- previous perinatal loss
- diabetes.

In these groups (which would apply to CKD), treatment to attain blood pressures of less than 140/90 mmHg is suggested. These thresholds are thus very similar to those recommended for people with CKD outside pregnancy.

Severe hypertension

Severe hypertension (blood pressure above 160/100 mmHg), particularly if associated with signs of early hypertensive encephalopathy, should be treated to protect the mother from serious complications such as stroke, heart failure or renal failure.

Choice of drug

All antihypertensive drugs cross the placenta. There are no data from large well-designed randomised trials on which to base a recommendation for use of one drug over another. Data regarding both comparative efficacy in improving pregnancy outcome and fetal safety are inadequate for almost all antihypertensive drugs. The ranges of commonly used oral antihypertensive drugs (in women with renal disease) are indicated in Table 12.2.

The previous data presented (see earlier) indicate that in many studies of antihypertensive use in nonpregnant patients with hypertension and CKD, ACE inhibitors and ARBs appear to be beneficial. There is general agreement that ACE inhibitors and ARBs should not be administered in pregnancy; therefore, it is best to discontinue these agents in women planning pregnancy and switch to another agent. Exposure of the fetus to such maternal medication leads to excess risk of fetal growth restriction, oligohydramnios, neonatal renal failure and probably cardiac and neurological congenital anomalies.[43]

The common consensus from the literature is to start treatment with either methyldopa or labetalol. A long-acting calcium channel blocker (i.e. nifedipine) can be added as either second- or third-line treatment. These drugs have been used extensively during pregnancy and appear to be safe and effective.[44]

Methyldopa, one of the most widely used drugs in pregnant women, is a centrally acting compound and, with some small differences, the US, Canadian and Australasian consensus statements make note of the wealth of clinical experience that has led to this drug being the preferred antihypertensive for use during pregnancy.[1,41,45] It is well tolerated, does not alter uteroplacental or fetal haemodynamics and has the longest follow-up of childhood development following *in utero* exposure.[41,45] However, it is a mild antihypertensive agent.[41,45] Many women will not achieve blood pressure targets on this agent alone or are troubled by its adverse effects, especially the sedation.

Labetalol, the most widely used beta-adrenergic blocker in pregnancy, is not selective, having some alpha-blockade effects. The safety of beta-adrenergic blockers, particularly propranolol, is somewhat controversial owing to individual reports of

Table 12.2. Oral antihypertensive medication commonly used to treat chronic hypertension with renal disease in pregnancy; reproduced with permission from Umans[14]

Drug (FDA risk[a,b])	Dose	Concerns or comments
Most commonly used first-line agents		
Methyldopa (B)	0.5–3.0 g/day in 2–3 divided doses	Preferred agent of the NHBPEP working group; maternal side effects sometimes limit use
Labetalol (C) or other β receptor antagonists	200–2400 mg/day in 2–3 divided doses	Labetalol is preferred by NHBPEP working group as alternative to methyldopa. Atenolol most commonly used in Canada and β blockers with intrinsic sympathomimetic activity are preferred by some in Australia. May cause fetal growth restriction when started early.
Nifedipine (C)	30–120 mg/day of a slow-release preparation	Less experience with other calcium entry blockers
Adjunctive agents		
Hydralazine (C)	50–300 mg/day in 2–4 divided doses	Few controlled trials, long experience; used only in combination with sympatholytic agent (e.g. methyldopa or a β blocker) to prevent reflex tachycardia
Thiazide diuretics (C)	Depends on specific agent	Most studies in normotensive gravidas
Contraindicated		
ACE inhibitors and ARBs (D)		Use after first trimester can lead to fetopathy, oligohydramnios, growth restriction, and neonatal anuric renal failure, which may be fatal

ACE = angiotensin-converting enzyme; ARB = angiotensin II receptor blocker; NHBPEP = National High Blood Pressure Education Program

[a] No antihypertensive has been proven safe for use during the first trimester (i.e. FDA Category A)

[b] The US Food and Drug Administration (FDA) classifies risk for most agents as C: either studies in animals have revealed adverse effects on the fetus (teratogenic or embryocidal effects or others) and there are no controlled studies in women, or studies in women and animals are not available; drugs should only be given if the potential benefit justifies the potential risk to the fetus; this nearly useless classification unfortunately still applies to most drugs used during pregnancy

preterm labour and neonatal apnoea, fetal growth restriction, bradycardia and hypoglycaemia.[46] Beta-adrenergic blockers do not appear to be associated with an increased risk of congenital anomalies. Those that lack intrinsic sympathomimetic activity may decrease uterine perfusion, increase fetal vascular resistance, and lower placental and neonatal weight at delivery.[47] Furthermore, myometrial relaxation in pregnancy is a beta2-receptor-mediated process, and nonselective beta-adrenergic blockers (such as propranolol) may counteract the effect of beta2 stimulation. Beta-adrenergic blockers that lack alpha-blocking properties (such as atenolol) have been associated with lower placental and fetal weight at delivery when started early in pregnancy.[47–49] Labetalol has both alpha- and beta-adrenergic blocking activity, and may preserve uteroplacental blood flow to a greater extent.[50]

A meta-analysis of beta-adrenergic blockers for treatment of mild hypertension during pregnancy found that these drugs increased the risk of having a small-for-gestational-age infant compared with no therapy/placebo (RR 1.36, 95% CI 1.02–1.82),[49] but, in contrast to a previous analysis,[39] this risk was not significantly higher than with other antihypertensive drugs. A limitation of this analysis is that it did not distinguish among different beta-adrenergic blockers (i.e. labetalol versus atenolol).

Experience with calcium channel blockers has been accumulating over the last decade and these agents appear to be safe for use in pregnancy.[41,46] Long-acting nifedipine (30–90 mg once daily as sustained release tablet, increased at 7–14 day intervals to a maximum dose of 120 mg/day) has been used without major problems.[51–53] Although more contemporary calcium antagonists such as amlodipine are widely used in nonpregnant individuals with hypertension, we are unaware of any published reports of their use in pregnancy. Non-dihydropyridine calcium antagonists such as verapamil and diltiazem have also been used, although most reports in the literature are of small numbers of women.

The role of thiazide diuretics has been a source of controversy, although current recommendations suggest that these agents can be continued as long as volume depletion is avoided.[44,45,54] The latter problem is unlikely with chronic therapy, since all of the fluid loss occurs within the first 2 weeks of use, assuming that drug dose and dietary sodium intake are relatively constant. In a small study of 20 patients taking diuretics in the first trimester, the mean increase in plasma volume was 18% in women continued on diuretics and 52% when they were discontinued; however, there was no difference in perinatal outcome between the two groups.[55]

Blood pressure 'targets'

The goal of therapy in women without end-organ damage is systolic blood pressure between 140 and 150 mmHg and diastolic pressure between 90 and 100 mmHg.[40] However, in women with end-organ damage (and pre-existing CKD would fall into this category), it is desirable to keep the blood pressure below 140/90 mmHg,[40] or even down to 120/80 mmHg (although this is controversial). Currently unresolved is whether lowering blood pressure to the 'normal' range (i.e. 120/80 mm Hg) would confer either maternal or fetal benefits.

Other management issues

Antepartum assessment is directed toward monitoring for superimposed pre-eclampsia and detecting signs of fetal growth restriction. This is best accomplished by frequent antenatal visits for monitoring maternal blood pressure, proteinuria and fundal height and by periodic ultrasound assessments of fetal size, liquor volume and fetoplacental blood flow.[36,40]

Fetal evaluation

There is no consensus on the role of antepartum fetal assessment in management of pregnancies complicated by mild maternal hypertension. A baseline ultrasound examination in early pregnancy is recommended to confirm gestational age. This avoids uncertainty about a diagnosis of fetal growth restriction versus incorrect estimation of the time of conception, if a late pregnancy ultrasound examination shows a small fetus.[40] In the absence of pre-eclampsia or fetal growth restriction, the need for and the frequency of antepartum fetal assessment are controversial. Many clinicians perform a non-stress 'cardiotocogram' test with amniotic fluid index or biophysical profile weekly or twice per week in the later third trimester. The evidence for such assessment is weak.

Close fetal surveillance is warranted when there is a high potential for uteroplacental vasculopathy, as with pre-eclampsia or fetal growth restriction. In these cases, serial sonographic assessment of fetal growth is indicated, with additional tests of fetal wellbeing.

A meta-analysis (regression) has demonstrated that fetal growth was significantly impaired by the reduction in mean arterial pressure induced by antihypertensive therapy: a 10 mmHg fall in maternal mean arterial pressure was associated with a 176 g decrease in birthweight (Figure 12.3).[56] This effect appears to be unrelated to the type of hypertension or choice of medication. There appears to be some evidence that chronic antihypertensive use, although reducing the maternal effects of severe hypertension may compromise optimal fetal growth. This is one of the reasons for increased fetal surveillance in the prenatal period for women with CKD and hypertension treated with antihypertensive medication.

Conclusion

Women with CKD and hypertension are at significant risk of increased maternal morbidity (and mortality from the sequelae of severe hypertension and pre-eclampsia) and increased risk of perinatal morbidity and mortality. In this high-risk group, there appears to be a rationale to treat pregnant women with antihypertensive medication to lower blood pressure to levels of below 140/90 mmHg, which is less 'tight' than blood pressure control outside pregnancy. In women with uncomplicated mild essential hypertension already on antihypertensive medication who have early pregnancy blood pressures of less than 120/80 mmHg, the medication should be tapered or discontinued and the blood pressure closely monitored. However, the use of antihypertensive therapy to lower blood pressure to levels of 130–125/80–85 mmHg (as outside pregnancy) requires further evaluation, bearing in mind that the pharmacological armamentarium is significantly limited in pregnancy. There is a need for a randomised controlled trial to evaluate the effects of 'tight' blood pressure control (dBP below 85 mmHg) as compared with less 'tight' control (dBP below 100 mmHg) for women with renal disease and hypertension in pregnancy.

For control of hypertension (remote form delivery) in women with CKD, therapy with either methyldopa or labetalol is first line. A long-acting calcium antagonist such as nifedipine may be added if necessary.

In particular, the drugs which demonstrate best long-term outcome (ARBs and ACE inhibitors) are contraindicated in pregnancy. In addition, lowering maternal blood pressure may adversely affect uteroplacental perfusion and fetal growth. Careful monitoring of the maternal and fetal conditions is thus required during pregnancy.

Acknowledgements

The data relating to systematic reviews of the literature on the treatment of pre-existing hypertension in pregnancy was obtained from 'Management of hypertension in pregnancy' by Dr Phyllis August (www.uptodate.com; 2007).

(a)

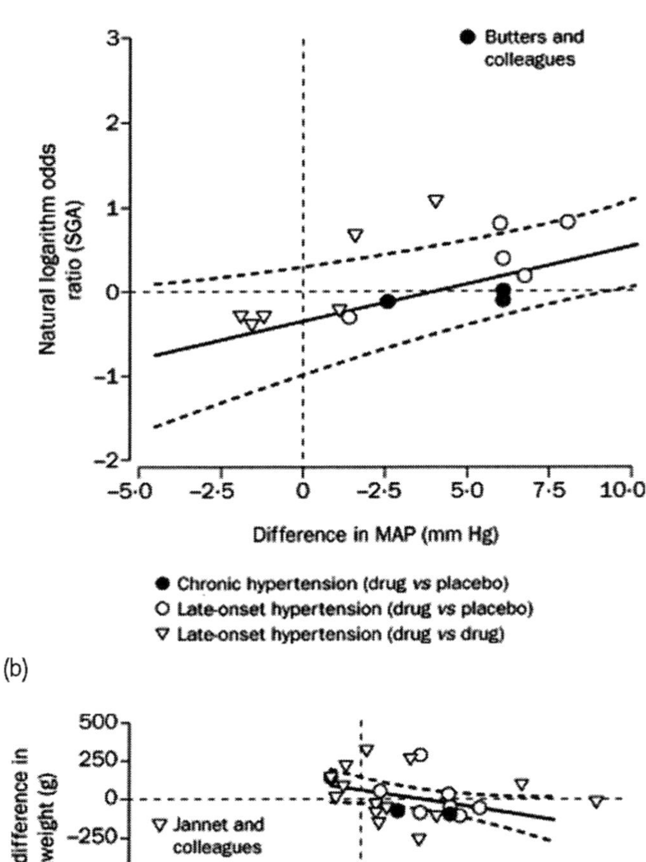

(b)

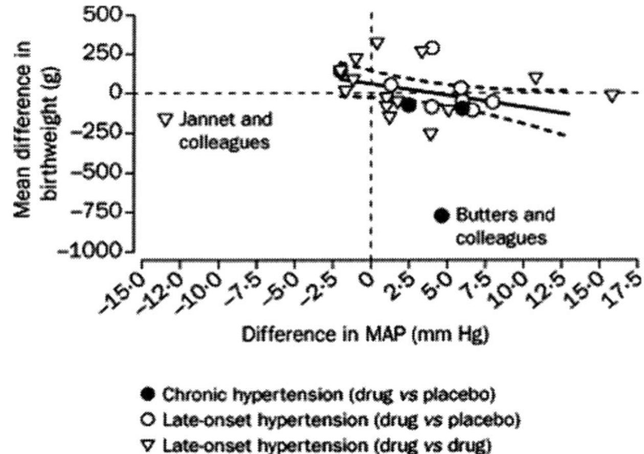

Figure 12.3. (a) Relation between fall in mean arterial pressure (MAP) induced by antihypertensive therapy and proportion of small-for-gestational-age (SGA) infants; Spearman's $\rho = 0{\cdot}69$ ($P = 0{\cdot}007$) without the Butters *et al.*[48] trial, and $\rho = 0{\cdot}64$ ($P = 0{\cdot}01$) with that trial; (b) Relation between fall in MAP induced by antihypertensive therapy and low birthweight; Spearman's $\rho = -0.46$ ($P = 0.021$) without both outlier trials; $\rho = -0.31$ ($P = 0.122$) with both outlier trials; $\rho = 0.44$ ($P = 0.025$) without the Jannet *et al.*[58] trial; $\rho = -0.30$ ($P = 0.14$) without the Butters *et al.*[48] trial; reproduced with permission from von Dadelszen *et al.*[56]

The CORD group is acknowledged and consists of the following clinicians: Alastair J Ferraro, Reem Al-Jayyousi, Nigel J Brunskill, Susan J Carr, Mark D Kilby, Liz Lightstone and Graham W Lipkin.

References

1. K/DOQI clinical practice guidelines on hypertension and antihypertensive agents in chronic kidney disease. *Am J Kidney Dis* 2004;43 (5 Suppl 2):1–290.
2. Tomson CR, Lamb EJ, Griffith K, O'Donoghue D, Feehally J. eGFR and chronic kidney disease: Time to move forward. *BMJ* 2007;335:111.
3. Delbaere I, Verstraelen H, Goetgeluk S, Martens G, De Backer G, Temmerman M. Pregnancy outcome in primiparae of advanced maternal age. *Eur J Obstet Gynecol Reprod Biol* 2007;135:41–6.
4. Coresh J, Astor BC, Greene T, Eknoyan G, Levey AS. Prevalence of chronic kidney disease and decreased kidney function in the adult US population: Third National Health and Nutrition Examination Survey *Am J Kidney Dis* 2003;41:1–12.
5. Mailloux LU, Haley WE. Hypertension in the end-stage renal disease patient : pathophysiology, therapy, outcomes and future directions. *Am J Kidney Dis* 1998;32:702–19.
6. Schwenger V, Ritz E. Audit of antihypertensive treatment in patients with renal failure. *Nephrol Dial Transplant* 1998;13:3091–5.
7. Shulman NB, Ford CE, Hall WD, Blaufox MD, Simon D, Langford HG, Schneider KA. Prognostic value of serum creatinine and effect of treatment of hypertension on renal function. Results from the hypertension detection and follow-up program. The Hypertension Detection and Follow-up Program Cooperative Group. *Hypertension* 1989;13(5 Suppl):I80–93.
8. Garg AX, Clark WF, Haynes RB, House AA. Moderate renal insufficiency and the risk of cardiovascular mortality: results from the NHANES I. *Kidney Int* 2002;61:1486–94.
9. Vanholder R, Massy Z, Argiles A, Spasovski G, Verbeke F, Lameire N; European Uremic Toxin Work Group. Chronic kidney disease as cause of cardiovascular morbidity and mortality. *Nephrol Dial Transplant* 2005;20:1048–56.
10. Baigent C, Burbury K, Wheeler D *et al.* Premature cardiovascular disease in chronic renal failure. *Lancet* 2000;356:147–52.
11. Klag MJ, Whelton PK, Randall BL, Neaton JD, Brancati FL, Ford CE, *et al.* Blood pressure and end stage renal failure. *N Engl J Med* 1996;334:13–18.
12. Confidential Enquiry into Maternal Death in the United Kingdom. *Saving Mothers' Lives: Reviewing Maternal Deaths to Make Motherhood Safer (2003–2005).* The Seventh Report of the Confidential Enquiries into Maternal Deaths in the United Kingdom. London: CEMACH; 2007.
13. Day C, Hewins P, Hildebrand S, Sheikh L, Taylor G, Kilby M, *et al.* The role of renal biopsy in women with kidney disease identified in pregnancy. *Nephrol Dial Transplant* 2008;23:201–6.
14. Umans JG. Hypertension in Pregnancy. In: *Comprehensive Hypertension.* Lip GYH, Hall JE, editors. Philadelphia: Mosby Elsevier; 2007. p. 669–92.
15. Fisher KA, Luger A, Spargo BH, Lindheimer MD. Hypertension in pregnancy: Clinicopathological correlations and remote diagnosis. *Medicine* 1981;60:267–76.
16. Maynard SE, Min JY, Merchan J, Lim KH, Li J, Mondal S, *et al.* Excess placental soluble fms-like tyrosine kinase-1 may contribute to endothelial dysfunction, hypertension and proteinuria in pre-eclampsia. *J Clin Invest* 2003;111:649–58.
17. Chobanian AV, Bakris GL, Black HR, Cushman WC, Green LA, Izzo JL Jr, *et al.*; Joint National Committee on Prevention, Detection, Evaluation, and Treatment of High Blood Pressure. National Heart, Lung, and Blood Institute; National High Blood Pressure Education Program Coordinating Committee. Seventh report of the Joint National Committee on Prevention, Detection, Evaluation, and Treatment of High Blood Pressure. *Hypertension* 2003;42:1206–52.
18. Hansson L, Zanchetti A, Carruthers SG, Dahlöf B, Elmfeldt D, Julius S, *et al.* Effects of intensive blood-pressure lowering and low-dose aspirin in patients with hypertension: principal results of the Hypertension Optimal Treatment (HOT) randomised trial. HOT Study Group. *Lancet* 1998;351:1755–62.

19. Tight blood pressure control and risk of macrovascular and microvascular complications in type 2 diabetes: UKPDS 38. UK Prospective Diabetes Study Group. *BMJ*. 1998;317:703–13. Erratum in: *BMJ* 1999;318:29.
20. European Society of Hypertension-European Society of Cardiology Guidelines Committee. 2003 European Society of Hypertension-European Society of Cardiology guidelines for the management of arterial hypertension. *J Hypertens* 2003;21:1011–53.
21. Zager PG, Nikolic J, Brown RH, Campbell MA, Hunt WC, Peterson D, *et al.* "U" curve association of blood pressure and mortality in hemodialysis patients. Medical Directors of Dialysis Clinic, Inc. *Kidney Int* 1998;54:561–9. Erratum in: *Kidney Int* 1998;54:1417.
22. Co-morbid conditions and correlations with mortality risk amongst 3,399 incident hemodialysis patients. *Am J Kidney Dis* 1992;20:32–8.
23. Ligtenberg G, Blankestijn PJ, Oey PL, Klein IH, Dijkhorst-Oei LT, Boomsma F, *et al.* Reduction of sympathetic hyperactivity by enalapril in patients with chronic renal failure. *N Engl J Med* 1999;340:1321–8.
24. Jafar TH, Stark PC, Schmid CH, Landa M, Maschio G, de Jong PE, *et al.*; AIPRD Study Group. Progression of chronic renal disease: the role of blood pressure control, proteinuria and angiotensin-converting enzyme inhibition. A patient level meta-analysis. *Ann Intern Med* 2003;139:244–52.
25. Galdo T, González F, Espinoza M, Quintero N, Espinoza O, Herrera S, *et al.* The impact of pregnancy on the function of transplanted kidneys. *Transplant Proc* 2005;37:1577–9.
26. Rey E, Couturier A. The prognosis pf pregnancy in women with chronic hypertension. *Am J Obstet Gynecol* 1994;171:410–16.
27. Ferrer RL, Sibai BM, Mulrow CD, Chiquette E, Stevens KR, Cornell J. Management of mild chronic hypertension during pregnancy: a review. *Obstet Gynecol* 2000;96:849–60.
28. Sibai BM, Lindheimer MD, Hauth J, Cartis S, VanDorsten P, Klebanoff M, *et al.* Risk factors for pre-eclampsia, abruption placentae, and adverse neonatal outcome amongst women with chronic hypertension. *N Eng J Med* 1998;339:667–71.
29. Ferraro A, Somerset DA, Lipkin G, Al-Jayyousi R, Carr S, Brunskill N, Kilby MD. Pregnancy in women with pre-existing renal diease: maternal and fetal outcomes. *J Obstet Gynaecol* 2005.25:S13.
30. Sibai BM, Cartis SN, Thom E, Klebanoff M, McNellis D, Rocco L, *et al.* Prevention of pre-eclampsia in healthy, nulliparous pregnant women. *N Eng J Med* 1993;329:1213–18.
31. CLASP: a randomised trial of low-dose aspirin for the prevention and treatment of pre-eclampsia among 9364 pregnant women. CLASP (Collaborative Low-dose Aspirin Study in Pregnancy) Collaborative Group. *Lancet* 1994;343:619–29.
32. Askie LM, Duley L, Henderson-Smart DJ, Stewart LA. PARIS Collaborative Group. *Lancet* 2007;369:1765–6.
33. Villar J, Abdel-Aleem H, Merialdi M, Mathia M, Ali MM, Zavaleta N, *et al.* WHO randomised controlled trial of calcium supplementation amongst low calcium intake pregnant women. *Am J Obstet Gynecol* 2006;194:639–49.
34. Poston L, Briley A, Seed P, Kelly FJ, Shennan AH. For the VIP trial consortium. Vitamin C and E in pregnant women at risk of pre-eclampsia: randomised controlled placebo-controlled trial. *Lancet* 2006;367:1016.
35. Rumbold AR, Crowther CA, Haslam RR, Dekker GA, Robinson JS for the ACTS study group. Vitamin C and E and the risks of pre-eclampsia and perinatal complications. *N Eng J Med* 2006;354:1796–806.
36. National Institutes of Health. *Working Group Report on High Blood Pressure in Pregnancy*. Washington, DC: National Institutes of Health; 2000.
37. Remuzzi, G, Ruggenenti, P. Prevention and treatment of pregnancy-associated hypertension: What have we learned in the last 10 years? *Am J Kidney Dis* 1991;18:285.
38. Magee, LA, Ornstein, MP, von Dadelszen, P. Fortnightly review: management of hypertension in pregnancy. *BMJ* 1999;318:1332.
39. Abalos E, Duley L, Steyn DW, Henderson-Smart DJ. Antihypertensive drug therapy for mild to moderate hypertension during pregnancy. *Cochrane Database Syst Rev* 2001;(2):CD002252.
40. Sibai, BM. Chronic hypertension in pregnancy. *Obstet Gynecol* 2002;100:369.

41. Redman CW. Controlled trials of antihypertensive drugs in pregnancy. *Am J Kidney Dis* 1991;17:149.
42. Magee LA, von Dadelszen P, Chan S, Gafni A, Gruslin A, Helewa M, *et al.*; CHIPS Pilot Trial Collaborative Group. The Control of Hypertension In Pregnancy Study pilot trial. *BJOG* 2007;114:770,e13–20.
43. Cooper WO, Hernandez-Diaz S, Arbogast PG, Dudley JA, Dyer S, Gideon PS, *et al.* Major congenital malformations after first-trimester exposure to ACE inhibitors. *N Engl J Med* 2006;8354:2443–51.
44. Cunningham FG, Lindheimer MD. Hypertension in pregnancy. *N Eng J Med* 1992;326:927.
45. Ferris TF. Hypertension in pregnancy. *Kidney* 1990;23:1.
46. Magee LA, Duley L. Oral beta-blockers for mild to moderate hypertension during pregnancy. *Cochrane Database Syst Rev* 2003;(3):CD002863.
47. Montan S, Ingemarsson I, Marsal K, Sjoberg N. Randomised controlled trial of atenolol and pindolol in human pregnancy: effects on fetal hemodynamics. *BMJ* 1992;304:946–8.
48. Butters L, Kennedy S, Rubin PC. Atenolol in essential hypertension during pregnancy. *BMJ* 1990;301:587–9.
49. Lydakis C, Lip GY, Beevers M, Beevers DG. Atenolol and fetal growth in pregnancies complicated by hypertension. *Am J Hypertens* 1999;12:541–7.
50. Pickles CJ, Symonds EM, Broughton Pipkin F. The fetal outcome in a randomized double-blind controlled trial of labetalol versus placebo in pregnancy-induced hypertension. *Br J Obstet Gynaecol* 1989;96:38–43.
51. Sibai BM, Barton JR, Akl S, Sarinoglu C, Mercer BM. A randomized prospective comparison of nifedipine and bed rest versus bed rest alone in the management of preeclampsia remote from term. *Am J Obstet Gynecol* 1992;167(4 Pt 1):879–84.
52. Fenakel K, Fenakel G, Appelman Z, Lurie S, Katz Z, Shoham Z. Nifedipine in the treatment of severe preeclampsia. *Obstet Gynecol* 1991;77:331–7.
53. Smith, P, Anthony, J, Johanson, R. Nifedipine in pregnancy. *BJOG* 2000;107:299–307.
54. Collins R, Yusuf S, Peto R. Overview of randomised controlled trials of diuretics in pregnancy. *BMJ* 1985;290:17–19.
55. Sibai BM, Grossman RA, Grossman HG. The effects of diuretics on plasma volume in pregnancy with long-term hypertension. *Am J Obstet Gynecol* 1984;150:831–5.
56. von Dadelszen P, Ornstein MP, Bull SB, Logan AG, Koren G, Magee LA. Fall in mean arterial pressure and fetal growth restriction in pregnancy hypertension: a meta-analysis. *Lancet* 2000;355:87–92.
57. Sarafidis PA, Bakris GL. Kidney disease and hypertension. In: *Comprehensive Hypertension*. Yip GY, Hall JE, editors. Mosby Elsevier; 2007. p. 607–19.
58. Jannet D, Carbonne B, Sebban E, Milliez J. Nicardipine versus metoprolol in the treatment of hypertension during pregnancy: a randomized comparative trial. *Obstet Gynecol* 1994;84:354–9.

Chapter 13

Assisted reproduction in women with renal disease

Jason Waugh

Introduction

Thirty years ago when Louise Brown was born, history was made as the first child conceived through *in vitro* fertilisation was delivered.[1] It is perhaps just as important to note that in 2008 it will be 50 years since the first child was born to a woman who had received a renal transplant.[2] There can be no doubt that advances in medical care have dramatically improved the quality of life and life expectancy of women with chronic kidney disease (CKD). With these changes have come improvements in fertility and as such it is now necessary to consider prepregnancy counselling for all women with renal disease who fall into a reproductive age group. For most women this counselling will centre on a risk assessment for pregnancy, a discussion about the likely outcomes of a pregnancy based on this risk assessment and then a consideration as to the timing of pregnancy, with advice being given regarding contraception. Prepregnancy optimisation of both renal function and general dietary supplementation and other factors such as smoking cessation should be discussed.

At the same time as advances have been seen in the medical management of renal disease, women will be aware of improvement in the management of subfertility, with many of these services being available through publicly funded healthcare systems or being affordable to many women through the private medical system.

It is therefore relevant to bring together in this chapter some of the issues that relate to the management of subfertility in women with renal disease. There will also be a small number who will seek advice on subfertility where there are other factors such as tubal occlusion or male factor infertility where, in the presence of mild or mild/moderate renal impairment, prepregnancy counselling may be similar to that for those couples who are planning for spontaneous conception. Additional advice will be necessary regarding complications of treatment and this is discussed below, as is the issue of the number of embryos which are returned in relation to the possible additional risk associated with multiple gestations (even twins).

Sexual dysfunction in CKD

In 1999, 41 056 women commenced therapy for end-stage renal disease (ESRD) in the USA and this is just the tip of the iceberg compared with the estimated 6 million people in the USA with reduced renal function who are often unaware of this as they remain completely asymptomatic.[3,4] Of the ESRD population, approximately 30% have a functioning renal transplant and this group may well have seen their renal function improve significantly.[5]

Disturbances in the hormonal milieu

Little is understood about the hormonal milieu in men and women with ESRD. Changes to dialysis regimens as well as the concomitant use of erythropoietin (EPO) have added to the variation seen in studies in this area over the past 30 years.

Derangements in the pituitary–gonadal axis occur in women on dialysis; luteinising hormone (LH) is increased and follicle-stimulating hormone (FSH) is normal or slightly increased. The exact pathophysiological mechanism for these changes is not clear but a hypothalamic defect in the regulation of gonadotrophin secretion is probably contributory. Early reports suggested that fewer than 10% of premenopausal women on dialysis have regular menstruation[6] (and probably ovulation) but later surveys have suggested menstruation rates of up to 42%.[7] There are no recent studies on ovulatory patterns in women on dialysis. Early studies reported anovulatory patterns in general and the presumed mechanism for this is a loss of the cyclic components of gonodotrophin secretion that are a feature of women with normal renal function. The low levels of estradiol and the loss of the pre-ovulatory peak in LH and estradiol are similar to patterns seen in anovulatory women without ESRD. While a disturbance in the positive feedback pathway of estradiol is almost certain, as supplementing exogenous estrogen fails to invoke an LH surge, an acquired hypothalamic defect in women with ESRD has been suggested and is supported by the loss of the LH surge and persistently low progesterone levels.[6]

Of interest, clomifene, a competitor for estrogen at the hypothalamus, increases LH and FSH, suggesting that the hypothalamus can respond to LH-releasing hormone. This would support the view that a defect at the hypothalamic level exists with an intact negative feedback of gonadotrophin release by low-dose estradiol contributing to the anovulatory mechanisms in these women.[8]

Elevated levels of endogenous endorphins secondary to reduced renal clearance in ESRD have also been implicated as they are also known to inhibit gonadotrophin release.[9]

The view that the negative feedback loop is intact is further supported by the observation that in postmenopausal women on dialysis FSH and LH levels are 'normal' (the same as postmenopausal women without ESRD). What is unknown is why the menopause tends to occur earlier in women with ESRD.[10]

Prolactin is commonly elevated in ESRD and this appears to be autonomous as it is resistant to interventions designed to inhibit or stimulate its release. This may contribute to hypothalamic–pituitary dysfunction as similar presentations are seen in women with elevated prolactin levels who do not have ESRD. The difference for women with ESRD is that when treated with bromocriptine they may normalise their prolactin levels but they will rarely resume normal menses and may continue to have galactorrhoea.[11]

More detailed studies in this area are required to explore these pathways and to elucidate the mechanisms for anovulation and menstrual disorders in ESRD as therapeutic interventions might significantly improve quality of life for dialysis patents.

Likewise, for those women who have had a successful renal transplant and who have normal or near-normal renal function and a stable graft, it would seem reasonable to consider requests for assisted conception favourably where all other criteria were met.

The situation is most complicated for those women who have severe renal impairment but are not yet on dialysis and those with an unstable graft post transplantation where any pregnancy could jeopardise any renal reserve. Under these circumstances it would seem difficult to justify assisted conception when most clinicians would be advocating contraception to preserve renal reserve. However, the window of opportunity for pregnancy might be getting smaller as these women are not yet 'sick' enough to be placed on the transplant waiting list.

Conclusion

Both nephrologists and obstetricians are likely to meet with requests from women/couples for advice regarding assisted conception. Few data exist nor are they likely to exist in the future.

The ethical dilemmas in this area have been explored and a woman's right to choose will mean such requests are forthcoming, but the majority of decisions can be made on clinical grounds based on data extrapolated from spontaneously conceived pregnancies which have been well described in ESRD.

The additional risks associated with superovulation mean that assisted conception should be reserved for women with the best and most stable renal function. Obstetricians and nephrologists may still be left caring for women where assisted conception has been used against the best medical advice. Despite assisted conception, termination of pregnancy may be the only way to preserve renal function or to prolong the mother's life expectancy. As in any such difficult situation, it is important that the mother's autonomy is respected and that she is supported in any decision she takes.

References

1. Steptoe PC, Edwards RG. Birth after the reimplantation of a human embryo. *Lancet* 1978;2:336.
2. Murray JE, Reid DE, Harrison JH, Merrill J. Successful pregnancies after human renal transplantation. *N Engl J Med* 1963;269:341–3.
3. US Renal Data System. *USRDS 2001 Annual Report*. Bethseda MD: National Institutes of Health, National Institute of Diabetes and Digestive and Kidney Diseases; 2001.
4. Jones CA, McQuillan GM, Kusek JW, Eberhardt MS, Herman WH, Coresh J, *et al.* Serum creatinine levels in the US population: third national health and nutrition examination survey. *Am J Kidney Dis* 1998;32:992–9.
5. Patel SS, Kimmel PI, Singh A. The new clinical practice guidelines for chronic renal disease: A framework for K/DOQI. *Semin Nephrol* 2002;22:449–58.
6. Lim VS, Henriquez C, Sievertsen G, Frohman LA. Ovarian function in chronic renal failure: Evidence suggesting hypothalamic anovulation. *Ann Intern Med* 1980;93:21–7.
7. Lim VS. Reproductive function in patients with renal insufficiency. *Am J Kidney Dis* 1987;9:363–7.
8. Holley JL, Schmidt RJ, Bender FH, Dumler F, Schiff M. Gynecologic and reproductive issues in women on dialysis. *Am J Kidney Dis* 1997;29:685–90.
9. Ginsberg ES, Owen WF Jr. Reproductive endocrinology and pregnancy in women on hemodialysis. *Nephron* 1984;37:195–9.
10. Schmidt RJ, Holley JL. Fertility and contraception in end stage renal disease. *Adv Ren Replace Ther* 1998;5:38–44.
11. Zingraff J, Jungers P, Pelissier C, Nahoul K, Feinstein MC, Scholler R. Pituitary and ovarian dysfunctions in women on haemodialysis. *Nephron* 1982;30:149–53.

12. Sacks CR, Peterson RA, Kimmel PL. Perception of illness and depressions in chronic renal disease. *Am J Kidney Dis* 1990;15:31–9.
13. Kimmel PL, Thamer M, Richard CM, Ray NF. Psychiatric illness in patients with end stage renal disease. *Am J Med* 1982;105:214–21.
14. Finkelstein FO, Finkelstein SH, Steele TE. Assessment of marital relationships of hemodialysis patients. *Am J Med Sci* 1976;271:21–8.
15. Wicks MN, Milstead EJ, Hathaway DK, Cetingok M. Subjective burden and quality of life in family caregivers of patients with end stage renal disease. *ANNA J* 1997;24:527–8,531–8.
16. Berkman AH, Katz LA, Weissman R. Sexuality and life style of home dialysis patients. *Arch Phys Med Rehabil* 1982;63:272–5.
17. Binik YM, Mah K. Sexuality and end stage renal disease: research and clinical recommendations. *Adv Renal Replace Ther* 1994;1:198–209.
18. Deneker B, Kimmel PL, Renich TP, Peterson RA. Depression and marital dissatisfaction in patients with ESRD and their spouses. *Am J Kidney Dis* 2001;38:839–46.
19. Rosas SE, Joffe M, Franklin E, Strom BL, Kotzker W, Brensinger C, *et al.* Prevalence and determinants of erectile dysfunction in hemodialysis patients. *Kidney Int* 2001;12:2654–63.
20. Procci WR, Goldstein DA, Adelstein J, Massry SG. Sexual dysfunction in the male patient with uremia: A reappraisal. *Kidney Int* 1981;19:317–23.
21. Gómez F, de la Cueva R, Wauters JP, Lemarchand-Béraud T. Endocrine abnormalities in patients undergoing long term hemodialysis. The role of prolactin. *Am J Med* 1980;68:522–30.
22. Armenti VT, Radomski JS, Moritz MJ, *et al.* Report from the National Transplant registry (NTPR): outcomes of pregnancy after transplantation. In: *Clinical Transplants 2002*. Los Angeles: UCLA Tissue Typing laboratory; 2002. p. 121–30.
23. Davison JM. Dialysis, transplantation and pregnancy. *Am J Kidney Dis* 1991;17:127–32.
24. Tendron A, Gouton J-B, Decramer S. *In utero* exposure to immunosuppressive drugs: experimental and clinical studies. *Paediatr Nephrol* 2002;17:121–30.
25. Bhutta AT, Cleves MA, Casey PH, Cradock MM, Anand KJ. Cognitive and behavioural outcomes of school age children who were born premature: a meta-analysis. *JAMA* 2002;288:728–37.
26. Ubel PA, Arnold RM, Caplan AL. Rationing failure: the ethical lessons lessons of the retransplantation of scarce vital organs. *JAMA* 1993;270:2469–74.
27. Veatch RM. *Transplantation Ethics*. Washington DC: Georgetown University Press; 2000.
28. Friedman Ross L. Ethical considerations related to pregnancy in transplant recipients. *N Engl J Med* 2006;354:1313–16.
29. McFaul PB, Patel N, Mills J. An audit of the obstetric outcome of 148 consecutive pregnancies from assisted conception: implications for neonatal services. *BJOG* 1993;100:820–5.
30. MRC Working Party. Births in Great Britain resulting from assisted conception, 1978–87. MRC working party on children conceived by *in vitro* fertilisation. *BMJ* 1990;300:1229–33.
31. Balasch J, Fabreques F, Arroyo V. Peripheral arterial vasodilatation hypothesis: a new insight into the pathogenesis of ovarian hyperstimulation syndrome. *Hum Reprod* 1999;13:2718–30.
32. Evbuomwan IO, Davison JM, Murdoch AP. Coexistent hemoconcentration and hypoosmolality during superovulation and in severe ovarian hyperstimulation syndrome: a volume homeostasis paradox. *Fertil Steril* 2000;74:67–72.

Section 5

Acute renal impairment

Chapter 14

Acute renal failure in pregna causes not due to pre-eclamp

David Williams

General

Acute renal failure is now a rare but serious complication of pregnancy. In early pregnancy, acute renal failure is associated with septic abortion (a complication now largely confined to the developing world) and dehydration related to hyperemesis gravidarum. Around the time of delivery, acute renal failure is most commonly caused by gestational syndromes such as pre-eclampsia and placental abruption (Box 14.1). Pregnancy is, however, a prothrombotic state, associated with heightened inflammation[1] and major changes to the vascular endothelium,[2] in particular the glomerular capillary endothelium.[3] These physiological changes predispose pregnant women to acute glomerular capillary thrombosis. Whereas nonpregnant patients who suffer an acute pre-renal insult, such as haemorrhage, dehydration or septic shock, may develop transient acute tubular necrosis if not adequately treated, the same pre-renal insult in pregnancy is more likely to develop into renal cortical necrosis with permanent renal impairment. This is even more likely to occur if a pre-renal insult coexists with a pregnancy-related condition that induces a consumptive coagulopathy and/or endothelial damage, for instance pre-eclampsia.

Box 14.1. Causes of acute renal failure in pregnancy

Most common causes	Placental abruption Severe pre-eclampsia/HELLP syndrome
Early pregnancy	Septic abortion Hyperemesis gravidarum Ovarian hyperstimulation syndrome
Rare causes	Amniotic fluid embolus Haemolytic uraemic syndrome (HUS)/thrombotic thrombocytopenic purpura (TTP) Acute fatty liver of pregnancy Acute obstruction of renal tracts

principles of management are aimed at identification and correction of precipitating insult and optimising fluid resuscitation, which is best guided by monitoring the central venous pressure and ideally pulmonary artery wedge pressure. If oliguria persists despite euvolaemia, with deteriorating renal function or fluid overload, then fluid restriction followed by renal replacement therapy is indicated.

Haemolytic uraemic syndrome/thrombotic thrombocytopenic purpura

Haemolytic uraemic syndrome (HUS) and thrombotic thrombocytopenic purpura (TTP) are very similar syndromes (from here on designated HUS/TTP). They are characterised by microangiopathic haemolytic anaemia and thrombocytopenia. Both congenital and acquired forms of HUS/TTP are more common in late pregnancy.[4] Women with HUS/TTP develop platelet thrombi attached to von Willebrand factor multimers in end-organ microvessels. This typically results in a multi-organ disorder with abdominal ischaemia and renal and/or neurological impairment.[5] A plasma metalloproteinase (ADAMTS13), which normally cleaves von Willebrand factor multimers to prevent microthrombi, is deficient in some women with congenital HUS/TTP[6] and antibodies that neutralise ADAMTS13 have been found in women with acquired HUS/TTP.[7]

HUS/TTP is more common in women (approximately 70% of all cases) and more common in association with pregnancy (approximately 13% of all cases).[4] During pregnancy, the levels of ADAMTS13 fall progressively,[8] which may explain why women with a congenital deficiency of ADAMTS13 or with other risk factors for thrombosis (e.g. obesity or a thrombophilia) are predisposed to peripartum HUS/TTP.

HUS/TTP and pre-eclampsia

Pre-eclampsia shares many similarities with HUS/TTP, not least that both syndromes occur most frequently in the third trimester or immediately postpartum. It is, however, most important to differentiate between them, because their management is different. Women with HUS/TTP often present with gastrointestinal or neurological abnormalities[4] and they are more likely to have severe renal impairment, haemolysis and thrombocytopenia compared with women who have pre-eclampsia. Disseminated intravascular coagulation (DIC) is rare in HUS/TTP, so prothrombin time and kaolin clotting time are usually normal.[5] Women with pre-eclampsia are more likely to have elevated hepatic transaminases, heavy proteinuria and abnormal clotting compared with women with HUS/TTP.[9] However, in many women the distinction between pre-eclampsia and HUS/TTP can only be determined by the course of the illness following delivery,[10] but here again acute renal failure due to pre-eclampsia usually gets transiently worse before improving.[11]

HUS/TTP management

Maternal survival from HUS/TTP has greatly improved since treatment with plasmapheresis – infusion of fresh plasma and removal of old plasma.[12] Until recently it was unclear why plasmapheresis was effective but the discovery of antibodies to ADAMTS13 (removed with old plasma) and a congenital deficiency of ADAMTS13 (replenished with infusion of fresh plasma) gives reason to this approach. However, a severe deficiency in ADAMTS13, which is not currently a routine laboratory measurement, is not present in all cases of HUS/TTP and plasmapheresis is effective in pregnant women who have milder deficiencies of ADAMTS13.[13]

Steroids are often added to the plasma exchange regimen and are a rational choice for acquired HUS/TTP with an autoimmune pathology, but there are no randomised controlled trials of their use. Antiplatelet regimens with aspirin and dipyridamole may also be beneficial in conjunction with plasma exchange.[14] Conversely, administration of platelets to thrombocytopenic patients with HUS/TTP can result in a precipitous decline in clinical status.

Acute renal cortical necrosis

In developed countries, acute renal cortical necrosis (ARCN) has become a rare complication of pregnancy. The reduced incidence of septic abortion and improved management of peripartum obstetric emergencies has prevented pre-renal impairment developing into acute tubular necrosis and then renal cortical necrosis. In developing countries, however, obstetric emergencies are still responsible for the majority of cases of ARCN.[15] Acute renal failure following septic abortion or peripartum obstetric emergencies developed into ARCN in 20% of women following a prolonged period of acute tubular necrosis.[16]

Acute renal cortical necrosis is most commonly caused by abruption of the placenta with haemorrhage, amniotic fluid embolus and sepsis associated with DIC.[17] Following haemorrhage or sepsis with hypotension, pre-renal failure will without adequate resuscitation lead to acute tubular necrosis. If anuria persists for longer than a week, ARCN should be suspected. A definitive diagnosis can be made with renal biopsy, but is often missed because of the patchy nature of cortical necrosis. Selective renal angiography will also confirm the diagnosis, but introduces another nephrotoxic agent and is usually unnecessary. Owing to the serious nature of the precipitating illness and the limited availability of renal replacement therapy in developing countries, maternal mortality is still high.[16] The indications for renal replacement therapy are as follows:

- hyperkalaemia (K more than 7.0 mmol/l), refractory to medical treatment
- pulmonary oedema, refractory to diuretics
- acidosis producing circulatory problems
- uraemia (there is no absolute level of uraemia above which dialysis is mandatory for new-onset acute renal failure, but a serum urea over 25–30 mmol/l or serum creatinine above 500–700 μmol/l (5.65–7.91 mg/dl), usually indicates a need for dialysis).

For those women who survive the acute illness, however, renal function usually returns slowly over the following 6–24 months. Long-term renal function depends on the extent of cortical necrosis, which is often incomplete or 'patchy'. Hyperfiltration through remnant glomeruli usually leads to a subsequent progressive decline in renal function.

Acute fatty liver of pregnancy

Acute fatty liver of pregnancy (AFLP) causes reversible peripartum liver and renal impairment in 1 in 5000 to 1 in 10 000 pregnancies.[18] The diagnosis is made on clinical and laboratory findings of impaired liver, renal and clotting function, rather than on histological or radiological evidence of a fatty liver.[18] Women with AFLP usually present with nausea, vomiting and abdominal cramps. Impaired renal function and reduced plasma antithrombin levels are early findings of AFLP that may precede liver dysfunction.[18] In established cases of AFLP, depressed function of the liver with prolonged prothrombin time, hypoglycaemia and DIC are more markedly abnormal than liver transaminases, which may only be moderately elevated.[18] In a series of 28 women with AFLP, other ubiquitous laboratory findings at the time of delivery were elevated serum total bilirubin (mean 7.5 mg/dl), serum creatinine (mean 205 μmol/l; 2.3 mg/dl) and uric acid levels (mean 11 mg/dl).[18]

A recessively inherited fetal inborn error of mitochondrial fatty acid oxidation may explain up to 20% of AFLP.[19] Mitochondrial fatty acid oxidation is important for both normal renal and liver function and may therefore explain the dual vulnerability of these organs in women with AFLP.

In women with AFLP, maternal renal impairment is aggravated by hypotension secondary to haemorrhage, which is itself most likely to follow an emergency operative delivery.[18,20] The combination of renal dysfunction, haemorrhage and DIC secondary to liver failure during pregnancy or postpartum requires intensive care with a multidisciplinary team of hepatologists, nephrologists, intensivists and obstetricians. Management is supportive, aimed at maintaining adequate fluid balance for renal perfusion, replacing blood, correcting the coagulopathy with fresh frozen plasma and possibly with antithrombin concentrate and fresh platelets. Hypoglycaemia should be corrected with 10% dextrose solutions. Temporary dialysis may be necessary but, with good supportive care, recovery of normal renal and liver function is usual.[18] Perinatal survival in association with AFLP is improving but is dependent on the early recognition of the maternal condition, close fetal surveillance, timely delivery and excellent neonatal care.

Nephrotoxic drugs during pregnancy

Nonsteroidal anti-inflammatory drugs (NSAIDs), including the more selective COX-2 inhibitors, reduce renal blood flow when given to the mother peripartum and can cause acute renal impairment, to both mother and fetus.[21,22] Women with reduced intravascular volume, especially with pre-existing renal impairment, are particularly vulnerable and should be prescribed NSAIDs with caution. Aminoglycosides are also nephrotoxic and feto-toxic and they should be prescribed with care and attention to drug plasma levels in women with mild renal impairment.[23]

Acute renal obstruction in pregnancy

Obstruction of the renal tracts during pregnancy may be due to renal calculi (see later), congenital renal tract abnormalities, a gestational over-distension syndrome or, very rarely, polyhydramnios. Women born with congenital obstructive uropathies at the pelvi- or vesicoureteric junction (PUJ or VUJ, respectively) are at increased risk of urine outflow obstruction in the second half of pregnancy, even if they have had surgical correction in childhood.[24] Congenital abnormalities of the lower urinary tracts including the bladder and urethra are varied and usually require extensive surgical correction in childhood. During pregnancy, these women are at increased risk of recurrent urine infections and, less commonly, of outflow obstruction requiring either temporary nephrostomy or ureteric stent.[25]

Women with a single kidney and urological abnormalities are particularly vulnerable to developing post-renal failure in relation to gestational obstruction of their solitary kidney. An incomplete obstruction can cause renal impairment with an apparently good urine output. High back-pressures compress and damage the renal medulla, leading to a loss of renal concentrating ability and production of dilute urine that is passed through an incomplete obstruction. It is also important for the obstetrician to remember that a congenitally single kidney is often associated with other abnormalities of the genital tracts, such as a unicornuate uterus.[26]

During pregnancy the renal tracts can rarely and spontaneously become grossly over-distended. If untreated, over-distension can occasionally lead to rupture of the kidney or renal tracts.[27] Women with over-distension of the renal tracts initially present with severe loin pain, most commonly on the right side and radiating to the lower abdomen. The pain is positional and inconstant; it is characteristically relieved by lying on the opposite side and tucking the knees up to the chest. A palpable tender flank mass may suggest renal tract rupture.[27] Rupture of the kidney almost always occurs in a previously diseased kidney, usually in association with a benign hamartoma or renal abscess.[27] Urinalysis will reveal either gross or microscopic haematuria. A renal ultrasound will detect a hydronephrotic kidney with a grossly dilated pelvicalyceal system, but up to 2 cm on the right side and up to 1 cm on the left is within normal limits for healthy pregnancy. Occasionally a urinoma will be evident around the kidney, indicating rupture of the renal pelvis that can sometimes seal spontaneously.

The pain from the over-distension syndrome varies from mild to very severe. Women with mild symptoms can usually be managed with advice on positional relief and regular analgesia. Women with severe unremitting pain, haematuria and grossly distended renal tracts on ultrasound, in the absence of structural or infected masses, usually have immediate pain relief following decompression of the system with either a ureteric stent or nephrostomy. Rupture of the kidney necessitates immediate surgery and almost invariably an emergency nephrectomy.[27]

Acute pyelonephritis

The same uropathogens that cause asymptomatic bacteriuria and cystitis are responsible for acute pyelonephritis.[28] Therefore the prevalence of asymptomatic bacteriuria in a pregnant population dictates the incidence of acute pyelonephritis. Screening and treating a high-risk population for asymptomatic bacteriuria (Box 14.2) reduces the incidence of acute pyelonephritis to less than 1%.[29,30] Unless acute pyelonephritis is treated promptly there is considerable maternal and fetal morbidity.[28]

Maternal symptoms and signs

Most women with acute pyelonephritis present in the second or third trimester.[28] Over 80% of women present with back ache, fever, rigors and costovertebral angle tenderness, while about half have lower urinary tract symptoms, nausea and vomiting.[28]

Box 14.2. Screening for asymptomatic bacteriuria in pregnant women

Screening for asymptomatic bacteriuria (every 4–6 weeks) is recommended for the following groups of pregnant women:

- past history of asymptomatic bacteriuria[41]
- previous recurrent urinary tract infections[41]
- pre-existing renal disease, especially scarred kidneys due to reflux nephropathy[42–44]
- structural and neuropathic abnormalities of the renal tracts[45,46]
- renal calculi[47]
- pre-existing diabetes mellitus[48] but **not** gestational diabetes[49]
- sickle cell disease and trait[41]
- low socio-economic group and less than 12 years of higher education.[29, 41]

Bacteraemia is present in 15–20% of pregnant women with acute pyelonephritis[28] and a small proportion of these women will develop septic shock and increased capillary leak, leading to pulmonary oedema.[31] It is important, however, to differentiate the hypotension due to reduced intravascular volume (fever, nausea and vomiting) from that due to septic shock. Women with pyelonephritis at risk of serious complications are those who present with the highest fever (above 39.4 °C), tachycardia (above 110 bpm), at more than 20 weeks of gestation and who have received tocolytic agents and injudicious fluid replacement.[32]

Fetal risks

Acute pyelonephritis can trigger uterine contractions and preterm labour.[33] Antibiotic treatment of pyelonephritis will reduce uterine activity, but those with recurrent infection or marked uterine activity are at increased risk of preterm labour.[33] As uterine activity is often present in the absence of cervical change and as tocolysis with beta mimetics aggravates the cardiovascular response to endotoxaemia,[32] tocolytic therapy should be used with care and only in those with cervical changes.[34]

Management of acute pyelonephritis

Women suspected of acute pyelonephritis from their history, symptoms and signs should be admitted to hospital. Laboratory tests should include full blood count, serum creatinine, electrolytes and urine culture. If there are systemic symptoms and/or septic shock, a blood culture may be useful. Pregnant women with pyelonephritis and septic shock need intensive care. In these women, assessment of the state of hydration is critical and often requires invasive haemodynamic monitoring with a central venous pressure line. This will optimise fluid balance, aiming for a urine output greater than 30 ml/hour to minimise renal impairment and reduce the risk of pulmonary oedema. Intravenous antibiotics should be started empirically (see below) until sensitivities of blood and urine cultures are known. These women often have transient renal impairment, thrombocytopenia and haemolysis, suggesting that the alveolar capillary endothelium is damaged by endotoxin.[31] A blood film and lactate dehydrogenase concentration will identify haemolysis.

Trials investigating the outpatient management of pyelonephritis in pregnancy have identified a group of women who can be managed at home.[34] These women should be at less than 24 weeks of gestation, be relatively healthy and understand the importance of compliance. They should have an initial period of observation in hospital to demonstrate ability to take oral fluids and receive intramuscular cefuroxime/ceftriaxone and, following satisfactory laboratory tests, can go home to be seen again within 24 hours for a second intramuscular dose of cephalosporin. They then start a 10 day course of oral cefalexin 500 mg four times daily or appropriate antibiotic with regular outpatient follow-up.[33] Following this outpatient regimen, 90% of women will improve but 10% will require hospital admission as a result of sepsis or recurrent pyelonephritis. Women with acute pyelonephritis over 24 weeks of gestation should be admitted for at least 24 hours to observe the maternal condition as above and to monitor uterine activity and fetal heart rate.[34]

Choice of antibiotic

Gram-negative bacteria causing pyelonephritis in pregnancy are often resistant to ampicillin;[35] therefore intravenous cefuroxime 0.75–1.5 mg (depending on severity of condition) every 8 hours is an effective first choice until sensitivities are known.[36] Women allergic to beta-lactam antibiotics can be given intravenous gentamicin (1.5 mg/kg every 8 hours) for the initial treatment of acute pyelonephritis. A single-dose regimen (7 mg/kg every 24 hours) should be avoided during pregnancy to reduce the very small risk of eighth nerve damage to the fetus.[37] Serum concentrations of gentamicin should be measured and dose adjustments made according to levels. Intravenous antibiotics should be continued until the woman has been afebrile for 24 hours. Oral antibiotics should then be given for 7–10 days, according to bacterial sensitivities or, if not available, as for symptomatic lower urinary tract infection (see above).[37]

Failure of these measures to improve the maternal clinical condition within 48–72 hours suggests an underlying structural abnormality. Ultrasonography is an easy but inconclusive way of excluding stones. If clinical suspicion is high, a plain abdominal X-ray will identify 90% of renal stones and a one-shot intravenous urogram at 20–30 minutes will identify the rest.[34] The risk to the fetus from radiation of one or two X-rays is minimal, especially when compared with the clinical benefit of identifying an obstructed, non-functioning kidney. Urinary tract obstruction can also be detected using magnetic resonance urography, especially during the second and third trimesters.[38]

Following one episode of pyelonephritis, pregnant women should have monthly urine cultures to screen for relapse or recurrence.[34] The risk of recurrent pyelonephritis can be reduced with antimicrobial prophylaxis, according to the sensitivities of initial bacterial infection[39,40] or with nitrofurantoin 100 mg nocte continued until 4–6 weeks postpartum.[34]

References

1. Redman CW, Sacks GP, Sargent IL. Preeclampsia: an excessive maternal inflammatory response to pregnancy. *Am J Obstet Gynecol* 1999;180:499–506.
2. Poston L, Williams DJ. Vascular function in normal pregnancy and pre-eclampsia. In: Hunt BJ, Poston L, Schachter M, Halliday A, editors. *An Introduction to Vascular Biology*. Cambridge: Cambridge University Press; 2002. p. 398–425.
3. Spargo B, McCartney CP, Winemiller R. Glomerular capillary endotheliosis in toxaemia of pregnancy. *Arch Pathol* 1959;593–9.
4. George JN. The association of pregnancy with thrombotic thrombocytopenic purpura-hemolytic uremic syndrome. *Current Opin Hematol* 2003;10:339–44.
5. Yarranton H, Machin SJ. An update on the pathogenesis and management of acquired thrombotic thrombocytopenic purpura. *Curr Opin Neurol* 2003;16:367–73.
6. Bianchi V, Robles R, Alberio L, Furlan M, Lämmle B. Von Willebrand factor-cleaving protease (ADAMTS13) in thrombocytopenic disorders: a severely deficient activity is specific for thrombotic thrombocytopenic purpura. *Blood* 2002;100:710–13.
7. Tsai HM, Lian EC. Antibodies to von Willebrand factor-cleaving protease in acute thrombotic thropurpura. *N Eng J Med* 1998;339:1585–94.
8. Mannucci PM, Canciani MT, Forza I, Lussana F, Lattuada A, Rossi E. Changes in health and disease of the metalloprotease that cleaves von Willebrand factor. *Blood* 2001;98:2730–5.
9. Williams DJ, de Swiet M. Pathophysiology of pre-eclampsia. *Intensive Care Med* 1997;23:620–9.
10. McMinn JR, George JN. Evaluation of women with clinically suspected thrombotic thrombocytopenic purpura-hemolytic uremic syndrome during pregnancy. *J Clin Apheresis* 2001;16:202–9.
11. Drakely AJ, Le Roux PA, Anthony J, Penny J. Acute renal failure complicating severe pre-eclampsia requiring admission to an obstetric intensive care unit. *Am J Obstet Gynecol* 2002;186:253–6.

12. Rock GA, Shumak KH, Buskard NA, Blanchette VS, Kelton JG, Nair RC, *et al.* Comparison of plasma exchange with plasma infusion in the treatment of thrombotic thrombocytopenic purpura. Canadian Apheresis Study Group. *N Engl J Med* 1991;325:393–7.
13. Vesely SK, George JN, Lämmle B, Studt JD, Alberio L, El-Harake MA, *et al.* ADAMTS13 activity in thrombotic thrombocytopenic purpura-hemolytic uremic syndrome: relation to presenting features and clinical outcomes in a prospective cohort of 142 patients. *Blood* 2003;102:60–8.
14. Bobbio-Pallavicini E, Gugliotta R, Centurioni R, Porta C, Vianelli N, Billio A, *et al.* Antiplatelet agents in thrombotic thrombocytopenic purpura (TTP): results of a randomised multicenter trial by the Italian Cooperative group for TTP. *Haematologica* 1997;82:429–35.
15. Chugh KS, Jha V, Sakhuja V, Joshi K. Acute renal cortical necrosis – a study of 113 patients. *Ren Fail* 1994;16:37–47.
16. Prakash J, Triathi K, Pandey LK, Gadela SR, Usha. Renal cortical necrosis in pregnancy-related acute renal failure. *J Indian Med Assoc* 1996;94:227–9.
17. Pertuiset N, Grunfeld JP. Acute renal failure in pregnancy. *Baillieres Clin Obstet Gynaecol* 1994;8:333–51.
18. Castro MA, Fassett MJ, Reynolds TB, Shaw KJ, Goodwin TM. Reversible peripartum liver failure: A new perspective on the diagnosis, treatment, and cause of acute fatty liver of pregnancy, based on 29 consecutive cases. *Am J Obstet Gynecol* 1999;181:389–95.
19. Yang Z, Yamada J, Zhao Y, Strauss AW, Ibdah JA. Prospective screening for pediatric mitochondrial trifunctional protein defects in pregnancies complicated by liver disease. *JAMA* 2002;288:2163–6.
20. Pereira SP, O'Donohue J, Wendon J, Williams R. Maternal and perinatal outcome in severe pregnancy-related liver disease. *Hepatology* 1997;26:1258–62.
21. Landau D, Shelef I, Polacheck H, Marks K, Holcberg G. perinatal vasoconstrictive renal insufficiency associated with maternal nimesulide use. *Am J Perinataol* 1999;16:441–4.
22. Steiger RM, Boyd EL, Powers DR, Nageotte MP, Towers CV. Acute maternal renal insufficiency in premature labor treated with indomethacin. *Am J Perinatol* 1993;10:381–3.
23. Williams DJ, Mayahi L. Maternal medicines and the fetus. In: Rodeck CH, Whittle MJ, editors. *Fetal Medicine: Basic Science and Clinical Practice.* 2nd ed. Edinburgh: Elsevier (in press).
24. Mor Y, Leibovitch I, Fridmans A, Farkas A, Jonas P, Ramon J. Late post-reimplantation ureteral obstruction during pregnancy: a transient phenomenon. *J Urol* 2003;170:845–8.
25. Greenwell TJ, Venn SN, Creighton S, Leaver RB, Woodhouse CR. Pregnancy after lower urinary tract reconstruction for congenital abnormalities. *BJU Int* 2003;92:773–7.
26. Bingham C, Ellard S, Cole TR, Jones KE, Allen LI, Goodship JA, *et al.* Solitary functioning kidney and diverse genital tract malformations associated with hepatocyte nuclear factor-1beta mutations. *Kidney Int* 2002;61:1243–51.
27. Meyers SJ, Lee RV, Munschauer RW. Dilatation and nontraumatic rupture of the urinary tract during pregnancy: a review. *Obstet Gynecol* 1985;66:809.
28. Gilstrap LC, Cunningham FG, Whalley PJ. Acute pyelonephritis in pregnancy: an anterospective study. *Obstet Gynecol* 1981;57:409–13.
29. Cunningham FG and Lucas MJ. Urinary tract infections complicating pregnancy. *Baillieres Clin Obstet Gynaecol* 1994;8:353–73.
30. Smaill F. Antibiotics for asymptomatic bacteriuria in pregnancy. *Cochrane Database Syst Rev* 2001;(2):CD000490.
31. Cunningham FG, Lucas MJ, Hankins GD. Pulmonary injury complicating antepartum pyelonephritis. *Am J Obstet Gynecol* 1987;156:797–807.
32. Towers CV, Kaminskas CM, Garite TJ, Nageotte MP, Dorchester W. Pulmonary injury associated with antepartum pyelonephritis: can patients at risk be identified? *Am J Obstet Gynecol* 1991;164:974–8.
33. Millar LK, DeBuque L, Wing DA. Uterine contraction frequency during treatment of pyelonephritis in pregnancy and subsequent risk of preterm birth. *J Perinat Med* 2003;31:41–6.
34. Wing DA. Pyelonephritis in pregnancy. Treatment options for optimal outcomes. *Drugs* 2001;61:2087–96.
35. Dunlow SG, Duff P. Prevalence of antibiotic-resistant uropathogens in obstetric patients with acute pyelonephritis. *Obstet Gynecol* 1990;76:241–5.

36. Vazquez JC, Villar J. Treatments for symptomatic urinary tract infections during pregnancy. *Cochrane Database Syst Rev* 2003;(4):CD002256.
37. Duff P. Antibiotic selection in obstetrics: making cost-effective choices. *Clin Obstet Gynaecol* 2002;45:59–72.
38. Spencer JA, Chahal R, Kelly A, Taylor K, Eardley I, Lloyd SN. Evaluation of painful hydronephrosis in pregnancy: magnetic resonance urographic patterns in physiological dilatation versus calculous obstruction. *J Urol* 2004;171:256–60.
39. Dwyer PL, O'Reilly M. Recurrent urinary tract infection in the female. *Curr Opin Obstet Gynecol* 2002;14:537–43.
40. Sandberg T, Brorson JE. Efficacy of long-term antimicrobial prophylaxis after acute pyelonephritis in pregnancy. *Scand J Infect Dis* 1991;23:221–3.
41. Pastore LM, Savitz DA, Thorp JM Jr. Predictors of urinary tract infection at the first prenatal visit. *Epidemiology* 1999;10:282–7.
42. McGladdery SL, Aparicio S, Verrier-Jones K, Roberts R, Sacks SH. Outcome of pregnancy in an Oxford-Cardiff cohort of women with previous bacteriuria. *Q J Med* 1992;303:533–9.
43. Smellie JM, Prescod NP, Shaw PJ, Risdon RA, Bryant TN. Childhood reflux and urinary infection: a follow up of 10–41 years in 226 adults. *Pediatr Nephr* 1998;12:727–36.
44. Bukowski TP, Betrus GG, Aquilina JW, Perlmutter AD. Urinary tract infections and pregnancy in women who underwent anti-reflux surgery in childhood. *J Urol* 1998;159:1286–9.
45. Natarajan V, Kapur D, Sharma S, Singh G. Pregnancy in patients with spina bifida and urinary diversion. *Int Urogynecol J Pelvic Floor Dysfunct* 2002;13:383–5.
46. Kincaid Smith P, Bullen M. Bacteriuria in pregnancy. *Lancet* 1965;191:359–99.
47. Abrahams HM, Stoller ML. Infection and urinary stones. *Curr Opin Urol* 2003;13:63–7.
48. Golan A, Wexler S, Amit A, Gordon D, David MP. Asymptomatic bacteriuria in normal and high-risk pregnancy. *Eur J Obstet Gynecol Reprod Biol* 1989;33:101–8.
49. Rizk DE, Mustafa N, Thomas L. The prevalence of urinary tract infections in patients with gestational diabetes mellitus. *Int Urogynecol J Pelvic Floor Dysfunct* 2001;12:317–21.

Chapter 15
Pre-eclampsia-related renal impairment

Louise Kenny

Introduction

Pre-eclampsia is the most common cause of impaired renal function arising *de novo* in late pregnancy. Pre-eclampsia typically presents in the third trimester with hypertension accompanied by proteinuria and is the most common cause of nephrotic syndrome in pregnancy. Pre-eclampsia remains a leading cause of maternal mortality. In recent years, an improved understanding of the renal pathophysiology of pre-eclampsia has improved clinical management of severe cases, particularly with respect to fluid balance, and this has had an appreciable impact on morbidity caused by fluid overload. In this chapter the renal pathophysiology of pre-eclampsia and the differential diagnosis of renal impairment, particularly in late pregnancy, are discussed. The investigation and management of renal impairment of pre-eclampsia, particularly with respect to intrapartum and immediate postpartum care, are described.

Renal pathophysiology in pre-eclampsia

In normal pregnancy, the glomerular filtration rate (GFR) increases by 40–60% during the first trimester,[1,2] resulting in a fall in serum markers of renal clearance, urea, creatinine and uric acid. In pre-eclampsia, both GFR and renal plasma flow are decreased by 30–40% compared with normal pregnancy of the same duration[3,4] and this results in a corresponding relative increase in serum urea and creatinine. However, it is important to note that, in pre-eclampsia, urea and creatinine often remain in the normal range for nonpregnant women despite a significant decrease in GFR from the high level of normal pregnancy.

Renal function is also impaired in pre-eclampsia and deteriorates in two stages. The first stage involves impairment of tubular function and this is reflected by a reduction in uric acid clearance and the development of hyperuricaemia.[5] Later, glomerular filtration becomes impaired and proteinuria develops.[6,7]

In normal pregnancy, there is a slight increase in urinary protein excretion. Significant proteinuria is defined by the International Society for the Study of Hypertension in Pregnancy (ISSHP) as 300 mg/day or more of protein in a 24 hour urine collection or a spot urine protein/creatinine ratio (PCR) of 30 mg/mmol or more.[8] Proteinuria in gestational hypertension heralds a poorer prognosis for both mother and baby.[9–11] Although the actual amount and the rate of increase of proteinuria have previously been found to be poor predictors of maternal or perinatal outcome,[12] a more recent study[13] suggested that there is a correlation between the degree of proteinuria and adverse maternal outcome: a high spot urine PCR in pre-eclamptic women of greater than

900 mg/mmol (approximately 9 g/day) or greater than 500 mg/mmol (approximately 5 g/day) in women over 35 years was found to be associated with a greatly increased likelihood of adverse maternal outcomes.

The proteinuria of pre-eclampsia is a relatively late sign, rarely preceding and more usually accompanying or following the development of hypertension. It is moderately selective in terms of the filtered proteins (mainly intermediate weight proteins such as albumin, transferrin and γ-globulin)[14,15] and it can vary from less than 1 g/day to 8–10 g/day. Pre-eclampsia is the leading cause of nephrotic syndrome in pregnancy. Recent data suggest that a loss of both size and charge selectivity of the glomerular barrier contribute to the development of albuminuria.[4]

Proteinuria reflects the involvement of the renal glomerulus in pre-eclampsia, which is associated with a characteristic non-inflammatory lesion commonly referred to as glomerular endotheliosis.[16–18] It primarily involves swelling and hypertrophy of the glomerular endothelial and mesangial cells, which encroach on and occlude the glomerular capillary lumina, giving rise to the typical bloodless appearance. Mesangial interposition may occur in severe cases or in the healing stages. Glomerular sub-endothelial and occasional mesangial electron-dense deposits can be seen. These likely relate to fibrin or related breakdown products. Immunofluorescence may reveal deposition of fibrin or fibrinogen derivatives, particularly in biopsies done within 2 weeks postpartum.[19] Electron microscopy demonstrates the loss of endothelial fenestrae (Figure 15.1).

Despite heavy proteinuria, the podocyte foot processes have traditionally been thought to be relatively preserved.[20] Recent data, however, suggest pre-eclampsia is associated with subtle damage to the foot process as evidenced by the appearance of podocyturia – the excretion of glomerular visceral epithelial cells or podoctyes into the urine of women with pre-eclampsia.[21] It has been speculated that subtle damage to the foot processes may actually be a significant pathological event in pre-eclampsia[22] as the epithelial podocyte secretes vascular endothelial growth factor (VEGF) and at least certain VEGF receptors, such as neuropilins, are expressed on podocytes.[23] Increasing sFlt1 (a soluble VEGF antagonist) levels in rodents produces a renal lesion similar in appearance to glomerular endotheliosis characteristic of pre-eclampsia, which suggests that impairment of VEGF signalling in the kidney may be responsible for this lesion.[24] Indeed, genetic deficiency of VEGF production in the podocytes also leads to glomerular endotheliosis.[25] Finally, dramatic decreases in nephrin (a podocyte marker) have been noted both in the glomerular podocytes of animals that are exposed to sFlt1 or VEGF antibody and in the glomeruli that are obtained from human pre-eclamptic renal biopsy specimens.[26]

It has been claimed[16] and refuted[27,28] that glomerular endotheliosis is pathognomonic. The former view would suggest that pre-eclampsia is primarily a renal disease. It is now accepted that renal involvement in pre-eclampsia can vary markedly and always occurs secondary to the primary uteroplacental pathology. In support of this, normal renal histology has been found in some cases of eclampsia[29] and previous biopsy studies have found biopsy-proven glomerular capillary endotheliosis in only 84% of nulliparae with a clinical diagnosis of pre-eclampsia and in only 38% of multiparae.[16,18] Interestingly, a recent study reported that glomerular endotheliosis is present in the kidneys of approximately 40% of normotensive pregnant women.[28] This study was unique for several reasons but particularly because of the major ethical debate triggered by its publication and then the authors' republishing without reference at all to the earlier publication. The role of renal biopsy in pregnancy is discussed in detail in Chapter 16. Suffice it to say that renal biopsy is rarely helpful in the differential diagnosis of pre-eclampsia, least of all in the nulliparous woman in the third trimester.

Glomerular enlargement and endothelial swelling usually disappear within 8 weeks of delivery, coinciding with resolution of the hypertension and proteinuria. Further investigation, including renal biopsy, may be indicated in women with persisting signs in the puerperium (see Chapter 16).

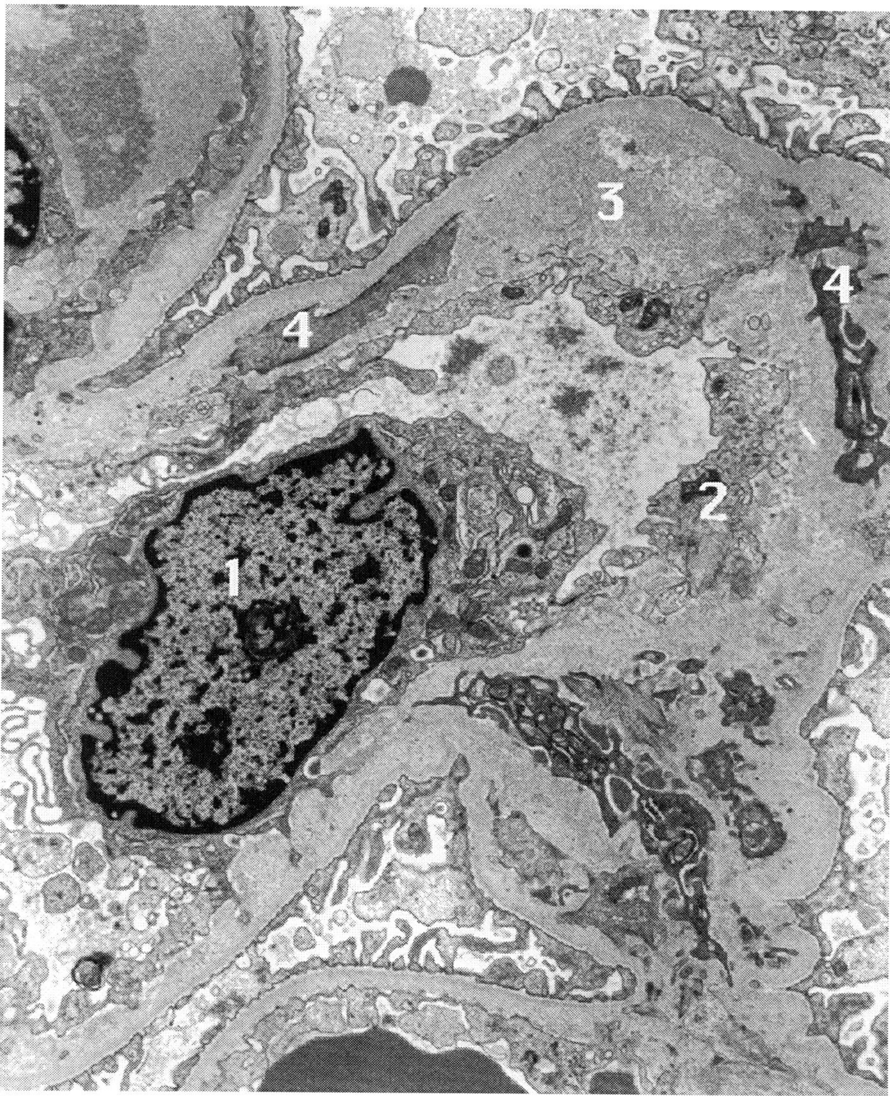

Figure 15.1. Transmission electron microscopy of a representative glomerular capillary enumerating pathological changes associated with pre-eclampsia; these include: (1) hypertrophied endothelial cells, (2) swollen segments of endothelial cytoplasmic rim in which fenestrae are not discernible, (3) sub-endothelial fibrinoid and granular deposits, and (4) interposition of mesangial cells; reproduced by permission from Macmillan Publishers Ltd: *Kidney International*, Lafayette *et al.*[3] © 1998

Differential diagnosis of pre-eclampsia-related renal impairment

Pre-existing renal disease and pre-eclampsia

In a primigravid woman with no antecedent history, the onset of hypertension and proteinuria during the third trimester is almost synonymous with pre-eclampsia. However, pre-eclampsia can mimic a variety of conditions that can manifest with the same symptoms and signs. Thus, on occasion the presentation of proteinuric hypertension in pregnancy may pose a diagnostic dilemma. This is particularly true in the case of an unbooked woman without a clearly documented normal blood pressure and urinalysis in whom hypertension and proteinuria may represent an exacerbation or onset of an underlying renal condition. The issue is further complicated by the fact that pre-eclampsia can be superimposed on pre-existing renal disorders and it can be difficult to distinguish between the two. It is imperative, wherever possible, to make a rapid diagnosis of pre-eclampsia as the condition remains a leading cause of maternal mortality in the developed world and delayed diagnosis and inappropriate clinical management continue to contribute to mortality rates.

In women of childbearing age, the most common causes of renal impairment are:

- reflux nephropathy
- diabetic nephropathy
- systemic lupus erythematosus (SLE)
- other forms of glomerulonephritis
- polycystic kidney disease.

All of the above predispose to the development of superimposed pre-eclampsia. In women presenting with renal impairment in late pregnancy, the aggressive nature and attendant morbidity of pre-eclampsia may render it dangerous and inadvisable to conduct an exhaustive search for an underlying renal disorder. If there is doubt about the diagnosis, pre-eclampsia should be overdiagnosed[30] and a search for a definitive diagnosis delayed until the postpartum period.

The one possible exception to this rule is lupus nephritis (see Chapter 9). This is a common cause of renal insufficiency in women of childbearing age. Exacerbations increase the risk of renal failure. Approximately half of women experience an exacerbation of lupus during pregnancy (although it is much less common in women who have been in remission for more than 6 months). Fetal loss rates are high. Wherever possible, a full history and investigation should seek to exclude (or implicate) this from the list of differential diagnoses of renal impairment in pregnancy because the treatment, particularly remote from term, is different from that of other forms of renal impairment. Treatment for lupus flares, aimed at inducing remission, includes prednisolone or azathioprine. It is important to have a high degree of confidence that worsening renal function in a woman with lupus reflects an exacerbation of the underlying disease and not the development of superimposed pre-eclampsia because prednisolone, although usually well tolerated, may worsen hypertension and lead to further complications. Furthermore, continuing the pregnancy in the presence of established pre-eclampsia may be fatal for mother and infant.

The presence of lupus anticoagulant and/or anticardiolipin antibodies increases the risk and the likelihood of renal lupus flares; therefore all women with lupus should be screened for these antibodies. There is some evidence that falling complement levels (C3 and C4) are helpful in distinguishing the worsening renal function of a lupus flare from that of superimposed pre-eclampsia.

Acute renal failure and pre-eclampsia

Acute renal failure in the presence of pre-eclampsia is rare and, when it occurs, it is usually precipitated by HELLP syndrome (haemolytic anaemia, elevated liver enzymes and low platelet count) or significant obstetric haemorrhage. Acute renal failure caused by hypovolaemic states is often reversible if renal perfusion is restored. Acute tubular necrosis follows more prolonged ischaemia. It is also reversible and damage is limited to the metabolically active tubular cells. More prolonged or severe renal ischaemia gives rise to acute cortical necrosis characterised by disintegration of both glomeruli and tubules in the renal cortex. Although the process is irreversible, it is the incomplete or 'patchy' variety that occurs more often in pregnancy.

There are several rare but important and difficult differential diagnoses of oliguric acute renal failure in late pregnancy and the puerperium. These include acute fatty liver of pregnancy (AFLP), thrombotic thrombocytopenic purpura (TTP) and haemolytic uraemic syndrome (HUS) (Table 15.1) (see Chapter 14). Differentiating among these conditions is critical because they respond to different therapeutic modalities. However, the clinical and histological features are so similar that establishing the correct diagnosis is often difficult. Most important is the history (for example, preceding proteinuria and hypertension favour pre-eclampsia) and time of onset.

Pre-eclampsia typically develops in the third trimester, but may rarely present before 20 weeks with only a few percent of cases developing postpartum, usually in the first 2 days. TTP almost always occurs antepartum; many cases begin before 24 weeks but the disease also occurs in the third trimester.

HUS is generally a postpartum disease. Symptoms can begin before delivery, but the onset in most cases is delayed for 48 hours or more after delivery (mean about 4 days). AFLP is characterised by acute hepatic failure with a significant elevation of liver function tests and renal function abnormalities tend to be mild unless disseminated intravascular coagulation (DIC) and haemorrhage intervene. These conditions will often share clinical and laboratory features and, at times, progress from one to another.

Antenatal and intrapartum management of renal impairment in pre-eclampsia

Management of hypertension

Antenatal control of blood pressure

The pharmacological prevention of pre-eclampsia in women with pre-existing renal disease and chronic hypertension is an important issue. Little evidence exists that the

Table 15.1. Laboratory differential diagnosis in pregnancy-associated thrombotic microangiopathies

Abnormality	HUS/TTP	AFLP	Pre-eclampsia/HELLP syndrome
Abnormal PT/PTT	No	Yes	No
Haemolysis	Yes	Yes	Yes
Thrombocytopenia	Yes	Yes	Yes
Abnormal liver function tests	No	Yes	Yes
Abnormal renal function tests	Yes	No/Yes	No/Yes

AFLP = acute fatty liver of pregnancy; HELLP syndrome = haemolytic anaemia, elevated liver enzymes and low platelet count; HUS = haemolytic uraemic syndrome; PT = prothrombin time; PTT = partial thromboplastin time; TTP = thrombotic thrombocytopenic purpura treatment of hypertension early in pregnancy reduces the incidence of superimposed pre-eclampsia and recent reviews concluded that data are insufficient to determine the benefits and risks of antihypertensive therapy for mild-to-moderate hypertension.[31,32]

Because most women with chronic hypertension in pregnancy have modest elevations in blood pressure, they can often be managed without medication. No large clinical trial has addressed the optimal level of blood pressure in a pregnant woman with hypertension. Guidelines vary, with recommendations to treat ranging from thresholds of 140/90 mmHg, 160/90 mmHg and 160/105 mmHg in Canada, Australia and the USA, respectively.[30,33,34] Recommendations in accord with those of the National High Blood Pressure Education Program (NHBPEP) Working Group on High Blood Pressure in Pregnancy[30] are that when maternal systolic blood pressure reaches levels of 150–160 mmHg or higher and diastolic 100–110 mmHg or higher, treatment may be started. However, many clinicians believe that women with evidence of end-organ disease (e.g. cardiac, renal or ocular) should be treated as aggressively as nonpregnant women to achieve blood pressures averaging below 140/80 mmHg.

One may consider discontinuing antihypertensive therapy in women who experience the physiological decrements in pressure that occur during the first half of pregnancy. Therapy can then be initiated at a blood pressure of 150/90–100 mmHg, regardless of the type of hypertension, and a variety of antihypertensive agents are available for use in pregnant women.[35] Orally administered antihypertensive agents should be used in standard doses in pregnancy. A detailed discussion of these agents, focusing on their pharmacokinetics and dynamics can be found elsewhere.[36] A summary of commonly used agents is provided in Table 15.2. Treatment of hypertension is also discussed in Chapter 12.

Table 15.2. Drugs for the treatment of chronic hypertension in pregnancy

Preferred agents	Concerns or comments
Indicated	
Methyldopa	Drug of choice according to NHBPEP working group; safety after first trimester well documented, including 7 year follow-up of offspring.
Labetalol	May be associated with fetal growth restriction and neonatal bradycardia.
Nifedipine	Possible interference with labour; may interact synergistically with magnesium sulphate.
Hydralazine	Few controlled trials, but long experience with few adverse events documented; useful only in combination with sympatholytic agent. May cause neonatal thrombocytopenia.
Beta blockers	May cause fetal bradycardia and decrease uteroplacental blood flow; this effect may be less for agents with partial agonist activity. May impair fetal response to hypoxic stress; risk of growth restriction when started in first or second trimester (especially atenolol).
Contraindicated	
ACE inhibitors and AT1 receptor antagonists	Lead to fetal loss in animals; human first-trimester use associated with fetal abnormalities; use in second and third trimester associated with fetopathy, oligohydramnios, growth restriction and neonatal anuric renal failure, which may be fatal.

NHBPEP = National High Blood Pressure Education Program

Control of blood pressure in severe pre-eclampsia

Lowering blood pressure does not cure pre-eclampsia but may permit prolongation of pregnancy, because uncontrolled hypertension is frequently an indication for delivery. Before delivery and even after delivery, the blood pressure can remain dangerously high and be labile for days. The main reason to lower blood pressure in a woman with pre-eclampsia is to prevent maternal cerebrovascular and cardiovascular complications of elevated blood pressure, and lowering blood pressure leads to a decrease in maternal death.[30,37] Indeed, the most recent triennial report of The Confidential Enquiry into Maternal and Child Health[38] highlights that underestimation of blood pressure and suboptimal management of hypertension remains a leading cause of death in women with pre-eclampsia in the UK.

The aim of stabilisation of blood pressure is to reduce the blood pressure to below 160/105 mmHg in the first instance (mean arterial pressure below 125 mmHg) and maintain the blood pressure at or below that level. There are two agents of choice: labetalol and hydralazine.

If the woman can tolerate oral therapy, an initial 200 mg oral dose of labetalol can be given. This can be done immediately before venous access is obtained and so can achieve as quick a result as an initial intravenous dose. This should lead to a reduction in blood pressure in about half an hour. A second oral dose can be given if needed.

If there is no initial response to oral therapy or if it cannot be tolerated, control should be with repeated boluses of labetalol followed by a labetalol infusion. A bolus infusion of 50 mg should be given over at least 5 minutes. This should have an effect by 10 minutes and should be repeated if diastolic blood pressure has not been reduced to below 160/105 mmHg. This can be repeated in doses of 50 mg, to a maximum dose of 200 mg, at 10 minute intervals. Following this or as initial treatment in moderate hypertension, a labetalol infusion should be commenced. An infusion of labetalol (20 mg/hour) should be started and the infusion rate should be doubled every half hour to a maximum of 160 mg/hour until the blood pressure has dropped and then stabilised at an acceptable level. Labetalol is contraindicated in women with asthma and should be used with caution in women with pre-existing cardiac disease.

If labetalol is contraindicated or fails to control the blood pressure then hydralazine is an alternative agent. A second agent should be considered where the mean arterial pressure is persistently over 120 mmHg. In such cases it is normally appropriate to continue the first drug, i.e. labetalol, while administering the second.

Hydralazine is given as a bolus infusion of 5 mg over 5 minutes measuring the blood pressure every 5 minutes. This can be repeated every 20 minutes to a maximum dose of 20 mg. This may be followed by an infusion of 40 mg of hydralazine at a rate of 1–5 mg/hour. However, if the labetalol infusion is continued, a hydralazine infusion may not be required as the blood pressure will probably settle with the bolus doses.

Fluid balance

Inappropriate management of renal impairment in pre-eclampsia can be fatal. Left ventricular dysfunction and capillary leak complicate fluid management in severe pre-eclampsia. A review of the last five triennial reports of The Confidential Enquiries into Maternal and Child Health[38] illustrates the declining mortality rates from acute respiratory distress syndrome and pulmonary oedema as awareness of the importance of appropriate fluid management has grown.

Clinical guidelines, both national and local, regarding the management of pre-eclampsia emphasise the need for careful fluid balance aimed at avoiding fluid overload.

While there is some variation, there is a consensus that in severe pre-eclampsia, total input should be limited to 80 ml/hour of a crystalloid solution. If oxytocin is used then it should be at high concentration (30 iu in 500 ml, as per NICE guidelines) and the volume of fluid included in the total input. Such a 'dry' regimen may provoke oliguria, particularly if the woman is still undelivered or labouring. This should not precipitate any specific intervention except to encourage early delivery. Even with this 'dry' approach, acute renal shutdown is extremely unlikely unless there is concomitant hypotension, coagulopathy or the use of nonsteroidal anti-inflammatory agents such as diclofenac.

As women with pre-eclampsia tend to maintain their blood pressure, despite regional blockade, fluid load prior to regional anaesthesia is unnecessary and may complicate fluid balance. For this reason, fluid loading in pre-eclampsia should always be controlled and should never be done prophylactically or routinely. Hypotension, when it occurs, can be easily controlled with very small doses of ephedrine.

Following delivery, fluid restriction should continue until a natural diuresis occurs (usually around 36–48 hours post delivery). The total amount of fluid (the total of intravenous and oral fluids) should be given at 80 ml/hour. It is important to remember that this must include the volume of fluid in drug infusions such as magnesium and labetalol.

Urine output should be recorded hourly and each 4 hour block should be summated and recorded. Each 4 hour block should total in excess of 80 ml. If two consecutive blocks fail to achieve 80 ml, then further action is appropriate. This would either be:

- If total input is more than 750 ml in excess of output in the last 24 hours (or since starting the regimen) then 20 mg of intravenous furosemide should be given. Colloid should then be given as below if a diuresis of more than 200 ml in the next hour occurs.

or

- If total input is less than 750 ml in excess of output in the last 24 hours (or since starting the regimen) then an infusion of 250 ml of colloid over 20 minutes should be given. The urine output should then be watched until the end of the next 4 hour block. If the urine output is still low then individual unit policies for fluid management in pre-eclampsia should be followed and liaison with and referral to a renal physician would be advisable.

Central venous pressure monitoring

Central venous pressure (CVP) monitoring may mislead in pre-eclampsia as it does not correlate well with the pulmonary capillary wedge pressure in these women. Owing to the fact that the pulmonary wedge pressure may be high in the absence of an elevated CVP, assessment of whether the myocardium is handling the therapeutic volume expansion can only be assessed after placement of a pulmonary artery catheter. This is controversial and very rarely used nowadays; it will only be necessary in very selected cases. CVP monitoring may occasionally be useful to exclude volume depletion as a cause for severe or prolonged postpartum oliguria but requires careful interpretation.

Dialysis

Most of the problems linked to acute renal failure will respond to conservative management, but if this approach is unsuccessful, dialysis will be necessary. Both haemodialysis and peritoneal dialysis can be used in pregnant or recently delivered women. The main indications for dialysis are:

- volume overload with congestive heart failure (pulmonary oedema)
- severe hyperkalaemia (K more than 7.0 mmol/l)
- severe acidosis
- uraemic symptoms not manageable by conventional methods.

Seizure prophylaxis

The drug of choice for the treatment and prevention of eclampsia is magnesium sulphate, but 97% of magnesium is excreted in the urine and therefore the presence of oliguria can lead to toxic levels. In the presence of oliguria following the normal loading dose of magnesium, further administration should be reduced or withheld. If magnesium is not being excreted then the levels should not fall and no other anticonvulsant is needed. Magnesium should be reintroduced if urine output improves.

Postnatal follow-up

Hypertension frequently persists after delivery in women with antenatal hypertension or pre-eclampsia, and blood pressure may be labile in the initial postpartum days. Some of this lability may reflect the redistribution of fluids from the extracellular to the intravascular space. However, postpartum hypertension that persists beyond 12 weeks may represent previously undiagnosed chronic hypertension, which should be investigated, followed and treated appropriately.

Postpartum evaluation should also be considered for women with pre-eclampsia who developed the condition early (before 34 weeks of gestation), had severe or recurrent pre-eclampsia or who have persistent proteinuria. In these cases, underlying renal disease, secondary hypertension and thrombophilias (e.g. factor V Leiden, prothrombin 20210, anticardiolipin antibodies and lupus anticoagulant) may be considered. Studies report varying rates of underlying and previously undiagnosed renal disease in women with severe pre-eclampsia ranging from 12.1%[39] to 71.7%.[40]

Counselling for future pregnancies requires consideration of different recurrence rates for pre-eclampsia, depending on the pathogenesis and population characteristics. The earlier in gestation, the higher the risk of recurrence: before 30 weeks, recurrence rates may be as high as 40%.[41] If pre-eclampsia has developed in a nulliparous woman close to term (i.e. after 36 weeks), the risk of recurrence is thought to be about 10%. Women who have had HELLP syndrome have a high risk of subsequent obstetric complications, with pre-eclampsia occurring in 55%, although the rate of recurrent HELLP appears to be low at only 6%.[42]

Hypertensive diseases of pregnancy have been associated with an elevated risk of hypertension and stroke later in life. In one study, gestational hypertension was associated with a relative risk (RR) of 3.72 for subsequent hypertension and pre-eclampsia, with an RR of 3.98 for subsequent hypertension and 3.59 for stroke.[43] Pre-eclampsia associated with preterm birth is also a risk factor for ischaemic heart disease when studied retrospectively.[44] These associations may serve to increase awareness of the need to monitor for future hypertensive and cardiovascular disorders.[45]

References

1. Sims EA, Krantz KE. Serial studies of renal function during pregnancy and the puerperium in normal women. *J Clin Invest* 1958;37:1764–74.
2. Davison JM, Dunlop W. Renal hemodynamics and tubular function normal human pregnancy. *Kidney Int* 1980;18:152–61.
3. Lafayette RA, Druzin M, Sibley R, Derby G, Malik T, Huie P, *et al.* Nature of glomerular dysfunction in pre-eclampsia. *Kidney Int* 1998;54:1240–9.
4. Moran P, Baylis PH, Lindheimer MD, Davison JM. Glomerular ultrafiltration in normal and preeclamptic pregnancy. *J Am Soc Nephrol* 2003;14:648–52.
5. Schaffer NK, Dill LV, Cadden JF. Uric acid clearance in normal pregnancy and pre-eclampsia. *J Clin Invest* 1943;22:201–6.
6. Dunlop W, Davison JM. The effect of normal pregnancy upon the renal handling of uric acid. *Br J Obstet Gynaecol* 1977;84:13–21.
7. Dunlop W, Furness C, Hill LM. Maternal haemoglobin concentration, haematocrit and renal handling of urate in pregnancies ending in the births of small-for-dates infants. *Br J Obstet Gynaecol* 1978;85:938–40.
8. Brown MA, Lindheimer MD, de Swiet M, Van Assche A, Moutquin JM. The classification and diagnosis of the hypertensive disorders of pregnancy: statement from the International Society for the Study of Hypertension in Pregnancy (ISSHP). *Hypertens Pregnancy* 2001;20:IX-XIV.
9. Naeye RL, Friedman EA. Causes of perinatal death associated with gestational hypertension and proteinuria. *Am J Obstet Gynecol* 1979;133:8–10.
10. Ferrazzani S, Caruso A, De Carolis S, Martino IV, Mancuso S. Proteinuria and outcome of 444 pregnancies complicated by hypertension. *Am J Obstet Gynecol* 1990;162:366–71.
11. Chua S, Redman CW. Prognosis for pre-eclampsia complicated by 5 g or more of proteinuria in 24 hours. *Eur J Obstet Gynecol Reprod Biol* 1992;43:9–12.
12. Schiff E, Friedman SA, Kao L, Sibai BM. The importance of urinary protein excretion during conservative management of severe preeclampsia. *Am J Obstet Gynecol* 1996;175:1313–16.
13. Chan P, Brown M, Simpson JM, Davis G. Proteinuria in pre-eclampsia: how much matters? *BJOG* 2005;112:280–5.
14. MacLean PR, Paterson WG, Smart GE, Petrie JJ, Robson JS, Thomson D. Proteinuria in toxaemia and abruptio placentae. *J Obstet Gynaecol Br Commonw* 1972;79:321–6.
15. Simanowitz MD, MacGregor WG, Hobbs JR. Proteinuria in pre-eclampsia. *J Obstet Gynaecol Br Commonw* 1973;80:103–8.
16. Spargo B, McCartney CC, Winemiller R. Glomerular capillary endotheliosis in toxemia of pregnancy. *Arch Pathol* 1959;68:593–9.
17. Pollak VE, Nettles JB. The kidney in toxemia of pregnancy: a clinical and pathologic study based on renal biopsies. *Medicine (Baltimore)* 1960;39:469–526.
18. Fisher KA, Luger A, Spargo BH, Lindheimer MD. Hypertension in pregnancy: clinical-pathological correlations and remote prognosis. *Medicine (Baltimore)* 1981;60:267–76.
19. Morris RH, Vassalli P, Beller FK, McCluskey RT. Immunofluorescent studies of renal biopsies in the diagnosis of toxemia of pregnancy. *Obstet Gynecol* 1964;24:32–46.
20. Mautner W, Churg J, Grishman E, Dachs S. Preeclamptic nephropathy. An electron microscopic study. *Lab Invest* 1962;11:518–30.
21. Garovic VD, Wagner SJ, Turner ST, Rosenthal DW, Watson WJ, Brost BC, *et al.* Urinary podocyte excretion as a marker for preeclampsia. *Am J Obstet Gynecol* 2007;196:320.e1–7.
22. Karumanchi SA, Lindheimer MD. Preeclampsia and the kidney: footprints in the urine. *Am J Obstet Gynecol* 2007;196:287–8.
23. Harper SJ, Xing CY, Whittle C, Parry R, Gillatt D, Peat D, *et al.* Expression of neuropilin-1 by human glomerular epithelial cells *in vitro* and *in vivo*. *Clin Sci (Lond)* 2001;101:439–46.
24. Maynard SE, Min JY, Merchan J, Lim KH, Li J, Mondal S, *et al.* Excess placental soluble fms-like tyrosine kinase 1 (sFlt1) may contribute to endothelial dysfunction, hypertension, and proteinuria in preeclampsia. *J Clin Invest* 2003;111:649–58.

25. Eremina V, Sood M, Haigh J, Nagy A, Lajoie G, Ferrara N, *et al.* Glomerular-specific alterations of VEGF-A expression lead to distinct congenital and acquired renal diseases. *J Clin Invest* 2003;111:707–16.
26. Sugimoto H, Hamano Y, Charytan D, Cosgrove D, Kieran M, Sudhakar A, *et al.* Neutralization of circulating vascular endothelial growth factor (VEGF) by anti-VEGF antibodies and soluble VEGF receptor 1 (sFlt-1) induces proteinuria. *J Biol Chem* 2003;278:12605–8.
27. Fisher ER, Pardo V, Paul R, Hayashi TT. Ultrastructural studies in hypertension. IV. Toxemia of pregnancy. *Am J Pathol* 1969;55:109–31.
28. Strevens H, Wide-Swensson D, Hansen A, Horn T, Ingemarsson I, Larsen S, *et al.* Glomerular endotheliosis in normal pregnancy and pre-eclampsia. *BJOG* 2003;110:831–6.
29. Dennis EJ 3rd, Smythe CM, McIver FA, Howehg JR. Percutaneous renal biopsy in eclampsia. *Am J Obstet Gynecol* 1963;87:364–71.
30. Report of the National High Blood Pressure Education Program Working Group on high blood pressure in pregnancy. *Am J Obstet Gynecol* 2000;183:S1–22.
31. Magee LA, Ornstein MP, von Dadelszen P. Fortnightly review: management of hypertension in pregnancy. *BMJ* 1999;318:1332–6.
32. Abalos E, Duley L, Steyn D, Henderson-Smart D. Antihypertensive drug therapy for mild to moderate hypertension during pregnancy. *Cochrane Database Syst Rev* 2007;(1):CD002252.
33. Brown MA, Hague WM, Higgins J, Lowe S, McCowan L, Oats J, *et al.* The detection, investigation and management of hypertension in pregnancy: full consensus statement. *Aust N Z J Obstet Gynaecol* 2000;40:139–55.
34. Helewa ME, Burrows RF, Smith J, Williams K, Brain P, Rabkin SW. Report of the Canadian Hypertension Society Consensus Conference: 1. Definitions, evaluation and classification of hypertensive disorders in pregnancy. *CMAJ* 1997;157:715–25.
35. Magee LA. Drugs in pregnancy. Antihypertensives. *Best Pract Res Clin Obstet Gynaecol* 2001;15:827–45.
36. Umans JG. Medications during pregnancy: antihypertensives and immunosuppressives. *Adv Chronic Kidney Dis* 2007;14:191–8.
37. Rey E, Couturier A. The prognosis of pregnancy in women with chronic hypertension. *Am J Obstet Gynecol* 1994;171:410–16.
38. Lewis G, editor, CEMACH, *Why Mothers Die 2000–2002.* The Sixth Report of Confidential Enquiries into Maternal Deaths in the United Kingdom. London: RCOG Press; 2004.
39. Murakami S, Saitoh M, Kubo T, Koyama T, Kobayashi M. Renal disease in women with severe preeclampsia or gestational proteinuria. *Obstet Gynecol* 2000;96:945–9.
40. Beller FK, Dame WR, Witting C. Renal disease diagnosed by renal biopsy. Prognostic evaluation. *Contrib Nephrol* 1981;25:61–70.
41. Sibai BM, Mercer B, Sarinoglu C. Severe preeclampsia in the second trimester: recurrence risk and long-term prognosis. *Am J Obstet Gynecol* 1991;165(5 Pt 1):1408–12.
42. Sibai BM, Mercer BM, Schiff E, Friedman SA. Aggressive versus expectant management of severe preeclampsia at 28 to 32 weeks' gestation: a randomized controlled trial. *Am J Obstet Gynecol* 1994;171:818–22.
43. Wilson BJ, Watson MS, Prescott GJ, Sunderland S, Campbell DM, Hannaford P, *et al.* Hypertensive diseases of pregnancy and risk of hypertension and stroke in later life: results from cohort study. *BMJ* 2003;326:845.
44. Haukkamaa L, Salminen M, Laivuori H, Leinonen H, Hiilesmaa V, Kaaja R. Risk for subsequent coronary artery disease after preeclampsia. *Am J Cardiol* 2004;93:805–08.
45. Bellamy L, Casas JP, Hingorani AD, Williams DJ. Pre-eclampsia and risk of cardiovascular disease and cancer in later life: systematic review and meta-analysis. *BMJ* 2007;335:974.

Chapter 16

Renal biopsy in pregnancy

Nigel J Brunskill

Renal biopsy in general nephrological practice

Since its first description in the early 1950s,[1] percutaneous renal biopsy has evolved to become an indispensable tool in the management of patients with kidney disease. In general nephrological practice the most common indications for performing native kidney biopsy are nephrotic syndrome, unexplained urinary dipstick abnormalities, acute kidney injury, renal dysfunction in the setting of systemic immunological diseases such as lupus or vasculitis, unexplained chronic kidney disease and familial renal disease. Ideally, the biopsy should provide specific diagnostic and prognostic information and facilitate informed management decisions. Recent prospective studies show that the pathological diagnosis provided by kidney biopsy results in altered patient management in 50–80% of cases.[2]

In some situations renal biopsy may be unsafe or technically impossible. An uncorrectable bleeding diathesis is an absolute contraindication to percutaneous renal biopsy, whereas hypertension (blood pressure above 160/95 mmHg) or hypotension, urinary infection, low platelet count, single kidney, renal cysts or tumour, severe anaemia, uraemia, obesity and an uncooperative patient are relative contraindications.[2]

In general, renal biopsy is performed with the patient in the prone position using local anaesthesia. Ultrasonography is used to locate the lower pole of the kidney and the biopsy needle advanced to the kidney under direct ultrasound guidance. This may be more challenging in large or obese patients. The disposable biopsy needle is attached to a spring-loaded biopsy 'gun' with a trigger mechanism which, when released with the patient's breath held, instantly advances the needle tip into the kidney. The biopsy needle is then withdrawn and the sample of renal tissue removed from the sample notch of the needle. This procedure may need to be repeated to obtain sufficient tissue for analysis.

Renal biopsy is not an uncomplicated procedure.[3–6] Pain around the biopsy site is common but severe pain should raise the possibility of significant peri-renal haemorrhage. Bleeding may also occur into the urine with macroscopic haematuria (3%) and painful clot colic. Some degree of peri-renal bleeding is inevitable after every biopsy and a mean fall in haemoglobin of 1 g/dl has been reported.[2] More severe bleeding complications requiring transfusion, renal embolisation or surgery occur in approximately 0.1% of procedures. In addition to kidney bleeding complications, other organs (liver, spleen, pancreas, gallbladder, large and small bowel) may be inadvertently biopsied or injured. Haematoma may rupture into the peritoneal cavity or track along the psoas muscle into the groin. Trauma to renal, mesenteric and lumbar arteries are all described, as are pneumo- and haemothorax and calyceal-peritoneal fistula.[3] Renal arteriovenous fistulae are also described.[7] Death following severe haemorrhage is rare but reported.

Evidence suggests that serious biopsy complications are more likely to occur in patients with severe illness, particularly those with severe acute renal failure, poorly controlled blood pressure or other relative contraindications. In some series renal amyloidosis is associated with a greater bleeding tendency after renal biopsy.[6] Careful patient selection is suggested to minimise risks.[4] Therefore, although renal biopsy is regarded as a safe procedure, it should only be performed under the supervision of experienced operators after careful patient evaluation.

Experience of renal biopsy in pregnancy

Pregnancy in women with renal disease is associated with adverse maternal and fetal outcomes[8,9] and an understandable desire of carers to fully understand underlying nephrological conditions in these women. Despite the rarity of significant renal biopsy complications in nonpregnant women, most experienced clinicians will still have encountered these problems, and decisions around renal biopsy are often difficult and the source of considerable anxiety. These feelings of anxiety are exacerbated when the performance of a potentially morbid, invasive diagnostic intervention is considered in pregnancy when the 'stakes' may be higher. Therefore it is important when considering renal biopsy in the special situation of pregnancy to ask: (i) is renal biopsy safe with a complication rate no worse than that in the nonpregnant situation and (ii) does the information obtained by renal biopsy affect the management of the mother or the pregnancy?

A few studies have specifically evaluated indications for renal biopsy in pregnancy with its subsequent outcomes and it is useful to consider the evidence from this work in chronological sequence. Initial reports were encouraging. Macroscopic haematuria occurred in just 3.5% of several hundred renal biopsies performed in pregnancy or shortly thereafter in an effort to establish the importance of chronic renal disease as a cause of hypertension in pregnancy,[10] although the renal biopsy itself was not the focus of the author's interest. The first series concentrating on complications of renal biopsies in pregnancy was provided by Schewitz *et al.*[11] and is widely referenced. The complication rate in their series was unacceptably high – a greater than 16% rate of macroscopic haematuria, nearly 5% peri-renal haematomas and one maternal death. It must be borne in mind however that the women reported by these authors were biopsied during the formative years of the biopsy procedure and that biopsy techniques were much different from those in use today. Also, indications and contraindications were less well developed and therefore patient selection less stringent than may be the case currently. Indeed, other workers demonstrated that complications may be considerably less than indicated by the study of Schewitz *et al.*[11] and suggested guidelines for the use of renal biopsy in pregnancy.[12]

Packham and Fairley[13] reported the outcomes of 111 renal biopsies performed in the first or second trimester of pregnancy over a 21 year period up to 1985. Of these women, 22 (20%) had a pre-existing diagnosis of glomerulonephritis and were biopsied in pregnancy to assess progress of this condition. The most common indications for biopsy in the remainder were haematuria and proteinuria (36% of all biopsies), nephrotic syndrome (12%) haematuria, proteinuria and hypertension (10.5%) and impaired renal function (8%). Four women underwent renal biopsy because of severe early pre-eclampsia and fetal death in an earlier pregnancy but in the absence of hypertension or renal abnormalities in the index pregnancy, and none of these yielded a positive diagnosis of glomerulonephritis. In 80% of those biopsied in pregnancy for the first time, a positive diagnosis of glomerulonephritis was revealed. In nine nephrotic patients, seven had membranous nephropathy, one had focal segmental glomerulosclerosis and one had immunoglobulin A (IgA) nephropathy. How often this information altered clinical management was not discussed. The complication rate, including failure to obtain tissue, was very low at 7.2%. There were no serious complications. The authors concluded that renal biopsy was safe in pregnancy, advocated a relaxed approach to renal biopsy in pregnancy and proposed increasing its use. However, this suggestion was challenged in an accompanying editorial where a more moderate interventional approach was advanced.[14]

Kuller *et al.*[15] reported results collected from 18 women biopsied at up to 30 weeks or immediately postpartum (three biopsies). The complication rate was relatively high with seven identifiable haematomas and two women requiring blood transfusion as a consequence. Again, precisely how often biopsy diagnosis altered management is not clear although the absence of glomerular endotheliosis in some women may have resulted in prolongation of their pregnancy. In a series of 15 renal biopsies prior to 30 weeks of gestation performed because of renal impairment of obscure cause or nephrotic syndrome, the only complication was macroscopic haematuria in one woman. As a result of these interventions, 11 women were treated with glucocorticoids.[16] Experience of 20 renal biopsies in pregnancy from the Queen Elizabeth Hospital, Birmingham, UK, indicates that, in carefully selected women, the procedure yields a positive diagnosis of glomerular disease in 95%, a change in management in 40% and no serious complications.[17]

Strevens *et al.*[18] biopsied 36 women with hypertension in pregnancy to compare glomerular endothelial changes with those observed in contemporaneous biopsies from 12 women with normal control pregnancies. The mean blood pressure of the proteinuric hypertensive women in this study was 150/101 mmHg. One woman with early-onset severe pre-eclampsia developed a haemodynamically significant haematoma and required blood transfusion. Glomerular endotheliosis was found in most healthy controls in addition to all the hypertensive women and the authors concluded that this lesion is not specific for pre-eclampsia. This series was also re-reported as Wide-Swensson *et al.*,[19] who provided more details of biopsy-related complications. Three women complained of pain after their biopsy and one had a small peri-renal haematoma. One woman with severe pregnancy-induced hypertension, proteinuria, oliguria and pulmonary oedema at 25 weeks of a twin pregnancy suffered a large retroperitoneal bleed requiring renal embolisation following renal biopsy. This represents a 1.8% rate of serious complications and it is unsurprising that a woman with severe hypertension should be affected.

Serious questions exist about the ethics of the studies reported by these authors.[18,19] Few medical practitioners consider renal biopsy an appropriate diagnostic investigation in pre-eclampsia because management is insufficiently altered to justify the risks involved, regardless of any perceived uncertainties about underlying pathology. Women with poorly controlled blood pressure in the setting of pre-eclampsia, such as those deliberately enrolled in this study, fall into a group at high risk of complications. In fact, generally accepted clinical criteria (see above) contraindicate the renal biopsy procedure in individuals with this degree of hypertension. Generally speaking, given the unavoidable risks of renal biopsy, this author believes that subjecting normal controls to the procedure in any study is ethically unacceptable. Despite these concerns, the study has been reported twice by the same group, in 2003 and 2007. The data in the two papers are very similar although the latter publication[19] fails to reference the former.[18]

When should renal biopsy be performed in pregnancy?

Overall, the available published evidence from studies of contemporary practice suggests that the complication rate of renal biopsy in pregnancy is broadly similar to that encountered with this intervention in general nephrological practice. It is possible that the prothrombotic environment engendered by pregnancy may mitigate bleeding. Nonetheless, because the reported experience of renal biopsy in pregnancy in the modern era amounts to only a few hundred cases, compared with thousands in the nonpregnant setting, it is not possible to conclude with complete confidence that rates of unusual but serious complications are equivalent. Clearly, if enough biopsies of pregnant women are performed, then a serious complication will eventually follow. Therefore, in pregnancy, consideration should be given to the same absolute and relative contraindications to the biopsy procedure that apply to the nonpregnant situation (see above). Potential operators should not be tempted to perform a renal biopsy in an unfamiliar manner, for example with the woman seated rather than prone. This may be of particular relevance in pregnancies over 24 weeks of gestation when it may difficult or uncomfortable for women to lie prone. Also, as in the nonpregnant setting, renal biopsy should not be performed in the presence of hypertension (above 160/95 mmHg).[2]

Given the above caveats, what indications necessitate renal biopsy in pregnancy? It can be difficult to distinguish between pre-eclampsia and primary renal disease in pregnancy and often the two may coexist. However, it is usually possible to distinguish between the two conditions by observing other clinical parameters. In pre-eclampsia, proteinuria generally develops rapidly after 20 weeks of gestation and other features such as rising serum urate, falling platelet count and abnormal liver enzymes may point to this diagnosis. Considering this, and in the knowledge that those bleeding complications that have been observed with renal biopsy in pregnancy particularly afflict hypertensive women with pre-eclampsia, renal biopsy cannot be recommended routinely as an investigation for pre-eclampsia.

In non-pre-eclamptic women with nephrotic syndrome after 32 weeks of gestation delivery should be expedited and renal investigations postponed to the postpartum period. Before 28 weeks of gestation, renal biopsy should be performed to make a histological diagnosis and to guide therapy, since some lesions may be amenable to steroid therapy. Between 28 and 32 weeks of gestation the decision is less straightforward. The major question is whether the mother has a condition, predominantly minimal change disease, which may respond promptly to steroids. In adults of childbearing age, minimal change disease comprises only about 25% of all nephrotic syndrome and may respond more slowly to therapy than the same condition diagnosed in children. It may be difficult to justify antepartum biopsy simply in order to prolong pregnancy for a couple of weeks to improve fetal outcome, when any maternal intervention is unlikely to have had a therapeutic effect. A trial of steroids is a possibility but many clinicians are uncomfortable with blind glucocorticoid treatment given the potential maternal complications such as hypertension, infection and diabetes.[20] An emerging literature also suggests that the prenatal use of glucocorticoids may initiate in the fetus a programme of physiological changes resulting in cardiovascular and metabolic disease in adulthood.[21] Therefore, in a morbidly nephrotic woman after 28 weeks of gestation when fetal viability is likely to be good, delivery should be expedited and renal investigation pursued thereafter.

Acute kidney injury in pregnancy with no apparent cause may require renal biopsy. In some systemic disorders such as lupus, serological investigations may be helpful diagnostically and elucidation of renal histopathology may be a key determinant of therapy. Indeed, prompt therapeutic intervention may be required to preserve renal function. Therefore biopsy should be performed before 28 weeks, but at later gestational age the pregnancy should be brought to an end to facilitate subsequent renal biopsy.

The finding in pregnancy of stable chronic kidney disease and hypertension with an active urinary sediment suggestive of a renal parenchymal disease should provoke close supervision and blood pressure control, but not renal biopsy which would be unlikely to alter management. A similar approach should be applied to non-nephrotic proteinuria, with or without renal functional impairment.

Overall, renal biopsy in pregnancy appears to be safe. Definite indications for its use exist before 28 weeks of gestation but are unusual. Renal biopsy should thus only rarely be needed in pregnancy and not after 28 weeks of gestation.

References

1. Alwall N. Aspiration biopsy of the kidney, including a report of a case of amyloidosis diagnosed through aspiration biopsy of the kidney in 1944 and investigated at an autopsy in 1950. *Acta Med Scand* 1952;143:420–35.
2. Topham PS. Renal Biopsy. In: Johnson RJ, Floege J, Feehally J, editors. *Comprehensive Clinical Nephrology*. Oxford: Elsevier Health Sciences; 2007. p. 69–76.
3. Parrish AE. Complications of percutaneous renal biopsy: a review of 37 years' experience. *Clin Nephrol* 1992;38:135–41
4. Hergesell O, Felten H, Andrassy K, Kuhn K, Ritz E. Safety of ultrasound-guided percutaneous renal biopsy-retrospective analysis of 1090 consecutive cases. *Nephrol Dial Transplant* 1998;13:975–7.
5. Manno C, Strippoli GF, Arnesano L, Bonifati C, Campobasso N, Gesualdo L, *et al.* Predictors of bleeding complications in percutaneous ultrasound-guided renal biopsy. *Kidney Int* 2004;66:1570–7.
6. Eiro M, Katoh T, Watanabe T. Risk factors for bleeding complications in percutaneous renal biopsy. *Clin Exp Nephrol* 2005;9:40–5.
7. Bennett AR, Wiener SN. Intrarenal arteriovenous fistula and aneurysm. A complication of percutaneous renal biopsy. *Am J Roentgenol Radium Ther Nucl Med* 1965;95:372–82.
8. Jones DC, Hayslett JP. Outcome of pregnancy in women with moderate or severe renal insufficiency. *N Engl J Med* 1996;335:226–32.
9. Fischer MJ, Lehnerz SD, Hebert JR, Parikh CR. Kidney disease is an independent risk factor for adverse fetal and maternal outcomes in pregnancy. *Am J Kidney Dis* 2004;43:415–23.
10. McCartney CP. Pathological anatomy of acute hypertension of pregnancy. *Circulation* 1964;30 Suppl 2:37–42.
11. Schewitz LJ, Friedman IA, Pollak VE. Bleeding after renal biopsy in pregnancy. *Obstet Gynecol* 1965;26:295–304.
12. Lindheimer MD, Spargo BH, Katz AI. Renal biopsy in pregnancy-induced hypertension. *J Reprod Med* 1975;15:189–94.
13. Packham D, Fairley KF. Renal biopsy: indications and complications in pregnancy. *Br J Obstet Gynaecol* 1987;94:935–9.
14. Lindheimer MD, Davison JM. Renal biopsy during pregnancy: 'to b . . . or not to b . . .?' *Br J Obstet Gynaecol* 1987;94:932–4.
15. Kuller JA, D'Andrea NM, McMahon MJ. Renal biopsy and pregnancy. *Am J Obstet Gynecol* 2001;184:1093–6.

16. Chen HH, Lin HC, Yeh JC, Chen CP. Renal biopsy in pregnancies complicated by undetermined renal disease. *Acta Obstet Gynecol Scand* 2001;80:888–93.
17. G Lipkin, personal communication.
18. Strevens H, Wide-Swensson D, Hansen A, Horn T, Ingemarsson I, Larsen S, *et al.* Glomerular endotheliosis in normal pregnancy and pre-eclampsia. *Br J Obstet Gynaecol* 2003;110:831–6.
19. Wide-Swensson D, Strevens H, Willner J. Antepartum percutaneous renal biopsy. *Int J Gynaecol Obstet* 2007;98:88–92.
20. Petri M. Immunosuppressive drug use in pregnancy. Autoimmunity 2003;36:51–6.
21. Seckl JR, Holmes MC. Mechanisms of disease: glucocorticoids, their placental metabolism and fetal programming of adult pathophysiology. *Nat Clin Pract Endocrinol Metab* 2007;3:479–88.

Section 6

Urology and pregnancy

Chapter 17
Urological problems in pregnancy

Jonathon Olsburgh

The most common urological symptoms in pregnancy are a consequence of pregnancy on a normal urinary tract rather than specific urological diseases presenting in pregnancy. However, both the diagnosis and management of urological diseases in pregnancy can be complex. This review will discuss aetiology and management of loin pain, urinary frequency, urinary tract infection (UTI) and haematuria. Additionally, imaging of the renal tract, renal stone disease, urinary tract malignancy and the management of women with urinary tract diversion or reconstruction in pregnancy will be specifically addressed. Postpartum complications affecting the urinary tract, such as fistulae and urinary incontinence, are not in the remit of this review.

Physiological changes to the urinary tract in pregnancy

Upper tract

The increase in cardiac output, total vascular volume and renal blood flow in the first and second trimesters of pregnancy leads to a 40–65% increase in glomerular filtration rate (GFR).[1] As a result, the kidneys increase by up to 1 cm in length and 30% in volume. The increase in urine production coincides with hormonal and mechanical changes to the maternal renal pelvis and ureter. A 'physiological hydronephrosis' of pregnancy occurs in more than half of pregnancies in the middle trimester. Less commonly, ureteric dilation has been observed as early as 7 weeks of pregnancy and may be due to a relaxant effect of progesterone. At this early stage of pregnancy, ureteric dilation does not equate with obstruction, whereas mechanical extrinsic compression can occur from second trimester onwards owing to both the gravid uterus and the engorged ovarian vein plexus crossing the ureter at the level of the pelvic brim. The ureter is usually dilated to the level of the true pelvis and of normal calibre at the level of the bladder. A fetus in the breech position in the third trimester may compress and obstruct the mid- or upper ureter. Dextrorotation of the gravid uterus may account for hydronephrosis being more common on the right side and the left ureter is also protected by the sigmoid colon.

Lower tract

From early pregnancy there is an increase in GFR and urine production. As the gravid anteverted uterus enlarges, it increasingly indents the superior aspect or dome of the bladder. This changes the bladder shape and increases resistance to bladder stretching.[2] In early pregnancy the functional bladder capacity remains fairly similar to the nonpregnant state but, by the third trimester, crowding of the pelvis decreases the functional bladder capacity. These factors explain much of the increase in daytime urinary frequency and nocturia that are seen from early pregnancy onwards.

Lower urinary tract symptoms

Urinary frequency and nocturia can be considered normal physiological consequences of a healthy pregnancy. Urinary tract infection and glycosuria (from gestational diabetes) must be excluded on urine dipstick examination. Urinary urgency is common (in over half of pregnant women) and, if severe, can lead to urinary urge incontinence, although this resolves postpartum in most women and, if incontinence persists, should be differentiated from stress urinary incontinence.

Stress urinary incontinence is also common, with between half and three-quarters of multiparous women having an episode during pregnancy.[3] Rates of stress urinary incontinence increase with increasing parity, previous vaginal delivery and obesity. Management should be supportive during pregnancy, with pelvic floor exercises and full evaluation for persistence of symptoms carried out in the postnatal period.

Urine retention in pregnancy is uncommon, occurring in less than 1 in 3000 pregnancies. However, it presents as an emergency with pain and anuria. In early pregnancy, urinary catheterisation for urine retention is described as easy as the cause of retention may be due to failure of urethral relaxation and detrusor contractility secondary to progesterone. This might be more common following ovarian hyperstimulation with *in vitro* fertilisation (IVF).

The retroverted uterus is more commonly associated with urine retention that classically occurs at 12–14 weeks. It is more common in women with a fibroid uterus or uterine abnormalities. In the third trimester, urine retention may occur if the uterus is incarcerated in the pelvis. This is associated with fibroids, uterine abnormalities and abnormal placentation such as placenta accreta. In the second and third trimester with a retroverted uterus, the bladder base may be elevated, distracting the bladder and leading to a functional rather than compressive retention. Management includes catheterisation, intermittent self-catheterisation and bimanual manipulation of a retroverted uterus to an anteverted position, which may require anaesthesia. Occasionally a Smith–Hodge lever pessary is needed temporarily to maintain the anteverted uterine position.

Urinary tract infection

Bacterial UTI in pregnancy should be classified as asymptomatic bacteriuria (ASB), symptomatic lower tract UTI (cystitis) or symptomatic upper tract UTI (pyelonephritis). UTI is a urological emergency when coexistent with urinary tract obstruction.

Although the incidence of ASB in pregnancy is similar to that in age-matched nonpregnant women, the rates of cystitis and pyelonephritis in pregnancy are three- to four-fold higher than in the nonpregnant state.[4,5] Furthermore, the consequences of pyelonephritis in pregnancy for both mother and fetus can be significant and include preterm birth and low birthweight. Haemorrhagic cystitis is also associated with preterm labour.

Meta-analysis of randomised controlled study data has shown that treating ASB with antibiotics leads to a 77% (95% CI 59–87%) relative risk reduction of pyelonephritis, with seven patients needing to be treated for one benefit.[6] Therefore it is widely accepted that screening for ASB in early pregnancy is beneficial, although the number needed to be screened to prevent one episode of pyelonephritis is 114. In the UK, screening occurs at the booking visit at approximately 12–16 weeks. Maternal risk factors for UTI include previous UTI, urinary tract abnormalities including reflux and reconstruction, diabetes and immunosuppression.

Gram-negative bacteria, especially Enterobacteriaceae including *Escherichia coli*, *Enterobacter* and *Klebsiella*, are the most common organisms causing UTI in pregnancy. Less commonly, other Gram-negative organisms such as *Pseudomonas*, *Proteus* and *Citrobacter* and Gram-positive organisms such as group B streptococcus are implicated. Other organisms that also need to be considered include *Chlamydia trachomatis*, *Gardnerella vaginalis*, *Ureaplasma urealyticum* and lactobacilli.

ASB is defined on midstream urine (MSU) culture as 10^5 colony-forming units (or greater) per millilitre of urine without symptoms. It should be confirmed on a second MSU culture.

A 3 day antibiotic course for ASB is as effective as a 7 day course, with both regimens having a 70% eradication rate, and a single dose closely approximates this.[5] A repeat MSU should be done 1 week later and any persistence or recurrence should be treated with culture-specific antibiotics for 7–10 days. Following treatment of ASB, women with low risk and successful treatment with a 3 day antibiotic course should have regular repeat MSU cultures to detect recurrent ASB. Women with low risk and recurrent ASB or with high risk of UTI should receive prophylaxis throughout pregnancy and an upper renal tract ultrasound scan. Women with high risk of UTI in pregnancy but a clear first MSU should have regular repeat MSUs to ensure that ASB does not go untreated.

Cystitis should be treated with empirical antibiotic therapy pending the results of an MSU collected prior to commencing treatment. In women in low-risk groups, an initial 3 day course and a repeat MSU a week later is appropriate, followed by regular screening for ASB. In high-risk patients, a baseline upper renal tract ultrasound scan should be arranged and consideration given to prophylaxis throughout pregnancy.

Occasionally, severe macroscopic haematuria can occur in pregnancy with cystitis (haemorrhagic cystitis), perhaps owing to the engorgement of the bladder mucosa in pregnancy. It may require parenteral antibiotics, bladder irrigation and cystoscopy to evacuate blood clot in the bladder.

Pyelonephritis should be managed initially with hospital admission for blood and urine cultures and 48–72 hours of parenteral antibiotics. If there has been clinical improvement, antibiotic therapy can be switched to a further 11–12 day oral antibiotic course. This should be followed by a repeat MSU a week later to ensure eradication of infection and then consideration given to low-dose antibiotic therapy for the remainder of pregnancy.

A renal tract ultrasound scan should be performed to exclude perinephric abscess. This should be managed with a percutaneous drain. As most pyelonephritis occurs in the third trimester, hydronephrosis is likely to be present. If systemic features are prominent (tachycardia, hypotension) then pyonephrosis should be suspected and percutaneous aspiration for culture and nephrostomy placement advised. Management should focus on the causes and relief of urinary tract obstruction (see below).

Loin pain, hydronephrosis and imaging

Loin pain in pregnancy has a variety of aetiologies. Ureteric obstruction may be due to the fetus, urolithiasis or a number of less common causes such as intrinsic pelviureteric junction obstruction (PUJO). Loin pain may occur with a bleed into a renal angiomyolipoma (AML), renal vein compressive hypertension, rupture of a renal artery aneurysm and non-urinary tract conditions.

Loin pain in pregnancy may be associated with hydronephrosis and, conversely, asymptomatic maternal hydronephrosis may be observed on routine ultrasound imaging.

Non-radiation-based imaging of the urinary tract is clearly the preferred choice in pregnancy, with ultrasound scanning being the first-line investigation.[7,8] A comparison of fetal exposure doses from urinary tract imaging is provided in Table 17.1.

A transabdominal ultrasound scan can detect dilation of the maternal renal pelvis and collecting system and an antero-posterior (AP) diameter of 1 cm or more together with calyceal dilation is defined as hydronephrosis. However, dilation does not equate with obstruction. In physiological hydronephrosis of pregnancy, dilation of the upper ureter should also be seen. If dilation is confined to the renal pelvis, it may be due to a renal pelvis calculus or PUJO that may be pre-existent or that has manifested itself as a result of the increase urine volume of pregnancy.

Table 17.1. Fetal exposure doses from urinary tract imaging

Examination	Fetal radiation dose	mSv equivalent	Reference
Ultrasound	nil	nil	
MRU	nil	nil	
CXR	0.02 rad	0.2	Loughlin (2007)[7]
KUB X-ray	0.05 rad 1.4–4.2 mGy	0.5 1.4–4.2	Loughlin (2007)[7], Biyani and Joyce (2002)[8], NRPB (1998)[18]
Limited IVU (3–4 films)	0.2–0.25 rad 1–2 cGy	2.0–2.5 10–20	Loughlin (2007)[7], Pais *et al.* (2007)[12]
Standard IVU	0.4–0.5 rad 1.7–10 mGy	4–5 1.7–10	Loughlin (2007)[7], Biyani and Joyce (2002)[8], NRPB (1998)[18]
Fluoroscopy	1.5–2 rad/minute	15–20/minute	Loughlin (2007)[7]
CT standard	2–2.5 rad	20–25	Loughlin (2007)[7]
CT abdomen	8–49 mGy	8–49	Biyani and Joyce (2002)[8], NRPB (1998)[18]
CT pelvis	25–79 mGy	25–79	Biyani and Joyce (2002)[8], NRPB (1998)[18]
Conventional CT KUB	3.5 cGy	35	Pais *et al.* (2007)[12]
Multidetector CT KUB	0.8–1.2 cGy	8–12	Pais *et al.* (2007)[12]
Low-dose/ultra low-dose CT KUB	0.721 cGy	7	Pais *et al.* (2007)[12]
Tc-99m DTPA	1.5–4 mGy	1.5–4	Biyani and Joyce (2002)[8], NRPB (1998)[18]
Tc-99m MAG-3	0.7 mGy	0.7	Biyani and Joyce (2002)[8], NRPB (1998)[18]
Lethal fetal dose (conception to first trimester)	100–500 mGy	100–500	Biyani and Joyce (2002)[8], NRPB (1998)[18]

CT = computed tomography; CXR = chest X-ray; DTPA = diethylenetriamine pentaacetic acid; IVU = intravenous urogram; KUB = kidneys, ureters and bladder; MAG-3 = mercaptoacetyltriglycine; MSU = midstream urine; NRPB = National Radiological Protection Board

The National Radiological Protection Board (now Health Protection Agency HPA) gives fetal doses in mGy (milliGray) whereas the standard international unit for X-ray exposure is now the mSv (milliSievert). The conversion factor to equivalent dose is 1, i.e. 1 mGy = 1 mSv for X-rays. Older and overseas literature report dose exposure in other units for which the conversion is 1 rad = 1 cGy = 10 mGy = 10 mSv.

The common scenario on transabdominal ultrasound is dilation to the mid- or lower ureter. The differential diagnosis is an obstruction either from an intraluminal cause, most commonly a calculus, or an extrinsic cause such as the gravid uterus, fibroids, ovarian hyperstimulation after IVF and, rarely, uterine artery aneurysm or non-obstructive hydronephrosis (physiological hydronephrosis of pregnancy).

The specificity of (B mode) ultrasound in pregnancy to diagnose a ureteric stone is poor (around 50%) and may be increased by a number of techniques. Firstly, use colour flow Doppler to determine the level of the iliac vessels in relation to the dilated ureter. Secondly, scan initially in a supine position and then rescan after 30 minutes in an 'all fours' position (in physiological hydronephrosis the AP renal diameter should be less than 1 cm after this manoeuvre). Thirdly, use transvaginal scanning to help to determine the level of the dilated ureter and detection of distal ureteric calculi. A 5 MHz vaginal transducer with a 90° sector angle and 30° off-axis beam is used. The renal resistive index (RI) has been investigated for its sensitivity to predict urinary tract obstruction in pregnancy. The RI is best at separating obstructed from non-obstructed systems but may also help to differentiate acute from chronic obstruction. In an obstructing process that develops over weeks, such as the enlarging uterus, adaptive processes in the renal vasculature maintain a near normal RI, whereas in an acute process such as a complete obstruction from a ureteric stone the RI is likely to be raised above 0.7. The limitation of these ultrasound techniques is that they are operator dependent.

Magnetic resonance urography (MRU) comprises an overview fast T2-weighted examination of the abdomen and pelvis, and thick-slab, heavily T2-weighted MRU images, followed by focused, high-resolution T2-weighted sequences obtained in an axial and coronal oblique plane through the level of ureteric calibre change.[9] MRU does not require Gadolinium contrast. MRU provides high-quality images that permits identification of and differentiation between extrinsic and luminal causes of ureteric obstruction. MRU also permits identification of other non-urinary tract causes of pain such as ovarian torsion or appendicitis. The exact cause of an intraluminal obstructing lesion is not specific with MRU as it appears as a 'filling defect' and could be either stone, clot or sloughed papilla (in a patient with diabetes or sickle cell disease). Another limitation of MRU is that most magnetic resonance imaging (MRI) scanners are closed ring systems with an internal radius of approximately 60 cm. Therefore, some women in the third trimester may not fit inside a closed-ring system; there are a small number of open-ring MRI scanners in the UK. A further limitation is a potential safety issue in the first trimester with the magnetic field generated by the MRI. Safety data are not yet available on the effect of exposing a fetus to 15 minutes in a 1.5 (or greater) tesla magnet. Currently, after a non-diagnostic ultrasound scan in the second or third trimester, MRU should be considered the second-line investigation of choice.

Access to MRU may not be available in all UK centres and, as the next investigations involve limited fetal exposure to radiation, discussion between urologist, obstetrician and patient is advised regarding the treatment plan.

Dynamic radionucleotide renography, such as technetium-labelled MAG-3, exposes the fetus to very low radiation doses and is a widely available test. It is best at diagnosing obstruction in the upper rather than lower ureter and requires an overall GFR of greater than 16 ml/minute/1.73 m^2.

Standard intravenous urogram (IVU) may expose the fetus to an unacceptably high radiation dose, particularly if a comprehensive series of follow-up plain films are required to delineate a level of ureteric obstruction. Prior to the advent of colour Doppler ultrasound and MRU, a modified and limited IVU series was performed, including a control and 15 minute film and then up to a maximum of two further delayed films. Use of a limited IVU is still advocated by the joint European and US guidelines.[10] A further problem with IVU is that intravenously administered iodinated contrast material crosses the placenta and may suppress fetal thyroid function. If a limited IVU is performed, fetal thyroid function must be checked in the first postnatal week.

Cystoscopy with retrograde ureteropyelography is generally performed under general anaesthesia, although in women it can be performed under local anaesthetic. It is important to limit fluoroscopy to the minimum required using coned beam and to shield the fetus. General anaesthesia in pregnancy is associated with increased risks of gastric aspiration, decreased respiratory reserve and increased risk of thromboembolic events. To improve venous return the patient should be placed in a modified Trendelenburg position with left uterine displacement.

The advantages of retrograde ureteropyelography are that it allows both diagnosis of obstruction, definition of the level of obstruction and the opportunity to insert a double-J ureteric stent without the trauma to the kidney associated with percutaneous nephrostomy (PCN). This is a particularly important consideration in a patient with a solitary kidney. Retrograde ureteropyelography will diagnose or refute suspected obstruction if there is minimal or no pelvicalyceal dilation on ultrasound. Many units suggest that to limit the fluoroscopic dose renal ultrasound be used to check the renal stent position. So although retrograde ureteropyelography is a basic routine investigation for urologists, in pregnancy there are a number of factors that make it a less familiar method. A further disadvantage is that the success rate of retrograde double-J stenting is slightly lower than in the nonpregnant patient.

While conventional unenhanced helical computed tomography (CT) has the greatest sensitivity and specificity for detecting renal tract calculi it delivers too high a dose of radiation to permit its use in pregnancy. However, new multidetector CT scanners with protocols for low-dose imaging of the renal tract can detect renal tract calculi while exposing the fetus to approximately half the amount of radiation as a limited IVU series. Further technical developments may lead to CT becoming an acceptable, sensitive and widely available technique for imaging the renal tract in pregnancy.

Urolithiasis

The incidence of renal calculus disease in pregnancy is reported to be no greater than in the general population. However, in the general population, stones are often diagnosed incidentally by X-ray or scan for another condition. Incidental presentation in pregnancy is less frequent and most renal stones present when symptomatic. An exact comparison of incidence and prevalence rates is thus difficult. Stones tend to present in the second or third trimester.

There are significant metabolic changes in pregnancy that relate to stone disease:

- circulating 1,25-dihydroxyvitamin D concentration increases, which results in a higher gastrointestinal absorption of calcium
- renal calcium excretion therefore increases up to twice the normal concentration; there is reduced renal tubular reabsorption of calcium
- a combination of these two above events leads to a physiological hypercalciuria with normocalcaemia
- filtered sodium and uric acid increase

- sodium excretion is unchanged as there is increased tubular reabsorption
- the filtered load of urinary citrate and magnesium stone inhibitors increases
- increased urinary excretion of glycosaminoglycans and acidic glycoproteins inhibits oxalate stone formation
- respiratory alkalosis, which leads to relatively alkaline urine, inhibits uric acid stone formation.

The overall situation is an increase in both stone-promoting and stone-inhibiting factors so that there is probably no increase in stone formation. However, there does appear to be an increase in the rate of encrustation of urinary tract stents and nephrostomy tubes compared with the nonpregnant state, with encrustation seen within 3 months of placement.

The severe pain of renal/ureteric colic has been associated with preterm labour in the second and third trimester. Renal/ureteric colic should not be treated with nonsteroidal anti-inflammatory drugs (NSAIDs) in pregnancy if at all possible and especially not in the third trimester. Options include paracetamol, opiate analgesia and epidural anaesthesia.

Painful hydronephrosis that does not settle with the above measures may require urinary tract decompression with a PCN. Sepsis associated with renal tract obstruction is a surgical emergency and a PCN should be placed promptly under ultrasound guidance by an experienced interventional radiologist.

The majority of stones are smaller than 5 mm and will pass spontaneously with analgesia, bed rest and hydration. Expulsive therapy with the use of alpha blockers and calcium channel antagonists is not recommended in pregnancy, although epidural anaesthesia placed for pain relief may give additional benefit by allowing smooth muscle relaxation of the lower ureter facilitating stone passage.

The management of symptomatic stones that do not respond to conservative measures needs to be based on a number of factors: size, number and location of stone(s) and the stage of pregnancy.[11,12] The options include temporising measures (until after delivery) and definitive treatment during pregnancy. Extracorporeal shockwave lithotripsy is contraindicated in pregnancy due to its potentially damaging effects to the fetus.

The most direct temporising method is external urinary drainage with a PCN. PCN is safe, placed under local anaesthetic and ultrasound guidance, relieves the pain of obstruction and allows immediate drainage and culture of infected urine and it avoids manipulation of the obstructed ureter with associated risks of perforation and further sepsis.

However, patients tolerate an external PCN tube only moderately well and often only for a few weeks. PCN tubes can become blocked, requiring flushing, or dislodged or encrusted, requiring replacement. Consideration should therefore be given to PCN as a route for subsequent antegrade internal double-J stent placement and an appropriately placed PCN track can be dilated to permit access for percutaneous nephrolithotomy (PCNL) or antegrade ureteroscopic stone removal. PCNL requires prolonged general anaesthesia and is generally not recommended in pregnancy but a number of centres have reported successful stone treatment with healthy maternal and fetal outcome.

A further possible technique for use with a PCN is stone dissolution therapy with irrigation of solutions via the nephrostomy tube. This technique is uncommonly used in urology but can help treat infection and cystine stones with appropriate solutions, usually after an initial therapy to fragment the stone to increase the surface area. This technique has not been fully evaluated in pregnant women.

Limitations of PCN are that placement is operator dependent and requires an experienced interventional radiologist and there is potential for bleeding both at the time of PCN insertion and exchange.

Cystoscopy, retrograde imaging and double-J stent placement have been discussed above. An impacted stone may not be able to be stented from below, requiring PCN placement. Stent encrustation can be fairly rapid in pregnancy and stents should be exchanged at approximately 8 weekly intervals. This can be a significant inconvenience and undertaking.

Advances in instrument design and fibre-optic technology have permitted the development of small-calibre, semi-rigid and flexible ureteroscopes that have revolutionised endourological stone management. New semi-rigid scopes are 7.5 F calibre and flexible scopes 8.2 F calibre. Ureteroscopy permits definitive stone removal (with baskets) and fragmentation using both pneumatic and laser technologies. The current most efficient technique using holmium laser appears to be safe in pregnancy.[10]

However, ureteroscopy in pregnancy is difficult and should only be undertaken by expert operators. Ureteroscopy is mainly performed retrograde under general anaesthesia but occasionally antegrade ureteroscopy via a dilated PCN track into the dilated ureter above a stone is more appropriate using flexible instruments. Stones in the lower third of the ureter are most amenable to treatment and the ureteric orifice may not require dilation owing to the dilating effects of progesterone. Following successful ureteroscopic stone fragmentation it was conventional to place a double-J stent. However, if there has been minimal ureteric wall trauma, it may be possible either not to place a double-J stent or to place a 'stent on a string' that can be removed 24 hours later on the ward.

Ureteroscopy in pregnancy is contraindicated with multiple stones, stones greater than 1 cm and in the presence of sepsis, when placement of a double-J stent or PCN with treatment of infection is the first priority.

Women with a known history of renal disease, for example those with cystinuria, who are contemplating pregnancy should be seen by their urologist. An up-to-date CT KUB (kidneys, ureters and bladder), MSU and metabolic stone profile should be arranged to determine stone burden, urine infection and a baseline metabolic risk profile prior to pregnancy. There is benefit in treating asymptomatic stones prior to pregnancy that otherwise might be observed. Advice should be given regarding fluid intake. Depending on type of previous stones and urine culture results consideration given to low-dose antibiotic prophylaxis throughout pregnancy. Women with previous struvite 'infection' stones should have antibiotic prophylaxis throughout pregnancy.

Haematuria and urinary tract tumours

Microscopic

In the study by Brown *et al.*,[13] asymptomatic dipstick haematuria (ADH) was found to be common, occurring on at least two occasions in 3–20% of pregnant women, microscopic haematuria being confirmed in the majority and ADH resolving postpartum in the majority. Ultrasound evaluation of the renal tract was normal in all cases and ADH did not confer any additional risk of gestational hypertension. There may be a two-fold risk of pre-eclampsia in nulliparous but not in multiparous women with ADH. Retesting at 3 month postpartum is recommended to detect the small minority who may have mild glomerular disease or who may require further urological investigation. Clearly the presence of dipstick haematuria and proteinuria, in the absence of infection, requires a complete nephrological assessment. Renal stone disease is associated with microscopic haematuria in approximately 90% of cases.

Macroscopic

Frank haematuria in pregnancy should be differentiated from vaginal bleeding and renal tract ultrasound scan is the investigation of choice together with MSU. Consideration should be given to both the upper and lower urinary tract as the source of the bleeding.

Upper tract

Significant renal trauma can cause haematuria and the leading cause of fetal demise from renal trauma in pregnancy is maternal demise. Therefore for renal trauma in pregnancy associated with hypotension the preferred imaging modality remains contrast-enhanced CT scan.

The benign renal tumour angiomyolipoma (AML) may grow rapidly in pregnancy with increased risk of rupture. This can present as frank haematuria, loin pain and can be life threatening. Ruptured AML in pregnancy requires either selective renal embolisation[14] or nephrectomy. A women contemplating pregnancy with a 4 cm AML would be best advised to have selective renal embolisation before pregnancy.

Malignant renal tumours are not more common in pregnancy.[15] However, a teenage pregnant woman with macroscopic haematuria has been reported to have had a Wilm's tumour and there are at least 50 reported cases of renal cell carcinoma (RCC) in pregnancy. Depending on the size of the lesion and the stage of pregnancy when the tumour is detected, management may be either observation with postpartum treatment (for a 4 cm or smaller lesion found in the third trimester) or nephrectomy. Laparoscopic nephrectomy for RCC has been described in both first and second trimesters with favourable maternal and fetal outcomes.

Occasionally, renal vein compression occurs secondary to the gravid uterus leading to profuse haematuria and loin pain. On the left side this is an aggravation of the classic 'nutcracker syndrome' in which the left renal vein lies between the aorta and superior mesenteric artery.

Lower tract

Pregnant women are typically younger than the age range in which bladder cancer occurs. However, as women are having babies at older ages and more women are smoking, the likelihood of bladder cancer developing during pregnancy is increased. Occupational exposure to aromatic amines in permanent hair dyes may occur in women's hairdressing and an occupational history should be taken. Bladder tumours usually present with haematuria that may be confused by the patient as 'vaginal bleeding'. Another confounding factor is that carcinoma *in situ* of the bladder presents with urine frequency and urgency that are typically present in pregnancy. Carcinoma of the bladder may be transitional cell, squamous cell or adenocarcinoma. Tumours greater than 0.5 cm can be visualised on transabdominal ultrasound scan with a full bladder. Flexible cystoscopy is safe at all stages of pregnancy. The majority of bladder tumours are superficial, i.e. papillary non-invasive or papillary superficially invasive. However, poorly differentiated superficial and muscle-invasive transitional cell carcinomas have a rapid tumour doubling time and a poor prognosis. An initial transurethral resection of bladder tumour (TURBT) under general anaesthesia appears to be safe in pregnancy and allows accurate staging and grading of the disease so that an appropriate diagnostic and management plan can be formulated, depending on histology results and what stage of pregnancy has been reached. These decisions need to be individualised but maternal health and safety are paramount and delaying definitive treatment for aggressive transitional cell carcinoma beyond 8–12 weeks from TURBT may have poor long-term prognostic implications. Follow-up cystoscopy for non-invasive transitional cell carcinoma may be delayed until after delivery.

Pregnancy in women with urinary tract reconstruction

Vesicoureteric reflux is considered in Chapter 8. However, distal obstruction at the site of previous ureteric re-implantation has been reported as presenting in pregnancy. The timing of this presentation may relate to the increased urine output in pregnancy revealing a previously subclinical narrowing. Therefore, it has been suggested that women with a history of ureteric re-implantation who are considering pregnancy should be evaluated with either a dynamic radionucleotide renogram or cystoscopy and retrograde ureteropyelogram to exclude obstruction prior to conception.

The indications for urinary tract diversion or reconstruction in women of childbearing age are due to benign rather than malignant disease.[16] These include congenital disease such as spina bifida (including myelomeningocele) and bladder extrophy or acquired neurological or fibrotic (including tuberculosis and schistosomiasis) diseases. The congenital diseases may be associated with other urogenital abnormalities including solitary kidney and uterine abnormalities. Furthermore, many of the conditions may be associated with some degree of renal impairment and all are associated with bacterial UTI. Nevertheless, the majority of these women are fertile. It is important to note that urine-based pregnancy tests in women with a bowel segment incorporated into the urinary tract are likely to give a false positive result and it is recommended that serum human chorionic gonadotrophin is used instead. Pregnancy should be managed in a joint obstetric–urology clinic with intensive monitoring and easy access to specialist help.

There is a diverse range of urinary tract reconstructions that a pregnant woman may have, including incontinent urinary diversion (ileal or colonic conduit), continent urinary diversion that may be either to the colon (ureterosigmoidostomy or Mainz II pouch) or continent catheterisable bowel pouch (Koch and Indiana pouch), enterocystoplasty (native bladder augmented with bowel that drains either via the urethra or via a continent catheterisable stoma (Mitrofanoff) or orthotopic neobladder.[16]

ASB is present in all patients with a bowel segment incorporated into the urinary tract. Some of the above configurations are also freely refluxing to the upper tract. It is, therefore, preferable that all these women have low-dose prophylactic antibiotic therapy throughout pregnancy.

Vaginal delivery may be possible and should be judged on the merits of both obstetric and urological factors. Breech presentation is very common in women with history of bladder extrophy. Neurological conditions that affect the bladder may also affect coordinated muscle activity required in the final stage of vaginal delivery.

Vaginal delivery is contraindicated in women with an artificial urinary sphincter and cautioned against in patients with orthotopic neobladder and ureterosigmoidostomy. Ureterosigmoidostomy or Mainz II pouch depend on an intact anal sphincter for continence and, if a vaginal delivery is attempted, care must be taken to make lateral episiotomies. For all women with complex urinary tract reconstruction, if caesarean section is likely, it should be anticipated and performed electively with an experienced urologist present. Some myelomeningocele patients may have a ventricular-peritoneal shunt to treat hydrocephalus – the shunt can be compressed by the gravid uterus and is at risk of bacterial infection if the peritoneum is opened during caesarean section.

An important mechanical factor that needs to be considered during pregnancy is the points of fixation of the ureters, the mesentery (that supplies the urinary tract reconstruction) and the efferent drainage. The mesentery stretches and is lateralised as the gravid uterus enlarges and can usually be safely moved laterally during upper-segment caesarean section.

An ileal conduit in a woman of childbearing age when formed should be fixed to the retroperitoneum. The enlarging uterus may compress the conduit leading to dilation of the upper tracts but this is rarely seen. Retroperitonealising the conduit prevents the conduit from being stretched, which may return to prepregnancy size postpartum and require self-catheterisation or revision. The conduit skin appliances may require adjustment to maintain a watertight seal as the position of the stoma changes with uterine enlargement. A pouch or Mitrofanoff catheterisable stoma can be stretched during pregnancy, leading to difficulties with self-catheterisation, which usually resolves postpartum.

The leading British experience in this field reports that there are no long-term adverse effects of pregnancy on renal function or the reconstructed urinary tract in 29 live births in 20 women.[17] Pregnancy-related complications were encountered, particularly UTI in at least half and upper tract obstruction and pre-eclampsia in 10%. The majority of babies were delivered by caesarean section.

Conclusion

The most common urological symptoms in pregnancy are urinary frequency and urgency but the most common reason for a urological consultation is loin pain associated with hydronephrosis. There is often difficulty in diagnosing the specific cause of hydronephrosis in pregnancy. Ultrasound scanning remains the first investigation and a number of specific measures to increase the sensitivity to differentiate between non-obstructive physiological hydronephrosis of pregnancy, obstruction by the gravid uterus and ureteric calculus are described. New ureteroscope instrument design and fibre-optic technology has permitted ureteroscopy to be used in expert hands during pregnancy to provide definitive stone treatment and reduce the problems associated with a number of temporising measures.

Macroscopic and persisting microscopic haematuria should be investigated initially with ultrasound scan and, when indicated, flexible cystoscopy, which is safe throughout pregnancy.

The rate of pyelonephritis in pregnancy can be reduced by screening and treating ASB and this is recommended. Certain at-risk groups benefit from low-dose antibiotic prophylaxis during pregnancy to reduce their risk of UTI.

Careful planning of pregnancy with joint urology and obstetric care is recommended for women with previous urinary tract reconstruction. Experience suggests that the majority can have healthy, successful pregnancies without compromise to the urinary tract reconstruction or renal function.

Acknowledgements

I would like to thank my colleagues Dr Caron Sandhu (consultant radiologist, Guy's and St Thomas' NHS Foundation Trust, London), Mr Jonathan Glass (consultant urologist, Guy's and St Thomas' NHS Foundation Trust, London) and Mr Adrian Joyce (consultant urologist, The Leeds Teaching Hospitals NHS Trust, Leeds) for their helpful discussions and advice.

References

1. Jeyabalan A, Lain KY. Anatomic and functional changes of the upper urinary tract during pregnancy. *Urol Clin North Am* 2007;34:1–6.
2. FitzGerald MP, Graziano S. Anatomic and functional changes of the lower urinary tract during pregnancy. *Urol Clin North Am* 2007;34:7–12.
3. Chaliha C, Stanton SL. Urological problems in pregnancy. *BJU Int* 2002;89:469–76.
4. Macejko AM, Schaeffer AJ. Asymptomatic bacteriuria and symptomatic urinary tract infections during pregnancy. *Urol Clin North Am* 2007;34:35–42.
5. Nicolle L.E. Screening for asymptomatic bacteriuria in pregnancy. In: *Canadian Guide to Clinical Preventive Health Care*. Ottawa: Health Canada; 1994. p. 100–6.
6. Smaill F, Vazquez JC. Antibiotics for asymptomatic bacteriuria in pregnancy. *Cochrane Database Syst Rev* 2007;(2):CD000490.
7. Loughlin KR. Urologic radiology during pregnancy. *Urol Clin North Am* 2007;34:23–6.
8. Biyani CS, Joyce AD. Urolithiasis in pregnancy. I: pathophysiology, fetal considerations and diagnosis. *BJU Int* 2002:89;811–18.
9. Spencer JA, Chahal R, Kelly A, Taylor K, Eardley I, Lloyd SN. Evaluation of painful hydronephrosis in pregnancy: magnetic resonance urographic patterns in physiological dilatation versus calculous obstruction. *J Urol* 2004;171:256–60.
10. EAU/AUA Nephrolithiasis Guideline Panel. *2007 Guideline for the Management of Ureteral Calculi*. Linthicum: American Urological Association and European Association of Urology; 2007. p. 46–7 [www.auanet.org/guidelines/uretcal07.cfm].
11. Biyani CS, Joyce AD. Urolithiasis in pregnancy. II: management. *BJU Int* 2002;89:819–23.
12. Pais VM, Payton AL, LaGrange CA. Urolithiasis in pregnancy. *Urol Clin North Am* 2007;34:43–52.
13. Brown MA, Holt JL, Mangos GJ, Murray N, Curtis J, Homer C. Microscopic hematuria in pregnancy: relevance to pregnancy outcome. *Am J Kidney Dis* 2005;45:667–73.
14. Morales JP, Georganas M, Khan MS, Dasgupta P, Reidy JF. Embolization of a bleeding renal angiomyolipoma in pregnancy: case report and review. *Cardiovasc Intervent Radiol* 2005;28:265–8.
15. Martin FM, Rowland RG. Urologic malignancies in pregnancy. *Urol Clin North Am* 2007;34:53–9.
16. Hautmann RE, Volkmer BG. Pregnancy and urinary diversion. *Urol Clin North Am* 2007;34:71–88.
17. Greenwell TJ, Venn SN, Creighton S, Leaver RB, Woodhouse CR. Pregnancy after lower urinary tract reconstruction for congenital abnormalities. *BJU Int* 2003;92:773–7. Erratum in: *BJU Int* 2004;93:655.
18. National Radiological Protection Board (NRPB, now Health Protection Agency HPA). *Advice on Exposure to Ionising Radiation During Pregnancy*. Didcot: NRPB; 1998.

Section 7

Surgical and medical issues specific to renal transplant patients

Chapter 18

Surgical issues of renal and renal/pancreas transplantation in pregnancy

John Taylor

Introduction

Both renal and pancreatic transplantation have increased during the past few decades and thus the potential complications associated with pregnancy, and indeed the care of women during pregnancy and delivery, requires careful management. In 2006 within the UK there were 416 cases of renal transplantation in women of childbearing age and 51 cases of renal/pancreas transplantation. Knowledge of the surgical procedures performed at transplantation can have important implications for the woman's care, particularly if a caesarean section is required.

Renal transplantation

The transplanted kidney is placed extraperitoneally in the false pelvis, lying lateral or anterior to the iliac vessels. The renal artery and vein are commonly anastomosed to the external iliac vessels in an end-to-side configuration. The transplant ureter crosses the external iliac vessels, usually close to the inguinal ligament and anastomosed to the most convenient place on the bladder, i.e. anterior and lateral.

In paediatric renal transplantation for recipients of less than 20 kg, the kidney is anastomosed to the aorta and vena cava. The transplant is placed behind the ascending colon and the ureter runs down to the bladder adjacent to the native ureter above the pelvic brim. The vesicoureteric anastomosis, though, is likely to be closer to the midline and more anterior on the bladder. Thus the transplant ureter is at a greater risk with subsequent pelvic surgery.

At least 10% of renal transplants will have two renal arteries. These can both be anastomosed end-to-side on the external iliac artery. A common variation is to divide the internal iliac artery and anastomose this end-to-end with a renal artery. The renal transplant vessels are not usually an issue during pregnancy. In the event of surgical dissection along the external iliac vessels or towards the renal transplant hilum, the renal vessels are at risk and great care and experience are essential.

Ureteric obstruction

A normal ultrasound without urinary obstruction before pregnancy is recommended. A dilated ureter in the absence of obstruction is not a contraindication to pregnancy.

However, it is important to know the state of the ureter prior to pregnancy, as the presence of hydronephrosis prepregnancy is associated with an increase in infections and lithiasis.[1] During pregnancy, hydronephrosis is expected and can worsen pre-existing dilation.

Despite its pelvic location, obstruction of the transplant ureter by the expanding uterus is unusual but has been reported and may be a consideration if polyhydramnios is present. A rise in serum creatinine is the essential feature of an obstructed renal transplant and in suspected obstruction an ultrasound of the transplanted kidney and bladder will facilitate achieving a diagnosis. However, pre-existing hydronephrosis of the transplanted kidney together with pregnancy-induced hydronephrosis can make ultrasonographic interpretation difficult. Clinical signs such as pain and renal colic normally associated with obstruction are not as reliable, as the transplanted kidney is denervated and symptoms absent or modified. The diagnosis is confirmed by improvement in renal function after relief of the obstruction. Renal obstruction can occur without hydronephrosis, where the ureter and renal pelvis are surrounded by fibrosis, which may be secondary to earlier urine leakage or infection.

Treatment depends on the extent of the deterioration in renal function and other complicating factors such as urinary tract infection. Aggressive intervention in cases of mild obstruction may cause more harm when compared with careful monitoring of the situation. A partial obstruction in the absence of urinary infection is not damaging in the 12–24 hour time frame, allowing time for thought. However, a low threshold for intervention is needed if the obstruction worsens. Simple interventions such as turning the patient onto the side away from the transplant kidney or the reduction of amniotic fluid volume can alleviate the obstruction.

The distinction between partial and significant obstruction is based on serial observation of renal function and input from the attending nephrologist.

In the presence of significant obstruction with hydronephrosis, a nephrostomy, an antegrade pyelogram and subsequent J stent placement is the most appropriate intervention.[2] Retrograde examination and the insertion of a stent can be attempted, but there is often difficulty accessing the transplant ureter owing its anterior location. It is important to note that obstruction can still occur with a J stent in place, especially if the stent is a tight fit in the ureter or becomes kinked, blocking the internal lumen.

The time of delivery for women with renal transplants is usually delayed until the onset of labour if maternal and fetal conditions remain satisfactory.[3] Despite its pelvic location, the transplanted kidney rarely produces dystocia and is not injured during vaginal delivery.[4] Caesarean section is usually performed only for standard obstetric reasons. A lower segment approach is usually feasible but previous urological surgery may make it difficult.

Renal/pancreas transplantation

The aim of pancreas transplantation is to produce complete insulin independence and ameliorate the complications of diabetes. The first successful pancreas transplant was performed by Lillehei and colleagues at the University of Minnesota in 1966. About 1400 pancreas transplants are performed annually in the USA.[5]

In 2006, for women of childbearing age in the UK, 41 pancreas transplants were performed with kidney transplantation (both organs from the same donor) in women with renal failure who were insulin dependent.[6] This is referred to as simultaneous pancreas/kidney transplantation. Eight pancreas transplants were performed after a previously successful kidney transplant in what is known as pancreas after kidney transplantation. Two pancreas transplants alone were done in non-uraemic women with labile diabetes and hypoglycaemic unawareness.

The principles of pancreas transplant surgery include providing adequate arterial blood flow to the pancreas and duodenal segment, adequate venous outflow of the pancreas via the portal vein and management of the pancreatic exocrine secretions.[7] The native pancreas is not removed. Pancreas graft arterial revascularisation is typically accomplished using the recipient right common or external iliac artery. Systemic venous revascularisation usually involves the right common iliac vein or the right external iliac vein following suture ligation and division of the internal iliac veins. The kidney is based on the recipient left iliac vessels. Both organs may be transplanted through a midline incision and placed intraperitoneally.

Pancreatic exocrine drainage is handled by means of anastomosis of the duodenal segment to the bladder or anastomosis to the small intestine (Figure 18.1).

Diet

Following successful pancreas transplantation, no dietary restrictions are required. In fact, the diet can be liberalised to include virtually anything because blood sugar control is restored to normal, as is the HbA_{1c}.

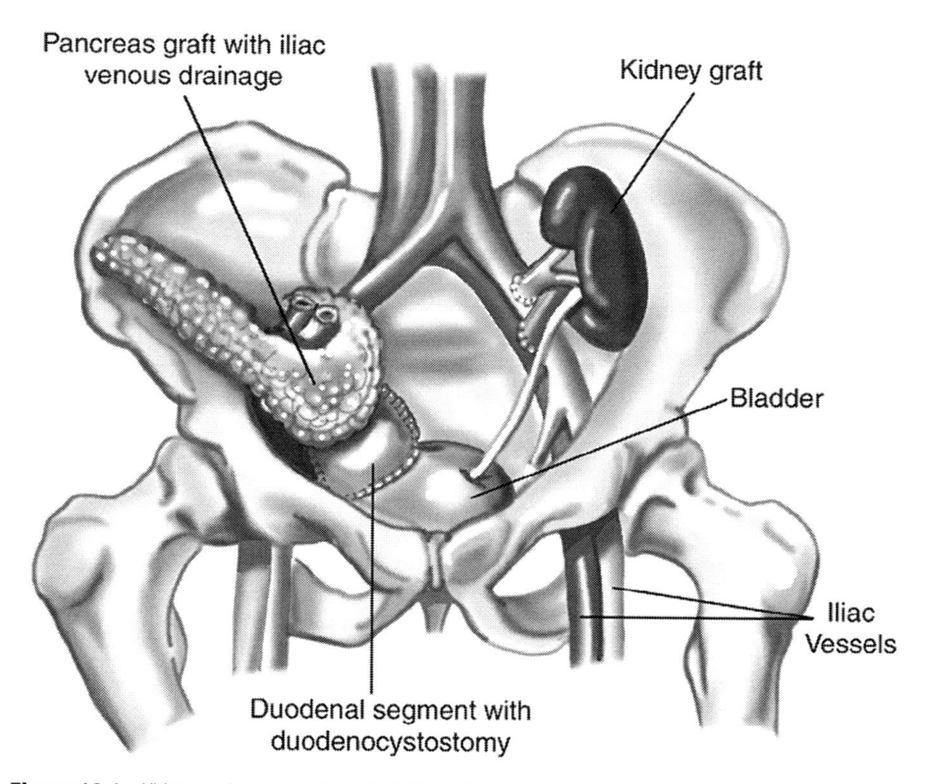

Figure 18.1. Kidney and pancreas transplantation with bladder drainage of exocrine secretions and systemic venous drainage – relationship to pelvis; reproduced with permission from Larsen[8]

Prognosis

The 2002 survival rates of kidney and pancreatic grafts and for patients (the most recent era analysed by the Scientific Registry of Transplant Recipients and International Pancreas Transplant Registry) were the best outcomes reported to date.[8] Survival rates at 1 year were 95% for patients, 91% for kidney grafts and 86% for pancreas grafts. Statistically and clinically, the outcome of kidney transplantation is significantly superior in patients receiving simultaneous pancreas/kidney transplant versus patients with type 1 diabetes receiving kidney transplant alone.[9] The anticipated half-life for insulin independence is 13 years.[10] The major benefit for these patients is improvement in quality of life through stabilisation of blood sugars, as beneficial effects on diabetic complications do not emerge for 5–10 years.[8]

Fertility and pregnancy after transplantation

Hypogonadism and fertility can improve after transplantation. Menstrual irregularity is still common after renal/pancreas transplantation and it is not clear whether this is due to the continued stress and morbidity of the first postoperative year, direct effects of the immunosuppressive agents on the reproductive axis, weight gain or aggravated insulin resistance in some already predisposed women. Pelvic surgery may compromise ovarian blood supply, resulting in primary hypogonadism after transplantation. Stress, including operations or infections, can temporarily disrupt the reproductive system in women in particular. Thus, there are many causes that are likely to contribute to the continuing reproductive dysfunction in women after transplantation. In one study evaluating hypogonadism in women before and after renal/pancreas transplantation, half of the women had hypogonadism prior to the transplantation, both primary and secondary, but 70% still had abnormal reproductive hormones 1 year later; these included one new case of primary hypogonadism, thought to be unrelated to surgery, and one case of ovarian hyperstimulation that improved with lowering the ciclosporin dose. Changes in reproductive function were unrelated to changes in prolactin concentration, but hyperprolactinaemia was still present at 1 year after transplantation in some women.[11]

The National Transplantation Pregnancy Registry (NTPR) was established to track the outcomes of all self-reported pregnancies in women who had had transplants in North America.[12] Listed in Box 18.1 are the 38 female renal/pancreas recipients who have reported 56 post-transplant pregnancies with 58 outcomes. Only one recipient reported gestational diabetes; regular insulin coverage was started at 24 weeks but was discontinued postpartum. Rejection occurred during three pregnancies; all three recipients went on to lose their grafts.

There were 46 liveborn among the renal/pancreas recipients, of which 25 were delivered by caesarean section. One caesarean section was complicated by a tear to the duodenal portion of the graft and required repair. Although the renal/pancreas offspring had lower mean gestational ages and birthweights compared with kidney-alone recipients, at a mean follow-up of 5.5 years all 45 children were reported healthy and developing well.

There were six graft losses within 2 years postpartum among the renal/pancreas recipients. Three recipients lost kidney function (two treated with transplantation, one with dialysis), one lost pancreas function (treated with insulin) and two recipients lost both pancreas and kidney function (one treated with re-transplantation, both subsequently died). Adequate graft function was reported by 26/37 (70%) of recipients,

Box 18.1. Pregnancy outcomes in 38 female renal/pancreas recipients with 56 pregnancies reported to the National Transplantation Pregnancy Registry (NTPR); reproduced with permission from Armenti *et al.*[12]

Maternal factors	
Mean transplant to conception interval	3.7 years
Hypertension during pregnancy	75%
Diabetes during pregnancy	2%
Infection during pregnancy	55%
Rejection episode during pregnancy	6%
Pre-eclampsia	34%
Graft loss within 2 years of delivery	16%
Outcomes (n = 58)[a]	
Therapeutic abortions	5%
Miscarriage	14%
Ectopic	2%
Stillbirth	0%
Live births	79%
Live births (n = 46)	
Mean gestational age	34 weeks
Premature (< 37 weeks)	78%
Mean birthweight	2096 g
Low birthweight (< 2500 g)	63%
Caesarean section	57%
Newborn complications	57%
Neonatal deaths (within 30 days of birth)[b]	1 (2%)
Immunosuppression by pregnancy	
Ciclosporin, azathioprine and prednisone	19 (34%)
Ciclosporin and prednisone	6 (11%)
Neoral®, azathioprine and prednisone	13 (23%)
Neoral® and prednisone	3 (5%)
Tacrolimus, azathioprine and prednisone	5 (9%)
Tacrolimus and azathioprine	2 (4%)
Tacrolimus and prednisone	4 (7%)
Tacrolimus and sirolimus	1 (2%)
Tacrolimus	1 (2%)
Gengraf®, azathioprine and prednisone	2 (4%)

[a] Includes twins

[b] One neonatal death due to sepsis (26 weeks, 624 g)

with a mean follow-up of 8.4 years since the pregnancy. Of the remaining 11 renal/pancreas recipients, three died and eight had varying degrees of graft function.

The UK Transplant Pregnancy Registry has reported three pregnancies in renal/pancreas recipients, with live births reported in two.[13] The outcome in the other was not reported.

Based on these data, pregnancy in a female pancreas transplant recipient should be treated as a high-risk pregnancy. Adverse outcomes for the mother and the baby are greater in renal/pancreas transplant recipients than those reported after kidney transplantation alone. Graft failure and infections are the greatest concerns for the mother, whereas miscarriage, small size, preterm birth and neonatal complications are the greatest concern for the baby. No significant increase in fetal malformations has been reported to date.

References

1. Hou, S. Pregnancy in chronic renal insufficiency and end-stage renal disease. *Am J Kidney Dis* 1999;33:235–52.
2. Cranston D, Little D. Urological complications after renal transplantation. In: Morris PJ, editor. *Kidney Transplantation: Principles and Practice*. 5th ed. Philadelphia: WB Saunders Company; 2001. p. 435–44.
3. EBPG Expert Group on Renal Transplantation. European best practice guidelines for renal transplantation. Section IV: Long-term management of the transplant recipient. IV.10. Pregnancy in renal transplant recipients. *Nephrol Dial Transplant* 2002;17 Suppl 4:50–5.
4. Davison JM. Pregnancy in renal allograft recipients: problems, prognosis and practicalities. *Baillieres Clin Obstet Gynaecol* 1994;8:501–25.
5. International Pancreas Transplant Registry [www.iptr.umn.edu/IPTR/database.html].
6. UK Transplant [www.uktransplant.org.uk/ukt/statistics/statistics.jsp].
7. Kaufman DB. *Pancreas Transplantation* [www.emedicine.com/med/topic2605.htm].
8. Larsen JL. Pancreas transplantation: indications and consequences. *Endocr Rev* 2004;25:919–46.
9. Ojo AO, Meier-Kriesche HU, Hanson JA, Leichtman A, Magee JC, Cibrik D, *et al.* The impact of simultaneous pancreas-kidney transplantation on patient survival. *Transplantation* 2001;71:82–90.
10. Rogers J, Baliga PK, Chavin KD, Lin A, Pullatt RC, Emovon O, *et al.* Long-term pancreas graft survival exceeds long-term kidney graft survival in simultaneous kidney-pancreas transplantation: differential effect of chronic calcineurin inhibitor therapy? *Am J Transpl* 2003;3 Suppl 5:322.
11. Mack-Shipman LR, Ratanasuwan T, Leone JP, Miller SA, Lyden ER, Erickson JM, *et al.* Reproductive hormones after pancreas transplantation. *Transplantation* 2000;70:1180–3.
12. Armenti VT, Radomski JS, Moritz MJ, Gaughan WJ, Hecker WP, Lavelanet A, *et al.* Report from the National Transplantation Pregnancy Registry (NTPR): outcomes of pregnancy after transplantation. *Clin Transpl* 2004:103–14.
13. Sibanda N, Briggs JD, Davison JM, Johnson RJ, Rudge CJ. Pregnancy after organ transplantation: a report from the UK Transplant pregnancy registry. *Transplantation* 2007;83:1301–7.

19

Chapter 19

Comorbid conditions that can affect pregnancy outcome in the renal transplant patient

Sue Carr

Many renal transplant patients have coexisting comorbid conditions that could influence the outcome of a pregnancy. It is essential that each comorbid condition is recognised and a management plan made for each of these at every stage of pregnancy – from the time of prepregnancy counselling to postpartum care. An overall integrated management plan for the pregnancy can then be developed and followed by the patient and the multidisciplinary team (Table 19.1).

Some of the more common comorbid conditions found in renal transplant patients are considered below.

Hypertension

A high proportion of renal transplant recipients are hypertensive before pregnancy (47–73%).[1] A further 25% will become hypertensive during pregnancy[2,3] and indeed, in the later stages of pregnancy, superimposed pre-eclampsia develops in 15–37% of renal transplant recipients.[4] Ciclosporin is associated with an increased incidence of hypertension during pregnancy.[5]

The presence of hypertension is one of the most important factors contributing to fetal growth restriction and/or preterm delivery in renal transplant patients.[2]

In pregnancy, mild to moderately raised blood pressure requires treatment with one or more antihypertensive medications. The aim is to maintain a safe level of blood pressure for mother, graft and fetus. However, lowering of blood pressure has been reported by some, but not all, authors to have an adverse impact upon fetal growth.[6–8] One meta-analysis[7] demonstrated that lowering maternal blood pressure resulted in increased incidence of small-for-gestational age infants but another analysis showed no overall risk of a small baby in women taking antihypertensive medication.[6]

Treatment of high blood pressure in pregnancy may reduce the risk of severe hypertension compared with placebo treatment or no treatment[9] but it is not clear whether it delays the development or progression of pre-eclampsia.[6,10] Blood pressure treatment may reduce the risk of fetal or neonatal morbidity (respiratory distress syndrome)[9] by contributing to avoidance of early gestation delivery.

Table 19.1. Management plan for pregnant renal transplant patients with additional comorbidities

Comorbidity	Prepregnancy	First trimester	Second trimester	Third trimester	Postpartum
General antenatal care in renal transplant patients	Confirm rubella antibody status. Hb electrophoresis. Advice re stopping smoking. Folic acid.	Folic acid. Discuss Down syndrome testing options. GTT in high-risk cases.	GTT at 24–28 weeks if indicated. Fetal USS monitoring.	Consider steroid cover in labour. Fetal USS monitoring.	
Renal transplant	Discuss implications of pregnancy on: • graft function • BP • proteinuria • risk of pre-eclampsia • obstetric risks. Immunosuppression: review current regimen and discuss/plan modification or conversion to alternative drugs, e.g azathioprine. Review other medications, e.g. statins, diuretics, ACE inhibitors.	Discuss prepregnancy issues if not seen before conception. Monitor BP. Monitor CNI levels. Monitor proteinuria. Monitor renal function. Advise re genetic issues: polycystic kidney disease or chronic pyelonephritis (baby will need a USS (record in maternal notes). Review other medications, e.g. statins, diuretics, ACE inhibitors.	Monitor BP. Monitor CNI levels. Monthly MSU. Monitor proteinuria. Monitor renal function. Consider GTT in tacrolimus-treated patients.	Monitor BP. Monitor CNI levels. Monthly MSU. Monitor proteinuria. Monitor renal function.	Monitor CNI levels. Monitor renal function. Arrange transplant OPD follow-up.
Recurrent UTIs	Discuss increased risk of UTIs and implications in pregnancy. Optimise immunosuppression and diabetic control. Advise re prevention of UTI. Plan monthly MSU and consider appropriate prophylaxis.	Monthly MSU. Treat infections promptly. Consider antibiotic prophylaxis if recurrent UTI. May require further investigation if additional pathology suspected clinically – USS.	Monthly MSU. Treat infections promptly. Consider antibiotic prophylaxis if recurrent UTI. May require further investigation if additional pathology suspected clinically – USS.	Monthly MSU. Treat infections promptly. Consider antibiotic prophylaxis if recurrent UTI. May require further investigation if additional pathology suspected clinically – USS.	Continue prophylaxis if previously prescribed. In mothers with chronic pyelonephritis and vesicoureteric reflux liaise with paediatricians re renal USS for the child.
Bone disease	Discuss and review current medication. Stop bisphosphonates and consider/convert phosphate binders.	Monitor bone biochemistry.	Monitor bone biochemistry.	Monitor bone biochemistry.	Monitor neonatal calcium levels if mother has marked hyperparathyroidism. Recommence the most suitable treatment for mother (depending on infant feeding). Avoid bisphosphonates if mother is planning further pregnancies.

Comorbidity	Prepregnancy	First trimester	Second trimester	Third trimester	Postpartum
Hypertension	Discuss implications of hypertension and safety of drugs in pregnancy. Plan conversion to alternative BP agents if required. Discuss risk of pre-eclampsia and consider aspirin prophylaxis.	Stop ACE inhibitors and ARBs, doxazosin etc. Convert other agents to methyldopa, labetalol or calcium channel blocker. Stop diuretics unless strong clinical indication to continue.	Monitor BP and titrate medication. Consider prophylactic aspirin.	Monitor BP and titrate medication.	Monitor BP. Depending on infant feeding, restart ACE inhibitors and ARBs, change methyldopa, labetalol to alternative antihypertensive agents.
Proteinuria	Discuss implications of proteinuria, possible thromboembolic risks and oedema.	Assess thromboembolic risk Assess need for LMWH prophylaxis or diuretics.	Monitor proteinuria. Assess thromboembolic risk. Assess need for LMWH prophylaxis. Monitor factor Xa levels in patients on LMWH.	Monitor proteinuria. Assess thromboembolic risk. Assess need for LMWH prophylaxis. Monitor factor Xa levels in patients on LMWH.	Continue LMWH prophylaxis for up to 6 weeks postpartum. Consider degree of proteinuria, mode of delivery, other risk factors for TED. Restart ACE inhibitors and/or ARBs.
Diabetes	Discuss risk in pregnancy and management plan. Increased risk of pre-eclampsia	Arrange liaison/combined follow-up with diabetes antenatal team. Monitor proteinuria. Monitor diabetes.	Aspirin prophylaxis. Monitor proteinuria. Monitor diabetes.	Aspirin prophylaxis. Monitor proteinuria. Monitor diabetes.	Monitor diabetes. Recommence ACE inhibitors and/or ARBs.
SLE	Discuss risks in pregnancy and increased risk of pre-eclampsia. Check anticardiolipin antibodies, lupus anti-coagulant. Check anti Ro and La antibodies.	Check and monitor lupus serology. Consider need for LMWH in antiphospholipid antibody-positive women. Plan fetal heart monitoring in Ro and La antibody-positive women.	Monitor factor Xa levels in patients on LMWH. Consider aspirin prophylaxis. Fetal heart scanning/monitoring in Ro and La antibody-positive women.	Monitor factor Xa levels in patients on LMWH. Fetal heart scanning/ monitoring in Ro and La antibody-positive women.	Review LMWH duration and whether there is a need to continue longer term. Depends on other factors: proteinuria, delivery, other risk factors, etc.
Anaemia	In women with CKD discuss possibility of anaemia requiring iron therapy and/or EPO. Check haematinics.	Monitor Hb: if < 11 g/dl consider Fe and or EPO on an individual patient basis.	Monitor Hb: if < 11 g/dl consider Fe and or EPO on an individual patient basis. Check haematinics.	Monitor Hb: if < 11 g/dl consider Fe and or EPO on an individual patient basis. Check haematinics.	Decide re continuation or discontinuation of therapy.

ACE = angiotensin-converting enzyme; ARB = angiotensin II receptor blocker; BP = blood pressure; CKD = chronic kidney disease; CNI = calcineurin inhibitor; EPO = erythropoietin; GTT = glucose tolerance test; Hb = haemoglobin; LMWH = low-molecular-weight heparin; MSU = midstream urine; OPD = outpatients department; SLE = systemic lupus erythematosus; TED = thromboembolic disease; USS = ultrasound scan; UTI = urinary tract infection

Renal transplant patients are at increased risk of cardiovascular disease and during pregnancy the impact of elevated blood pressure on long-term graft function and future maternal cardiovascular prognosis should be considered. It is well established that poorly controlled blood pressure leads to decline in renal function in native kidneys. Similarly, in renal transplant patients, lowering systolic blood pressure is associated with improved graft and patient survival.[11,12] As a result, numerous organisations have set target blood pressure levels for renal transplant patients.[13–15]

In general, in normal pregnancy, treatment is considered mandatory when blood pressure is above 160/100 mmHg. However, in the renal transplant patient there is often a degree of chronic kidney impairment and the consensus is to maintain the blood pressure at a lower level (less than 140/90 mmHg) to minimise progression of underlying renal impairment, to preserve graft function during pregnancy and to protect the maternal cardiovascular system. The ideal target level of blood pressure during pregnancy in the renal transplant patient is unknown.

Choice of antihypertensive agent

Methyldopa

In general, methyldopa (0.5–2.0 g/day) is the recommended first-line treatment for mild to moderate hypertension in renal transplant pregnancy.[13] Case–control studies have established the safety of methyldopa in pregnancy and long-term follow-up of children of mothers taking methyldopa showed no adverse effects.[9,16] Women should be warned of the potential adverse effects, including drowsiness and depression.

Beta blockers

Beta blockers (labetalol 0.2–1.2 g/day orally) are safe in pregnancy (although to be avoided in asthmatics) with the exception of atenolol, which is associated with an increase in small-for-gestational-age babies and should be avoided in pregnancy.[17]

Calcium channel blockers

Calcium channel blockers (nifedipine 40–80 mg/day orally) appear to be safe and well tolerated and are frequently used in pregnancy.

Diuretics

Diuretics may cause hypovolaemia and compromise in placental blood flow and should be avoided in pregnancy. However, some pregnant renal transplant patients with severe oedema due to the presence of proteinuria (from chronic allograft nephropathy or recurrent glomerular disease) may require diuretic therapy for treatment of severe fluid retention during pregnancy. In this situation, the risks versus the benefits of diuretic therapy should be assessed on an individual basis.

Angiotensin-converting enzyme inhibitors and angiotensin II receptor blockers

Angiotensin-converting enzyme (ACE) inhibitors and angiotensin II receptor blockers (ARBs) are contraindicated in pregnancy and should be discontinued.[18] In the second and third trimesters of pregnancy, ACE inhibitors have been associated with a fetopathy, comprising oligohydramnios, fetal growth restriction, hypocalvaria, renal dysplasia, anuria, renal failure and often intrauterine death.[4,18,19]

Previously, ACE inhibitors and ARBs were not considered teratogenic in early pregnancy but a recent study reported a 2.7 times greater risk of serious congenital malformation following exposure to ACE inhibitors in the first trimester of pregnancy. Malformations were reported in cardiovascular and central nervous systems (and in the renal tract on *post hoc* analysis).[18]

Reduction in risk of pre-eclampsia

There is no specific evidence relating to renal transplant patients, with most studies to date having investigated the general population.

Low-dose aspirin

Trials in the general population have shown conflicting results.[6,10] A meta-analysis in 1991 demonstrated that low-dose prophylactic aspirin reduced the risk of pre-eclampsia but two subsequent larger multicentre studies showed minimal effects. The secondary analyses identified that certain groups may derive some benefit from low-dose aspirin. Low-dose aspirin may be prescribed to women at high risk of pre-eclampsia (previous history of severe pre-eclampsia, diabetes, chronic hypertension, chronic kidney disease)[20,21] and is generally started after 12 weeks if there are no contraindications. Renal transplant patients are at increased risk of pre-eclampsia and may have additional comorbid factors such as diabetes or history of systemic lupus erythematosus (SLE) that increase this risk further. Hou[22] recommended treatment of women with renal insufficiency with prophylactic aspirin in the second trimester.

Dietary calcium supplementation

Initial reports were encouraging showing that supplementation with 1 g of calcium daily reduced the risk of pre-eclampsia. Subsequent trials were conflicting and secondary analyses have shown that this treatment may be beneficial in women with extremely low dietary calcium intake. Often renal transplant patients will have renal bone disease and may not be suitable candidates for supplemental calcium.[6]

Prophylactic antioxidants

There is some evidence that the prophylactic antioxidants vitamins C and E can reduce risk but the results of several large trials have failed to show any benefit and suggest an adverse effect on fetal growth. Vitamins C and E should thus not be used.

Infections in pregnancy

Urinary tract infections

Normal pregnancy-related changes in the urinary tract (diminished bladder tone and physiological dilation of ureter and renal pelvis) predispose all women to urinary tract infection (UTI) in pregnancy.

The risk of UTI in pregnancy is increased further in renal transplant patients owing to a number of factors:

- surgical factors, such as transplant surgery or re-implantation of ureters
- pre-existing urological abnormalities, such as bladder problems, calculi or reflux to native or transplant kidney

- underlying renal disease, such as reflux nephropathy
- immunosuppression
- comorbid diseases, such as diabetes.

The common pathogens include *Escherichia coli*, *Enterobacter*, *Klebsiella*, *Pseudomonas* and *Proteus*.[21,23,24]

UTI in pregnancy has been associated with preterm birth and low birthweight in some but not all studies.[23–26] One study reported increased incidence of atrial septal defect and another reported increased risk of developmental delay but further studies have not reported any increase in congenital malformation.[24]

In a transplant patient, it is important to ensure that immunosuppression is minimised and that diabetes, when present, is well controlled to reduce risk of infection.

Asymptomatic bacteriuria

As part of routine antenatal care, all women are screened for the presence of asymptomatic bacteriuria (ASB). In normal pregnancy, ASB affects 2–10% of women and 30% will develop a symptomatic UTI if left untreated. Antibiotic treatment should be prescribed, which will reduce the risk of symptomatic infections by up to 70%.

Commonly used antibiotics in renal transplant patients during pregnancy include cefalexin and trimethoprim (avoid in early pregnancy).[24,25]

It is important to perform a follow-up urine culture. The European Best Practice Guidelines (EBPG) recommendation is that all renal transplant patients should have a monthly midstream urine sample sent to screen for ASB and additional samples sent if symptoms develop.[13]

EBPG recommends 2 weeks of antibiotic treatment for ASB and prophylactic antibiotics for the remainder of the pregnancy following treatment of ASB.[13,27]

Symptomatic urinary tract infection

In renal transplant patients, the reported incidence of UTI varies from 19% to 42% in recent studies.[28–31] Thompson *et al.*[28] reported UTI in 26% of renal transplant pregnancies, Galdo *et al.*[29] 13.5%, Oliveira *et al.*[30] 42.3% and Hooi *et al.*[31] 13%.

In general, a pregnant renal transplant recipient with UTI should receive 7–10 days of antibiotic therapy[25] depending on local antibiotic policies. Pregnant renal transplant patients with a UTI in pregnancy should be considered for prophylactic antibiotic therapy for the remainder of the pregnancy with either low-dose cefalexin or trimethoprim (depending on stage of pregnancy and sensitivities) at night. Women receiving antibiotic prophylaxis for UTI prepregnancy should continue on an appropriate antibiotic through the pregnancy.

Pyelonephritis

The incidence of acute pyelonephritis in normal pregnancy is 1–2% and up to 40% in women with untreated bacteriuria in pregnancy. In a transplant patient, acute pyelonephritis can develop in either the native or transplanted kidney and, in view of the immunosuppressed state, the symptoms and signs may be difficult to ascertain. It is important to be alert to this possible diagnosis and to reduce the risk by monthly urinary screening and prompt treatment of urinary tract sepsis during pregnancy. Intravenous antibiotic therapy should be started promptly while awaiting specific urine culture and sensitivity results that will further guide management.

Viral and other infections

Cytomegalovirus

Following renal transplantation, patients are potentially at risk of cytomegalovirus (CMV) infection. or reactivation. At the time of transplantation, all transplant recipients and donor kidneys are tested for evidence of previous CMV infection. The presence of detectable immunoglobulin G (IgG) anti-CMV antibodies in the plasma indicates a previous CMV infection and is present in more than two-thirds of donors and recipients prior to transplantation.[32] A CMV-negative transplant recipient can be at risk of CMV infection from a CMV-positive transplant kidney and CMV-positive transplant recipients can be subject to reactivation of CMV virus or re-infection, usually related to high levels of immunosuppression. The risk of CMV infection is highest in the first year following renal transplantation. CMV-negative recipients of CMV-positive kidneys and CMV-positive recipients of CMV-positive kidneys who have been significantly immunosuppressed will receive prophylaxis against CMV infection in some units using ganciclovir or valganciclovir.[33]

In general, when patients delay pregnancy by 12–24 months, post-transplant CMV is unlikely to be a problem as the risk of acute rejection and the immunosuppressive drug levels are generally lower. However, in a pregnancy during the first 12 months following transplant, when the risk of acute rejection and immunosuppression levels are still quite high, CMV infection may occur.

In the fetus, approximately 90% of congenital infections are asymptomatic and affected children can present in later life with impaired psychomotor development and hearing, neurological, eye or dental abnormalities. In symptomatic congenital CMV, infants can develop splenomegaly, jaundice and a petechial rash. In the more severe form of the disease, cytomegalovirus inclusion disease, there can be multi-organ involvement with microcephaly, motor disability, chorioretinitis, cerebral calcifications, lethargy, respiratory distress and seizures.

When CMV infection is suspected, samples should be sent urgently for detection and quantification of CMV DNA using quantitative polymerase chain reaction (PCR).[33]

Rubella

Women with chronic kidney disease who may become pregnant should be vaccinated against rubella infection before renal transplant. The vaccine is a live vaccine and cannot be administered to an immunosuppressed patient.

Hepatitis C

The prevalence of hepatitis C virus (HCV) infection has increased in dialysis patients and hence there are an increasing number of HCV-positive patients who receive a renal transplant.

Worldwide, studies have reported 11–49% of renal transplant patients to be HCV-positive.[34,35] There is an increased risk of post-transplant liver disease in HCV-positive patients and immunosuppressive therapy can lead to an increased viral replication and increased viral load. The viral load, however, does not directly correlate with the presence of liver disease.

The effect of HCV infection on graft and patient survival following renal transplant is unclear as studies have shown conflicting results. Studies have shown that short-term patient survival is similar to that in non-HCV-positive patients but long-term outcomes are worse.[34,35] A recent large meta-analysis demonstrated increased mortality and reduced graft survival in over 6000 HCV antibody-positive patients.[34,35] This may be important in considering the impact of a pregnancy in an HCV-positive transplant patient with respect to a mother's long-term survival and ability to care for a child.

In pregnancy, vertical transmission of the HCV virus occurs in 5–10% of pregnancies of HCV RNA-positive mothers and is related to the viral load. Pregnancy should therefore be planned at a time of minimal viral load to reduce the risk of vertical transmission to the fetus. In non-transplant HCV-positive pregnancies, the outcome is usually good, with improvement in aminotransaminase levels during pregnancy reported in two studies.[34,36] However, one study revealed deterioration in histological findings in the liver following pregnancy. There appears to be no evidence of increased fetal malformation.

It is important that HCV infection is diagnosed early in infants of mothers who are HCV-positive using HCV DNA PCR as HCV antibodies are passively transferred from the mother. There is no evidence of transmission of HCV by breastfeeding.

There have been few reports of pregnancy in HCV-positive renal transplant patients (Table 19.2). Ventura *et al.*[36] recently reported three cases of pregnancy in HCV-positive renal transplant patients without chronic liver disease. In these three cases there was no evidence of progression of liver disease during follow-up 2 years postpartum.

Many patients with hepatitis C are treated with ribavirin, which is contraindicated in pregnancy because of teratogenicity in animal studies. It is advised that effective contraception be used during oral administration and for 6 months after treatment in women and in men.[37] Interferon is generally avoided in renal transplant patients.

Hepatitis B

The presence of hepatitis B virus (HBV) infection is increasing in the dialysis population and increasingly HBV-positive patients without evidence of liver disease on a liver biopsy are considered for renal transplantation. Some patients may acquire HBV following renal transplantation. Patients who are HBV DNA-positive require antiviral therapy following transplantation, which may need to be continued long term.

Table 19.2. Outcome of pregnancies reported in HCV-positive renal transplant recipients; data from Ventura *et al.*[36]

Years post-transplant	Serum creatinine (mg/dl)	HCV ELISA/HCV DNA PCR	Liver function and coagulation	Outcome (birthweight)
3	1.1	Positive/negative	Normal	Delivered at 38 weeks (3100 g) Infant HCV ELISA negative at 6 months
4	1.1 Normal blood pressure	Positive/positive	Normal	Delivered at 37 weeks (3020 g) Infant HCV ELISA negative at 6 months
3	0.8 High blood pressure 1 antihypertensive agent	Positive/positive	Normal	Delivered at 7 weeks (2450 g) Infant HCV ELISA negative at 6 months

ELISA = enzyme-linked immunosorbent assay; HCV = hepatitis C virus; PCR = polymerase chain reaction

Renal transplant patients with HBV infection have reduced survival and are at increased risk of graft loss. Outcomes are improving with improvements in antiviral therapies.[38] Lamivudine should be avoided in the first trimester of pregnancy.

In general, pregnancy is uneventful in women who are hepatitis B carriers and exacerbation of disease during pregnancy is uncommon. The most significant risk is of vertical transmission to the infant during delivery, which can occur in up to 80% of cases.[26,38,39] The administration of HBV immunoglobulin and vaccination is effective in reducing infection in the infant.

It is important that close liaison takes place between hepatologists, renal physicians and obstetricians when managing pregnancy in a renal transplant patient with hepatitis B or C positivity.

Herpes simplex

Persistent viral infections can occur in renal transplant patients, including herpes simplex infection. A child can be infected with herpes simplex as a result of spread due to contact at the time of birth. The risk of transmission can be reduced by caesarean delivery. Aciclovir is safe in pregnancy.[39]

Toxoplasmosis

Congenital toxoplasmosis has been reported following reactivation of this infection in an immunosuppressed mother.[26] The majority of infants with congenital toxoplasmosis (70–90%) are asymptomatic at birth but have a high risk of developing subsequent abnormalities, especially chorioretinitis with potential visual impairment, if adequate treatment is not given. Symptomatic infants may present the classic triad of chorioretinitis, hydrocephalus and intracranial calcification although other manifestations may include fever, rash, hepatosplenomegaly, microcephaly, seizures, jaundice, thrombocytopenia and sometimes lymphadenopathy. In addition, mental developmental delay, deafness, seizures and spasticity can be seen in a minority of untreated children.

This condition can be diagnosed pre- or postnatally using serology or PCR testing. Treatment is generally reported to improve prognosis in affected infants and is usually spiramycin (a macrolide antibiotic), pyrimethamine or sulfadiazine (unlicensed).[40] These agents may interact with immunosuppressive agents and some are renally excreted: specific advice should be sought from a pharmacist and infectious disease specialist.[40]

Haematological abnormalities

Anaemia

In normal pregnancy the red cell mass increases under the control of erythropoeitin (EPO) but, because the relative increase in plasma volume is greater, haemodilution occurs and there is a decrease in haemoglobin concentration. As a result of this a renal transplant patient may become anaemic as well as iron deficient or may have anaemia related to chronic renal impairment. Women with impaired transplant function may be receiving treatment with EPO before pregnancy or require this treatment during pregnancy if renal transplant function has deteriorated. It is important to exclude other causes of anaemia including vitamin deficiencies, bleeding and haemolysis in an anaemic renal transplant patient.[41]

In addition, immunosuppressive agents, particularly azathioprine (and mycophenolate, which is contraindicated in pregnancy), can cause bone marrow suppression.

Anaemia if untreated can cause both fetal and maternal morbidity. In the fetus, anaemia can lead to an increased risk of infections and is associated with growth restriction and preterm birth.[42,43] In the mother, cardiovascular symptoms may develop, including breathlessness and delayed wound healing and infection.[42]

Anaemia in pregnancy can be treated with oral iron supplementation but parenteral iron may be required in women who are unable to tolerate oral iron supplements or who are receiving EPO therapy. A recently published Cochrane review[44] concluded that intravenous iron enhanced haematological response compared with oral iron but concerns were expressed regarding lack of large good-quality trials and lack of information on adverse events.

Iron sucrose is reported to be effective in the treatment of severe anaemia in pregnancy, anaemia unresponsive to oral iron supplementation and women receiving EPO therapy with iron deficiency or functional iron deficiency.[45]

Iron dextran has been used in pregnancy owing to ease of administration but in view of the incidence of adverse reactions iron sucrose is generally preferred in women receiving EPO.

In general, for a pregnant transplant patient, the aim is to maintain the haemoglobin level at around 11 g/dl. If haemoglobin falls below this level, the following investigations should be considered:

- ferritin level, transferrin saturation ratio
- vitamin B12 and folate
- blood film to exclude red cell fragmentation
- haemolysis screen
- parvovirus infection test.

Anaemia in pregnancy may be exacerbated by anaemia of chronic kidney disease due to transplant dysfunction (above additional factors excluded). Magee *et al.*[46] found that serum EPO levels were inappropriately low and rate of erythropoiesis low in transplant patients in a study comparing 30 transplant patients with 30 normal pregnant controls.

Hou[39] suggested EPO should be started if haematocrit falls below 30% and the dose titrated to maintain haemoglobin at 10–12 g/dl.

There are several reports of the safe use of EPO in renal transplant pregnancies.[47–49] Goshorn and Yuell[48] reported successful use of darbepoetin-alpha in a woman with impaired renal function (serum creatinine 203 μmol/l) and haemoglobin 7.5 g/dl at 28 weeks of gestation. EPO does not appear to cross the placenta[48] and has not been reported to be teratogenic but it has been associated with increases in blood pressure which needs careful monitoring.[49]

Post-transplant erythrocytosis

Post-transplant erythrocytosis (PTE) is defined as a haematocrit of over 51% and occurs in up to 20% of transplant patients, usually within the first 2 years of transplantation. The aetiology of PTE remains uncertain but it may be due to an over-secretion of EPO by native kidneys, the transplanted kidney or the liver. Erythrocytosis, if untreated, is associated with increased incidence of vascular and thromboembolic disorders. This condition is often treated with ACE inhibitors or ARBs which are contraindicated in pregnancy. Pregnant transplant patients known to have PTE need regular monitoring of the haemocrit and assessment of thromboembolic risk. If haemocrit rises significantly, venesection could be considered.[50]

Hyperlipidaemia

An increasing number of renal transplant recipients are treated with statin therapy for hypercholesterolaemia and to reduce the risk of coronary events, stroke and cardiovascular morbidity following renal transplantation.[51]

Animal studies have suggested that statins are teratogenic and case reports in humans reported central nervous system and limb defects in newborns exposed to statins *in utero*.[19,52–54] The highly lipophilic statins such as atorvastatin and simvastatin reach concentrations in the fetal circulation that are similar to maternal levels. These agents are contraindicated in pregnancy. Pravastatin is more hydrophilic and to date has not been associated with abnormal pregnancy outcomes.[52] These drugs should be discontinued before conception.

Skeletal problems

Pre-existing bone problems are a common consideration in the pregnant renal transplant patient.

Seventy-seven percent of renal transplant patients have abnormal parathyroid hormone concentrations[55] owing to chronic renal impairment following renal transplantation or because of incomplete resolution of pre-transplant hyperparathyroidism. In addition, some patients may have had a previous parathyroidectomy.

Severe primary hyperparathyroidism is associated with poor pregnancy outcome, with increased neonatal death (31%) and hypocalcaemia (19%).[56] In the transplant patient, hyperparathyroidism is generally mild and asymptomatic but there are few published data regarding the outcome of pregnancy. In a single case report of a renal transplant patient with mild tertiary hyperparathyroidism (adjusted calcium 2.74 mmol/l, parathyroid hormone 14 pmol/l), serum calcium level remained stable during pregnancy despite deterioration in renal function. The infant developed mild neonatal hypocalcaemia requiring treatment with intravenous calcium gluconate.

It is important that infants of mothers with hyperparathyroidism are monitored for clinical signs of hypocalcaemia (irritability, jerking, grimacing and convulsions) and that serum calcium levels are checked regularly following delivery.

Renal transplant patients may be prescribed numerous medications for the management of skeletal problems, including: calcium supplements, alfacalcidol, phosphate binders, bisphosphonates and, more recently, cinacalcet. The use of these agents must be careful considered before and during pregnancy (Table 19.3). Calcium supplements and alfacalcidol are safe in pregnancy and should be continued. Some phosphate binders are safe, including calcium carbonate-based binders, but the newer phosphate binders, including sevelamer and lanthanum carbonate, should be avoided in pregnancy although there is little evidence at present and each case must be assessed individually.

As a result of steroid therapy pre- and/or post-transplantation, some young women who have had a transplant may have osteoporosis or osteopenia. Bisphosphonates used in the treatment and prevention of osteoporosis act to inhibit bone resorption. Bisphosphonates are known to cross the placenta[57] but very little is known about the safety of bisphosphonates in pregnancy.

Table 19.3. Management of skeletal problems in pregnant renal transplant patients

	Usual treatment	Treatment during pregnancy
Secondary hyperparathyroidism	Phosphate binders	Continue calcium carbonate Discontinue sevelamer or lanthanum
	Alfacalcidol	Continue alfacalcidol
Tertiary hyperparathyroidism	Parathyroidectomy	In very severe cases consider surgery in second trimester[55] Monitor calcium levels closely in pregnancy
	Cinacalcet	Discontinue cinacalcet
Previous parathyroidectomy	Alfacalcidol	Continue alfacalcidol
	Calcium supplements	Continue calcium supplements
Osteoporosis	Calcium supplements	Continue calcium supplements
	Bisphosphonates	Discontinue bisphosphonates
Osteopenia	Calcium supplements	Continue calcium supplements

Information is mainly from animal studies at present. Patlas *et al.*[57] reported fetal skeletal abnormalities with shortening of bony diaphyses in rats receiving alendronate compared with control animals. They concluded that alendronate probably accumulates in fetal bones.

Another study in rats reported an association between alendronate administration and maternal hypocalcaemia in late pregnancy that was proportional to the duration of treatment. Delivery in alendronate-treated animals was protracted, leading to fetal loss, but this effect was reversible with intravenous calcium. The authors concluded that maternal bisphosphonate therapy led to an inability to mobilise calcium via bone resorption.[58]

One report in humans found no adverse effect of bisphosphonates on the human fetus,[59] which was endorsed by the report of Onroy *et al.*[60] of no adverse effects on pregnancy outcome when alendronate was taken prepregnancy or in early pregnancy in 24 pregnancies.

At present there is little evidence available regarding the safety of these agents in pregnancy. In general, bisphosphonates should be discontinued prepregnancy or as soon as pregnancy is suspected and careful consideration should be given before these agents are prescribed to women of childbearing age.

Thromboembolic risk

Renal transplant patients often have proteinuria during pregnancy or other comorbid factors which may increase thromboembolic risk. In this situation a pregnant renal transplant patient may be prescribed prophylaxis with low-molecular-weight heparin (LMWH), which is not associated with an increased risk of osteoporosis in pregnancy.[61]

Other comorbid diseases

Diabetes

A renal transplant patient may have end-stage renal disease due to diabetic nephropathy or may have developed new-onset diabetes after transplant (NODAT). In addition, patients receiving steroids and tacrolimus are at increased risk of glucose intolerance. A meta-analysis reported that tacrolimus-treated patients had five times the risk of post-transplant diabetes compared with patients treated with ciclosporin.[62] Therefore, glucose tolerance testing may be warranted during pregnancy in tacrolimus-treated patients. A recent review reported that 3–12% of pregnant renal transplant patients had diabetes.[4,63]

There are several additional issues to consider in a diabetic renal transplant recipient who is pregnant. The risks of preterm delivery and pre-eclampsia are increased by both diabetes and renal transplantation. Fetal growth restriction is less common in diabetic pregnancies. Patients with diabetic nephropathy affecting the transplanted kidney may have significant proteinuria during pregnancy (especially if ACE inhibitors and ARBs have been discontinued at conception) and present an increased thromboembolic risk during pregnancy as previously described. In addition, oedema and severe nephrotic syndrome may require diuretic treatment during pregnancy.

The diabetic patient may be treated with oral hypoglycaemic agents but could require insulin treatment during pregnancy. Metformin has been used in pregnancy in Australasia and is currently the subject of a clinical trial.[19]

In the pregnant diabetic renal transplant patient, it is very important to maintain close liaison between specialist renal and diabetic obstetric teams throughout the pregnancy.

Systemic lupus erythematosus

One to two percent of patients on the renal transplant waiting list have lupus nephritis as a cause of end-stage renal disease. The success of renal transplantation in this group is comparable to that of other recipient groups, with graft survival of 70–90% at 1 year.[64] SLE is a disease that frequently affects young women and pregnancy is often a consideration for this group of renal transplant recipients. The transplant patient with an underlying diagnosis of SLE can face several additional problems during pregnancy, including recurrent miscarriages (see Chapter 9). A further consideration in this group is the potential presence of lupus anticoagulant and anticardiolipin antibody in some patients who may require prophylactic LMWH therapy during pregnancy. The presence of anti-Ro and anti-La antibodies leads to an increased risk of fetal cardiac problems. In this situation there is a risk of congenital heart block. SLE is associated with increased risk of preterm delivery and pre-eclampsia.

A recent publication of retrospective data from the National Transplantation Pregnancy Registry (NTPR) data reported on outcomes in 38 pregnancies of women with a renal transplant and previous lupus nephritis compared with 60 non-SLE transplant pregnancies.[63] McGrory *et al.*[64] reported no difference in live birth rate, transplant acute rejection, graft survival or mortality in SLE versus non-SLE transplant recipients.

The preterm birth rate was high in both SLE and non-SLE transplant pregnancies (42% versus 55%) as was the rate of low birthweight. The incidence of hypertension, diabetes and caesarean section was lower in SLE transplant patients in this study.

Post-transplant malignancy

Renal transplant patients are at increased risk of malignancy compared with the general population. In particular, the risks of skin cancers, lymphomas and *in situ* carcinomas including carcinoma of the cervix are increased.[65]

Cervical neoplasia

Several authors have reported increased incidence of cervical neoplasia in renal transplant recipients.[65–70] Kasiske *et al.*[70] reported the incidence of cervical cancer to be increased five-fold. However, Halpert *et al.*[67] reported a 17-fold increase and Ozsaran *et al.*[68] reported a 75% incidence in heavily immunosuppressed kidney transplant recipients.

The diagnosis of precancerous changes in the cervix was associated with an increased risk of preterm birth in an Australian study of 17 633 women between 1982 and 2000. The risk was increased in treated and untreated women compared with the general population.[69] In view of the increased risk it is important that renal transplant patients undergo annual cervical screening to detect early disease,[70,71] which can then be treated prepregnancy.

Abnormal smears should be followed by colposcopy but biopsies should be deferred until the second trimester to minimise the risk of pregnancy loss. If the diagnosis is made during pregnancy, definitive management with ablation or excision should be delayed until postpartum.[72] More aggressive lesions including carcinoma *in situ* may require more definitive management during pregnancy.[72]

Post-transplant lymphoproliferative disorder

Post-transplant lymphoproliferative disorder (PTLD) occurs in approximately 1–3% of renal transplant recipients, most commonly in the first year following transplantation.[73] The risk is related to the degree of immunosuppressive therapy and, because immunosuppressive regimes have become more aggressive, the incidence has increased in recent years. The risk is higher in patients under 25 years of age and in Caucasians. The survival rate depends upon the tumour type but it is generally between 25% and 35%. There are no published data on the outcome of pregnancy in renal transplant patients who have suffered PTLD.

References

1. Armenti VT, Ahlswede KM, Ahlswede BA, Jarrell BE, Mortitz MJ, Burke JF. National transplantation pregnancy registry outcomes of 154 pregnancies in cyclosporine treated female kidney transplant recipients. *Transplantation* 1994;57:502–5.
2. Sibanda N, Briggs D, Davison JM, Johnson RJ, Rudge CJ. Outcomes of pregnancies after renal transplantation: A report of the UK Transplant Registry. *Hypertens Pregnancy* 2004;23 Suppl 1:136.
3. Lindheimer MD, Davison JM, Katz AI. The kidney and hypertension in pregnancy: twenty exciting years. *Semin Nephrol* 2001;21:173–89.
4. McKay DB, Josephson MA. Pregnancy in recipients of solid organs: Effects on mother and child. *N Engl J Med* 2006;354:1281–93.
5. Fischer T, Neumayer HH, Fischer R, Barenbrock M, Schobel HP, Lattrell BC, *et al.* Effect of pregnancy on long term kidney function in renal transplant recipients treated with cyclosporine and with azathioprine. *Am J Transplant* 2005;5:2732–9.
6. Duley L, Meher S, Abalos E. Management of pre-eclampsia. *BMJ* 2006;332:463–8.
7. von Dadelszen P, Ornstein MP, Bull SB, Logan AG, Koren G, Magee LA. Fall in mean arterial pressure and fetal growth restriction in pregnancy hypertension. *Lancet* 2000;355:87–92.
8. Homuth V, Dechend R, Luft FC. When should pregnant women with an elevated blood pressure be treated? *Nephrol Dial Transplant* 2003;18:1456–7.
9. Magee LA, Ornstein MP, von Dadelszen P. Fortnightly review: management of hypertension in pregnancy. *BMJ* 1999;318:1332–6.
10. Broughton-Pipkin F, Roberts JM. Hypertension in pregnancy. *J Hum Hypertens* 2000;14:705–24.
11. Opelz G, Wujciak T, Ritz E. Association of chronic kidney graft failure with recipient blood pressure. Collaborative Transplant Study. *Kidney Int* 1998;53:217–22.
12. Opelz G, Dohler B, Collaborative Transplant Study. Improved long term outcomes after renal transplantation associated with blood pressure control. *Am J Transplant* 2005;5:2725–31.

13. EBPG Expert Group on Renal Transplantation. European best practice guidelines for renal transplantation. Long-term management of the transplant patient Section IV: Pregnancy in renal transplant patients. *Nephrol Dial Transplant* 2002;17 Suppl 4:50–5.
14. Abbud-Filho M, Adams PL, Alberú J, Cardella C, Chapman J, Cochat, P, *et al.* A report of the Lisbon Conference on the care of the kidney transplant recipient. *Transplantation* 2007;83(8 Suppl): S1–22.
15. Kidney Disease Outcomes Quality Initiative (K/DOQI). K/DOQI clinical practice guidelines on hypertension and antihypertensive agents in chronic kidney disease. *Am J Kidney Dis* 2004;43(5 Suppl 1):S1–290.
16. Sibai BM. Treatment of hypertension in pregnant women. *N Engl J Med* 1996;335:257–64.
17. Abalos E, Duley L, Steyn D, Henderson-Smart D. Antihypertensive drug therapy for mild to moderate hypertension during pregnancy. *Cochrane Database Syst Rev* 2001;(2):CD002252.
18. Cooper WO, Hernandez-Diaz S, Arbogast PG, *et al.* Major congenital malformations after first trimester exposure to ACE inhibitors. *N Engl J Med* 2006;354:2443–54.
19. Kyle PM. Drugs and the fetus. *Curr Opin Obstet Gynecol* 2006;18:93–9.
20. CLASP: a randomised trial of low-dose aspirin for the prevention and treatment of pre-eclampsia among 9364 pregnant women. *Lancet* 1994;343:619–29.
21. Royal College of Obstetrics and Gynaecologists. *Pre-eclampsia.* London: RCOG Press; 2003, p. 312.
22. Hou S. Pregnancy in chronic renal insufficiency and end-stage renal disease. *Am J Kidney Dis* 1999;33:235–52.
23. Davison JM. Renal complications that may occur in pregnancy. In: Davison AM, Cameron JS, Grunfeld JP, Ponticelli C, Ritz E, Winearls CG, *et al.*, editors. *Oxford Textbook of Clinical Nephrology.* 3rd ed. Oxford: Oxford University Press; 2005, p. 2233–42.
24. Davison JM. Renal disorders in pregnancy. *Curr Opin Obstet Gynecol* 2001;13:109–14.
25. Dwyer PL, O'Reilly M. Recurrent urinary tract infection in the female. *Curr Opin Obstet Gynecol* 2002;14:537–43.
26. Stratta P, Canavese C, Giacchino F, Mesiano P, Quaglia M, Rosetti M. pregnancy in kidney transplantation: Satisfactory outcomes and harsh realities. *J Nephrol* 2003;16:792–806.
27. Davison JM, Milne JEC. Pregnancy and renal transplantation. *Br J Urol* 1997;80 Suppl 1:29–32.
28. Thompson BC, Kingdon EJ, Tuck SM, Fernando ON, Sweny P. Pregnancy in renal transplant recipients: the Royal free Hospital experience. *Q J Med* 2003;96:837–44.
29. Galdo T, Gonzalez M, Espinoza N, Qunitero N, Espinoza O, Herrera S, *et al.* Impact of pregnancy on the function of transplanted kidneys. *Transplant Proc* 2005;37:1577–9.
30. Oliveira LG, Sass N, Sato JL, Osaki KS, Medina Pestana JO. Pregnancy after renal transplantation – a five-yr single-center experience. *Clin Transplant* 2007;21:301–4.
31. Hooi LS, Rozina G, Wan-Shaariah MY, Teo SM, Tan CHH, Bavanandan S, *et al.* Pregnancy in patients with renal transplants in Malaysia. *Med J Malaysia* 2003;58:27–36.
32. Vella J, Bennett W, Brennan DC. *Cytomegalovirus Infection in Renal Transplant Recipients.* UpToDate; 2008 [www.uptodate.com].
33. British Transplantation Society. *Guidelines for the prevention and management of cytomegalovirus disease after solid organ transplantation.* London: British Transplantation Society; 2004 [www.bts.org.uk/standards.htm].
34. Natov S, Pereira BJG. *Hepatitis C Virus Infection and Renal Transplantation.* UpToDate; 2007 [www.uptodate.com].
35. Bacq Y. *Pregnancy in Women with Underlying Chronic Liver Disease.* UpToDate; 2007 [www.uptodate.com].
36. Ventura AMG, Imperiali N, Dominguez B, del Pradoa Sierra M, Munoz MA, Morales JM. Successful pregnancies in female kidney transplant recipients with hepatitis C infection. *Transplant Proc* 2003;35:1078–80.
37. Joint Formulary Committee. *British National Formulary.* London: British Medical Association and Royal Pharmaceutical Society of Great Britain [bnf.org/bnf].
38. Rose BD, Lok ASF. *Hepatitis B Virus Infection in Renal Transplant Recipients.* UpToDate; 2007 [www.uptodate.com].
39. Hou S. Pregnancy in renal transplant patients. *Adv Ren Replace Ther* 2003;10:40–7.

40. Johnson KE. *Overview of TORCH Infections*. UpToDate; 2007 [www.uptodate.com].
41. Coyne DW, Brennan DC. *Anaemia in the Renal Transplant Recipient*. UpToDate; 2007 [www.uptodate.com].
42. Breymann C. The use of iron sucrose complex for anaemia in pregnancy and postpartum period. *Semin Hematol* 2006;43 Suppl 6:S28–31.
43. Sifakis S, Angelakis E, Vardaki E, Koumantaki Y, Matalliotakis I, Koumantakis E. Erythropoetin in the treatment of iron deficiency anaemia during pregnancy. *Gynecol Obstet Invest* 2001;51:150–6.
44. Reveiz L, Gyte GM, Cuervo LG. Treatments for iron-deficiency anaemia in pregnancy. *Cochrane Database Syst Rev* 2007;(2):CD003094.
45. Perewusnyk G, Huch R, Huch A, Breymann C. Parenteral iron therapy in obstetrics: 8 years experience with iron sucrose complex. *Br J Nutr* 2002;88:3–10.
46. Magee LA, von Dadelszen P, Darley J, Beguin Y. Erythropoiesis and renal transplant pregnancy. *Clin Transplant* 2000;14:127–35.
47. Thorp M, Pulliam J. Use of recombinant erythropoietin in a pregnant transplant recipient. *Am J Nephrol* 1998;18:448–51.
48. Goshorn J, Yuell T. Darbepoetin alfa treatment for post-renal transplantation anaemia during pregnancy. *Am J Kid Dis* 2005;46:E81–6.
49. Kashiwagi M, Breymann C, Huch R, Huch A. Hypertesnion in a pregnancy with renal anemia after recombinant human erythropoietin (rhEPO) therapy. *Arch Gynecol Obstet* 2002;267:54–6.
50. Rose BD, Brennan DC, Sayegh MH. *Erythrocytosis Following Renal Transplantation*. UpToDate; 2007 [www.uptodate.com].
51. Holdaas H, Fellström B, Cole E, Nyberg G, Olsson AG, Pedersen TR, *et al.* Long-term cardiac outcomes in renal transplant recipients receiving fluvastatin: the ALERT extension study. *Am J Transplant* 2005;5:2929–36.
52. Patel C, Edgerton L, Flake D. What precautions should we take with statins for women of child-bearing age? *J Fam Pract* 2006;55:75–7.
53. Edison RJ, Muenke M. Central nervous system and limb abnormalities in case report of first-trimester statin exposure. *New Engl J Med* 2004;350:1579–82.
54. Kenis I, Tartakover-Matalon S, Cherepin N, Drucker L, Fishman A, Pomeranz M, *et al.* Simvastatin has deleterious effects on human first trimester placental explants. *Hum Reprod* 2005;20:2866–72.
55. Morton A, Dalzell F, Isbel N, Prado T. Pregnancy outcome in a renal transplant patient with residual mild tertiary hyperparathyroidism. *Br J Obstet Gynaecol* 2005;112:124–5.
56. Schnatz PF, Curry SL. Primary hyperparathyroidism in pregnancy: evidence-based management. *Obstet Gynecol Surv* 2002;57:365–76.
57. Patlas N, Golomb G, Yaffe P, Pinto T, Breuer E, Ornoy A. Transplacental effects of bisphosphonates on fetal skeletal ossification and mineralization in rats. *Teratology* 1999;60:68–73.
58. Minsker DH, Manson JM, Peter CP. Effects of bisphosphonate, alendronate on parturition in the rat. *Toxicol Appl Pharmacol* 1993;121:217–23.
59. Rutgers-Verhage AR, deVries TW, Torringa MJL. No effects of bisphosphonates on the human fetus. *Birth Defects Res Part A Clin Mol Teratol* 2003;67:203–4.
60. Onroy A, Wajnberg R, Diav-Citrin O. The outcome of pregnancy following pre-pregnancy or early pregnancy alendronate treatment. *Reprod Toxicol* 2006;22:578–9.
61. Greer IA, Nelson-Piercy C. Low-molecular-weight heparins for thromboprophylaxis and treatment of venous thromboembolism in pregnancy: a systematic review of safety and efficacy. *Blood* 2005;106:401–7.
62. Knoll GA, Bell RC. Tacrolimus versus cyclosporin for immunosuppression in renal transplantation: meta-analysis of randomised trials. *BMJ* 1999;318:1104.
63. Armenti VT, Radomski JS, Moritz MJ, Gaughan WJ, Hecker WP, Lavelanet A, *et al.* Report from the National Transplantation Pregnancy Registry (NTPR): outcomes of pregnancy after transplantation. *Clin Transpl* 2004:103–14.
64. McGrory CH, McCloskey LJ,DeHoratius RJ, Dunn SR, Moritz MJ, Armenti VT. Pregnancy outcomes in female renal recipients: A comparison of systemic lupus erythematosus with other diagnoses. *Am J Transplant* 2003;3:35–42.

65. Brennan DC, Rodeheffer RJ, Ambinder RF. *Development of Malignancy Following Solid Organ Transplant.* UpToDate; 2007 [www.uptodate.com].
66. Stany M, Rose MD, Scott G, Zahn CM. Special situations: abnormal cervical cytology in immunocompromised patients. *Clin Obstet Gynecol* 2005;48:186–92.
67. Halpert R, Fruchter RG, Sedlis A, Butt K, Boyce JG, Sillman FH. Human papilloma virus and lower genital neoplasia in renal transplant recipients. *Obstet Gynecol* 1986;68:251–8.
68. Ozsaran AA, Ates T, Dikman Y, Zeytinoglu A, Terek C, Erhan Y, *et al.* Evaluation of the risk of cervical intraepithelial neoplasia and human papilloma virus in renal transplant patients receiving immunosuppression. *Eur J Gynaecol Oncol* 1999;20:127–30.
69. Bruinsma F, Lumley J, Tan J, Quinn M. Precancerous changes in the cervix and risk of subsequent preterm birth. *BJOG* 2007;114:70–80.
70. Kasiske BL, Snyder JJ, Gilbertson DT, Wang C. Cancer after kidney transplantation in the United States. *Am J Transplant* 2004;4:905.
71. Morath C, Mueller M, Goldschmidt H, Schwenger V, Opelz G, Zeier M. Malignancy in renal transplantation. *J Am Soc Nephrol* 2004;15:1582.
72. Ward R, Bristoe RE. Cancer and pregnancy: recent developments. *Curr Opin Obstet Gynecol* 2002;14:613–17.
73. Freiberg JW, Jessup M, Brennan DC. *Lymphoproliferative Disorders following Solid Organ Transplantation.* UpToDate; 2007 [www.uptodate.com].

Section 8

Consensus views

Chapter 20

Consensus views arising from the 54th Study Group: Renal Disease in Pregnancy

Service

General

1. Multidisciplinary clinics should be established to assess and care for pregnant women with kidney disease. including those women receiving dialysis and kidney transplant recipients.
2. Named experts, forming a multidisciplinary team (MDT), with appropriate facilities, need to be available to manage or advise on all women with kidney disease in pregnancy.
3. The MDT requires, as a minimum, an obstetrician, a renal/obstetric physician and a specialist midwife, all with expertise in the management of kidney disease in pregnancy.

Prepregnancy

4. Women of childbearing age with kidney disease* should be made aware of the implications regarding reproductive health and contraception.
5. Women with kidney disease* considering pregnancy should be offered prepregnancy counselling by the MDT. This active preparation for pregnancy should be individualised to each woman's needs and should involve her partner.
6. Prepregnancy counselling should allow discussion of and, where possible, modification of remediable risk factors, including consideration of familial conditions and optimisation of medications.
7. Women with kidney disease* considering *in vitro* fertilisation (IVF)/assisted reproduction should be referred for prepregnancy counselling to the MDT. Strong consideration should be given to recommending single-embryo transfer if IVF is required.
8. Women with normal or only mildly decreased prepregnancy renal function (serum creatinine below 125 μmol/l (1.4 mg/dl)) can be advised that obstetric outcome is usually successful without adverse effects on the long-term course of their disease, although there is an increased risk of antenatal complications including pre-eclampsia.

* Including those women receiving dialysis and kidney transplant recipients.

Antenatal

9. Women with kidney disease* should be offered low-dose aspirin as prophylaxis against pre-eclampsia, commencing within the first trimester.
10. The use of eGFR (estimated glomerular filtration rate) from the Modification of Diet in Renal Disease (MDRD) formula cannot be recommended for use in pregnancy.
11. Women found or suspected to have kidney disease in pregnancy should be referred to a nephrologist.
12. Women with greater than or equal to +1 dipstick positive proteinuria (in the absence of infection) should have this quantified.
13. Baseline quantification of proteinuria should be undertaken by accurate 24 hour collection for urine protein and by protein/creatinine ratio (PCR). Follow-up may then be undertaken with PCR.
14. Persistent proteinuria (above 500 mg/day) diagnosed before 20 weeks of gestation should prompt referral to a nephrologist.
15. Nephrotic syndrome is an indication for thromboprophylaxis with heparin in pregnancy and the puerperium.
16. Lesser degrees of proteinuria may constitute a risk for venous thromboembolism. This should inform the decision as to whether or not to deploy thromboprophylaxis in pregnancy.
17. Asymptomatic bacteriuria and urinary tract infection (UTI) in pregnancy should be treated.
18. Antibiotic prophylaxis should be given to women with recurrent bacteriuria/ UTIs and kidney disease*.
19. Women known to have lupus nephritis or suspected lupus flare should be referred to the MDT.
20. In pregnant women with kidney disease* the target blood pressure should be below 140/90 mmHg.
21. Prednisolone, azathioprine, ciclosporin or tacrolimus alone or in combination do not appear to be associated with fetal abnormality and should not be discontinued in pregnancy, whereas the safety of mycophenolate mofetil/ enteric-coated mycophenolic acid, sirolimus/everolimus or rituximab is yet to be determined.
22. Clinicians caring for women who have undergone renal transplantation and/or lower urological surgery should involve the appropriate surgical team, as part of the delivery plan, where considered necessary.
23. Renal units, in conjunction with obstetric units, should formulate a 'protocol for management of women receiving or starting dialysis in pregnancy' to be activated when a dialysis patient becomes pregnant or a pregnant woman requires new dialysis.

Postpartum

24. Women with known or newly identified kidney disease in pregnancy should resume their established care with a planned early postpartum renal review.

* Including those women receiving dialysis and kidney transplant recipients.

25. Women with known or newly identified kidney disease in pregnancy should be offered early contraceptive advice.
26. Postnatal evaluation of women with early-onset (necessitating delivery before 32 weeks of gestation) pre-eclampsia is important to identify women with underlying renal disease.
27. Isolated microscopic haematuria with structurally normal kidneys does not need to be investigated during pregnancy but should be evaluated if persistent postpartum.

Education

28. Educational programmes for healthcare professionals managing women of childbearing age with kidney disease* should be developed.
29. Educational resources should be made available to women themselves.

Research

30. Define biomarkers that will effectively predict those women with kidney disease who are at particular risk of specific complications or poor maternal/fetal outcome.
31. Establish and fund registry data collection and facilitate research on outcomes of women and their offspring with kidney disease*.
32. Provide level I evidence (randomised controlled trials) to inform discussion about 'tight blood pressure control' versus less tight control in pregnant women with kidney disease*.
33. Evaluate excretion into breast milk and relevance to wellbeing of the neonate of drugs used by women with kidney disease*.
34. Evaluate the use of imaging modalities to improve differentiation of physiological hydronephrosis of pregnancy from true urinary tract obstruction.
35. Define precisely the time course and mechanism(s) of renal and systemic haemodynamic alterations in health and disease, especially during early pregnancy.
36. Evaluate novel therapeutic strategies such as administration of relaxin in humans.
37. Investigate the altered gestational and postpartum natriuretic responses, and their relationship to plasma volume expansion, in normal pregnant women and in those with kidney disease*.
38. Establish precisely what degree of non-nephrotic proteinuria constitutes a risk for venous thromboembolic disease.
39. Validate the educational programmes for patients and healthcare professionals managing women of childbearing age with kidney disease*.

---

* Including those women receiving dialysis and kidney transplant recipients.

Index

Notes
Abbreviations used in index entries:
ACE = angiotensin-converting enzyme
ARB = angiotensin II receptor blocker
CKD = chronic kidney disease
ESRD = end-stage renal disease
HUS/TTP = haemolytic uraemic syndrome/thrombotic thrombocytopenic purpura
MCUG = micturating cystourethrogram
NO = nitric oxide
All index entries relate to renal disease and pregnancy unless otherwise indicated.
vs denotes differential diagnosis.

ACE inhibitors
  adverse fetal outcomes 232
  in CKD (nonpregnant women) 152
  congenital malformations associated 24, 113, 158, 233
  in diabetic nephropathy (prepregnancy) 112–13, 115
  discontinuation in pregnancy 22–3, 32, 34, 77, 158, 194
    prepregnancy counselling advice 24
    renal transplant recipients 232
  postpartum initiation 55
acute fatty liver of pregnancy (AFLP) 181–2, 193
acute renal cortical necrosis (ARCN) 179, 181, 193
acute renal failure, causes 179–87, 193
  acute fatty liver of pregnancy 182, 193
  differential diagnosis 193
  HUS/TTP 180, 193
  nephrotoxic drugs 182
  pre-eclampsia and 193
  renal cortical necrosis 181
  renal obstruction 182–3
  summary of causes 179
acute tubular necrosis 193
$ADAMTS_{13}$ 180
adrenal suppression, fetal 134
adult polycystic kidney disease (APKD) 56
age, maternal, chronic hypertension in CKD and 154
albumin
  excretion
    diabetic nephropathy 111, 112, 119
    normal pregnancy 33
  serum levels 35, 38
  tubular catabolism 37
aldosterone antagonists 144
alendronate, renal transplant recipients 240
alfacalcidol 239
'all or nothing' effect, drug use, pre-embryonic stage 130
alpha-fetoprotein 40
Alport syndrome 56
American College of Rheumatology (ACR), lupus definition 96–7
American Society of Transplantation (AST) 76
aminoglycosides 39, 182
amlodipine 160
amniotic fluid volume 63, 65
amoxicillin 39
amyloidosis, renal 202
anaemia
  CKD 26, 141, 143, 238
  fetal 139
  management in dialysis patients 66
  microangiopathic haemolytic 180
  in renal transplant recipients 143, 231, 237–8
ANCA
  cytoplasmic-staining (*c*-ANCA) 97
  perinuclear/nuclear-staining (*p*-ANCA) 97
ANCA-negative vasculitis 95
ANCA-positive vasculitis 95
  case study, midwifery role 50
  epidemiology 95
  pregnancy outcome 103

angiogenesis, eNOS system role 13
angiomyolipoma (AML) 212, 217
  ruptured 217
angiotensin-converting enzyme (ACE) inhibitors *see* ACE inhibitors
angiotensin II 9
angiotensin II receptor blockers (ARBs)
  in CKD (nonpregnant women) 152
  discontinuation in pregnancy 22–3, 24, 32, 34, 158, 194
    renal transplant recipients 232
  postpartum initiation 55
  teratogenicity 24
animal studies
  NO-dependent renal vasodilation 8
  renal haemodynamic changes 5
  renal sodium excretion control 9–10
  teratogenicity of drugs 130
  VEGF deficiency in pre-eclampsia model 13
anion gap 36
antenatal care
  in CKD 31–41
    case study 50
    fetal wellbeing assessment 40–1
    glomerular filtration rate 33
    guidelines 41
    hypertension 32–3
    key principles 31–2
    medication use 39
    models 41
    nephrotic syndrome 33–6
    by obstetrician and renal physician 41
    proteinuria 33–6
    renal tubular function assessment 36–7
    superimposed pre-eclampsia 39–40
    underlying renal disease 36
    urinary tract infections 37–8
    visit schedule 41
    volume homoeostasis management 38
  consensus views 250
  in lupus nephritis 36, 107
  in maternal hypertension 32–3, 154, 160
  in renal transplant recipients 84
  schedule, in CKD 41
  in vasculitic nephritis 50, 107
antenatal education, in renal disease 48
antibiotic therapy
  acute pyelonephritis 184–5, 211, 234
  asymptomatic bacteriuria 211, 234
  cystitis 211
  urinary tract infections 38, 39, 90
anti-C1q antibodies 97
anticardiolipin antibodies 192, 241
anti-CD20 antibodies (rituximab) 76, 106
anticoagulation, in dialysis 66
anti-dsDNA antibodies 97, 102
antihypertensive therapy 32, 39, 158–60, 194
  choice of drug 158–60, 194
  in CKD in nonpregnant women 151–3
  in CKD in pregnant women 156–60
  discontinuation/tapering in pregnancy 76, 156, 157, 158
    see also ACE inhibitors
  'double blockade' (ACE inhibitors/ARBs), in nonpregnant women 153
  drugs contraindicated in pregnancy 32, 34, 39, 159, 194, 232
    see also ACE inhibitors
  fetal growth restriction association 161, 162
  first-line agents 158, 159
  indications 156, 157, 160, 194
  mean arterial pressure fall induced by 161, 162
  in mild essential hypertension 156–7, 160, 194
  prepregnancy counselling review 24
  rationale for use 157, 161
  renal transplant recipients 232–3
  in severe pre-eclampsia 195
  transplacental transfer 158
  see also hypertension (maternal), management
anti-La antibodies 241
antineutrophil cytoplasmic antibody *see* ANCA
antioxidants
  renal transplant recipients 233
  superimposed pre-eclampsia prevention 156
antiplatelet agents
  HUS/TTP management 181
  see also aspirin, low-dose
anti-Ro antibodies 241
antithymocyte globulin (ATG) 76
anti-TNFα, lupus nephritis 106
anuria, acute renal cortical necrosis 181
arachidonic acid, metabolism 156
arginine vasopressin (AVP) osmoregulatory system 9
arteriolar resistance 5
aspirin, low-dose 39

in diabetic nephropathy 117
HUS/TTP management 181
pre-eclampsia prevention 25, 39, 117
renal transplant recipients 233
superimposed pre-eclampsia prevention 156
assisted reproduction 167–76
in CKD 27, 174–5
complications 173
in vitro fertilisation 83
pharmacology 172–3
in renal transplant recipients 82–3, 175
asymptomatic bacteriuria (ASB) *see* bacteriuria, asymptomatic (ASB)
atenolol 39, 159, 232
atorvastatin 239
atrial natriuretic peptide (ANP) 6, 9, 10
atrial septal defect 234
autoantibodies
in lupus nephritis 95, 97, 102
in renal transplant recipients 75
in SLE 75
azathioprine 39, 135–6
breastfeeding and 136
in lupus nephritis 105–6
metabolism 131, 135
serum creatinine levels in pregnancy and 71, 74
teratogenicity 135
transplacental transfer 135

bacteraemia 184
bacteriuria, asymptomatic (ASB) 90, 183, 210–11
antibiotic treatment 210–11, 234
bowel segment incorporation into urinary tract 218
detection/confirmation 37, 211
incidence/prevalence 183, 210
renal transplant recipient 234
screening 90, 183, 211, 234
barrier contraception, renal transplant recipients 82
beta-adrenergic blockers 158–60, 194
renal transplant recipients 232
beta-lactam antibiotics, in acute pyelonephritis 185
betamethasone 134
birth defects *see* congenital abnormalities
bisphosphonates, renal transplant recipients 239–40
bladder
cancer 217–18
carcinoma *in situ* 217
congenital abnormalities 182
physiological changes in pregnancy 209–10
in renal/pancreas transplantation 225
bleeding, renal biopsy complication 201–2, 203
blood pressure
antihypertensive drug indications 156, 157, 160, 194
automated recorders for 32
in diabetic nephropathy 117
hypertension definition 32
increase after delivery 33
increase in CKD 32
lability, after delivery 195, 197
lowering, adverse effect on fetal growth 229
measurement 32
mortality relationship, ESRD 152
normal changes in pregnancy 4, 5, 32, 150
prediction of worsening CKD 150
target
in CKD 32, 33, 151, 152
in diabetic nephropathy 117
in hypertension 156, 158, 160, 194, 195, 232
in severe pre-eclampsia 195
see also diastolic blood pressure; hypertension; systolic blood pressure
blood volume
multiple pregnancies 173
ovarian hyperstimulation syndrome 174
total, in normal pregnancy 141, 142
see also plasma volume expansion
B lymphocytes 80
bone disease, in renal transplant recipients 239–40
management plan 230
bone marrow suppression 135, 238
bone mineral density, loss, glucocorticosteroid use 134
breastfeeding
azathioprine use and 136
ciclosporin and tacrolimus use 139
corticosteroid use and 135
furosemide use and 144
guidelines on drug use whilst 133
mycophenolate mofetil use and 140
promotion and facilitation by midwives 49
risks and benefits 49
sirolimus/everolimus use 141
British National Formulary (BNF), drug use in pregnancy 132

bromocriptine 168
buserelin 172

C3 and C4 complement components, in lupus nephritis 97, 102
caesarean section
in chronic hypertension in CKD 153, 154
in diabetic nephropathy 115, 116, 117
renal transplant recipients 80, 224
after urinary tract reconstruction 218–19
calcineurin inhibitors (CNIs) 75, 76, 80
calcium
excretion 214
metabolism changes, dialysis associated 66
supplements 156, 233, 239
calcium channel blockers 158, 160, 232
calorie intake 66
captopril, in diabetic nephropathy 113
cardiovascular disease
CKD and 22, 149, 150
diabetic nephropathy with 113, 115, 120, 121
risk in renal transplant recipients 232
risk with renal abnormalities 55
care, patterns *see* antenatal care; prepregnancy care
caseload midwifery 46
case study, ANCA-positive vasculitis, midwifery care 50
CD20, antibodies (rituximab) 76, 106
cefalexin 38, 184, 234
cefuroxime 184–5
CellCept *see* mycophenolate mofetil
CEMACH study 112, 119, 195
central venous pressure monitoring 196
cephalosporins 39
cerebral palsy 122
cervical neoplasia, post-renal transplant 241–2
childbirth, normal, definition 46
children, of renal transplant recipients, outcome 80, 81
CHIP trial (blood pressure control in hypertension) 157, 161
cholestasis, obstetric 138
cholesterol, serum 35
chronic kidney disease (CKD)
anaemia 26, 142, 143, 238
animal models, VEGF role 13
antenatal care *see* antenatal care
assisted reproduction 27, 174–5
cardiovascular disease risk 22
cardiovascular mortality 149, 150
definition 149
deterioration, blood pressure for predicting 150
drug clearance 132–3
ethics of pregnancy 170–1
gestational GFR 4, 33, 40, 132–3, 149
haemoglobin decrease 142
hormonal disturbances 168
hypertension in 149–50
in nonpregnant women, treatment 151–3
in pregnancy *see under* hypertension (maternal)
management in pregnancy 36
drugs 39, 129–47
general principles 31–44
MDRD equation (eGFR) 22
prepregnancy renal function predictive of outcome 3
prevalence 22, 149
progression risk, blood pressure and protein excretion 152
progressive, ciclosporin *in utero* association 138
proteinuria 133
risk quantification 25–7
severity, classification 133
sexual dysfunction *see* sexual dysfunction, in CKD
stages, eGFR and 22
superimposed pre-eclampsia *see* pre-eclampsia
VEGF protective action 11
Churg–Strauss syndrome 99, 104
ciclosporin 39, 136–9
breastfeeding and 139
diabetes risk 241
in lupus nephritis 106
miscarriage association 136, 137
pharmacokinetics 138
pregnancy outcomes 136–9
renal transplant recipients 136–9
hypertension association 77, 138
levels in pregnancy, rejection 76
low birthweight and 79, 137, 139
perinatal mortality 78
serum creatinine levels and 71, 74
sirolimus use with 141
transplacental transfer 136
CKD *see* chronic kidney disease (CKD)
cleft palate, corticosteroids associated 134
clomifene citrate 168, 172
clonus 40
Cochrane review, continuity of care 46

Cockcroft–Gault formula 33
communication, facilitation, midwife's role 49
computed tomography (CT), renal tract calculi 214
Confidential Enquiry into Maternal and Child Health (CEMACH) 112, 119, 195
congenital abnormalities
  ACE inhibitors associated 24, 113, 158, 233
  azathioprine association 135, 136
  ciclosporin association 137
  corticosteroids associated 134
  drug use in first trimester 132
  mycophenolate mofetil 139, 140
  pregnancy in ESRD 170–1
  see also teratogenicity
congenital abnormalities of kidney and urinary tract (CAKUT) 89–90
  bladder/urethra 182
congenital obstructive uropathy 182
congenital toxoplasmosis 237
connective tissue disease
  postpartum follow-up 55–6
  see also systemic lupus erythematosus (SLE)
consensus views 249–51
continuity of care, midwifery 46–7
contraception methods 24
  renal transplant recipients 82
  see also intrauterine contraceptive device (IUCD)
cordocentesis 119
coronary artery disease, diabetic nephropathy with 113, 115, 120, 121
corticosteroids 134–5
  acute kidney rejection treatment 76
  breastfeeding and 135
  fetal risks 204–5
  HUS/TTP management 181
  maternal risks 134–5
  preterm birth in diabetic nephropathy and 118
  renal lupus flare control 105, 107
  risks/benefits of use 134
  transplacental passage 134
  trial, in minimal change disease 204
counselling
  after pre-eclampsia 197
  pregnancy outcome optimised in dialysis patients 64
  prepregnancy *see* prepregnancy counselling
COX-2 inhibitors 182
creatinine, serum
  abnormal level in pregnancy 33
  in chronic hypertension in CKD 153, 154
  in diabetic nephropathy 114
  eGFR *vs*, CKD prevalence 22
  elevated, in obstructed renal transplant 224
  fall, in normal pregnancy 71
  in lupus nephritis 96, 98, 102
  postpartum, renal transplant recipients 74
  postpartum follow-up and 53
  in reflux nephropathy 91
  in renal transplant recipients 71, 74, 224
  risks associated with renal impairment levels 25
creatinine clearance 33
  in diabetic nephropathy 120, 121
  measurement 33
  normal changes in pregnancy 4, 33
  renal impairment definition 96
Crohn's disease 136
crystalloid solutions, in severe pre-eclampsia 196
cyclic guanosine monophosphate (cGMP)
  increase in pregnancy 5–6
  renal sodium retention and 9
  renal tubular loss of responsiveness 9, 10
cyclophosphamide 39
  fetal abnormalities associated 106
  in lupus nephritis 100, 106
cystatin C 33
cystitis 210
  antibiotic treatment 211
  haemorrhagic 210, 211
cystoscopy 214
cytomegalovirus (CMV) infection 235
cytotoxic therapy, lupus nephritis 105–6

decision making
  advice against pregnancy and 27, 123
  in high-risk pregnancy 27
  loss of control in high-risk pregnancy 45
  see also informed decisions, by women
delivery
  indications in pre-eclampsia 40
  see also caesarean section; vaginal delivery
depression 169
dexamethasone 134
Diabetes Control and Complications Trial (DCCT) 122

diabetes mellitus
effect on pregnancy 112
new-onset after transplant (NODAT) 240–1
in renal transplant recipients 231, 240–1
tacrolimus/ciclosporin-related risk 240–1
type 1 112, 113
postpartum follow-up 55
renal/pancreas transplantation 224–7
type 2 111
presentation in pregnancy 55
diabetic nephropathy 111–25
ACE inhibitor use 112–13, 115
advice against pregnancy 123
blood pressure (target) 117
caesarean section 115, 116, 117
comorbidity 113–15, 120
cardiovascular disease 113, 115, 120, 121
screening for 115
creatinine levels 114
epidemiology 112–13
histology 111
long-term prognosis 119–22
maternal outcomes 119–22
neonatal/fetal outcomes 122
management 123, 151
microalbuminuria 111, 112
postpartum follow-up 55
pregnancy complications/outcome 111, 112, 115–19
factors affecting perinatal outcome 119
fetal growth restriction 116, 117
hypertension 112, 114, 117, 121
maternal death 120
perinatal death 111, 116, 117, 119
pre-eclampsia 117
preterm birth/delivery 116, 117, 118–19
proteinuria 114, 118, 121
thromboembolism 115, 117
pregnancy exacerbating 112, 119–22
pregnancy incidence in 112
progression risk, in pregnancy 119–20
renal transplant recipients 241
VEGF antagonism, protective action 13
diabetic retinopathy 113, 122
dialysis 61–8
assisted reproduction and 174–5
blood pressure target with 152
complications of pregnancy 63–4
early diagnosis of pregnancy 64
fetal/maternal monitoring 66–7
frequency/duration 63, 65
increased, problems associated 65–6
incidence of pregnancy 61–2
indications for, in pre-eclampsia 196–7
postmenopausal women, hormone levels 168
pregnancy outcomes 27, 61, 62–3, 170
fetal loss 27
strategies to optimise 64–7
pregnancy risks 23, 25, 27
prepregnancy counselling 23
protocol for pregnancy in 67
regimen changes to improve pregnancy outcome 65
see also haemodialysis; peritoneal dialysis
diastolic blood pressure
in chronic hypertension in CKD 153, 154
target, in hypertension 160, 194
diet, after pancreas transplantation 225
diltiazem 34, 160
dipyridamole, HUS/TTP management 181
disseminated intravascular coagulation (DIC)
in HUS/TTP 180
in lupus nephritis 101, 103
diuretics 143–4
avoidance in pregnancy 39
renal transplant recipients 232
thiazide 159, 160
transplacental transfer 144
dopamine-induced natriuresis 10
double-J ureteric stent 214, 215
drugs 129–47
to avoid in pregnancy 24, 32, 39, 236, 237
see also antihypertensive therapy
clearance, in CKD 133
dose–response relationship 131
factors affecting exposure and impact 130–1
in first trimester 130, 132
metabolism 131
nephrotoxic, acute renal failure due to 182
prepregnancy counselling 22–3, 24–5, 129, 132
in second/third trimesters 132
teratogenicity *see* teratogenicity

timing of use, fetal development 130
use in pregnancy 129–47
guidelines 132–3
prescribing principles 132
see also individual drugs and drug groups

eclampsia, prevention 197
ectopic pregnancy 173
EDTA registry 74
education
antenatal, in renal disease 48
consensus views 251
physicians, on risks of pregnancy 28
embryotoxicity, sirolimus 141
emotional needs of women, midwife's role in recognising 49
endoglin 13, 34
endorphins, endogenous 168
endothelial cells, VEGF role 11
endothelin 8
type B (ET_B) receptor 8
end-stage renal disease (ESRD)
blood pressure, mortality relationship 152
carers, men as, and psychosocial issues 169
in diabetes mellitus 111, 112, 120, 122
dialysis for *see* dialysis
effect on pregnancy/fertility treatment 170
ethics of pregnancy 170–1
postpartum follow-up to avoid 54
pregnancy/fertility treatment effect on 170
issues affecting child after 170–1
reflux nephropathy causing 89, 91
sexual dysfunction *see* sexual dysfunction, in CKD
systolic hypertension 149
epidural anaesthesia, in urolithiasis 215
erythrocyte sedimentation rate (ESR), vasculitic nephritis 103
erythrocytosis, post-transplant 238–9
erythropoietic-stimulating agents (ESA) 141–3
adverse effects, and doses 143
erythropoietin
increased plasma level 141–2
in normal pregnancy 237
requirement in dialysis 66
requirement in renal impairment 26
safety/efficacy in pregnancy 142–3, 238
Escherichia coli, urinary tract infection 38, 211.234

estimated glomerular filtration rate (eGFR) 22, 25, 149
estrogens, renal vasodilation trigger 6
ethics
of pregnancy in ESRD 170–1
of renal biopsy in pregnancy 203–4
EURODIAB study 112, 122
Euro-Lupus group 98, 99
Euro-Lupus group definitions
non-renal flare 99
proteinuria 96
renal flare 98
Euro-Lupus Nephritis trial 98
European Best Practice Guidelines (EBPG), Expert Group on Renal Transplantation 76, 234
everolimus 141

fatty acid oxidation, mitochondrial, inborn error 182
fatty liver of pregnancy *see* acute fatty liver of pregnancy (AFLP)
fertility
impairment, prepregnancy counselling 24
after renal/pancreas transplantation 226–7
see also infertility; subfertility
fertility treatment 171
effect on renal disease 170
pharmacology 172–3
renal disease effect on 170
fetal development, drug use timing 130
fetal growth
adverse effect of blood pressure reduction 229
in renal transplant recipients 79
fetal growth restriction 26
chronic hypertension in CKD 153, 161
diabetic nephropathy 116, 117
dialysis association 63
in renal impairment, risks 26
fetal heart-rate monitoring, maternal dialysis and 67
fetal loss
in diabetic nephropathy 111
dialysis and 27
in lupus nephritis (maternal) 101
in reflux nephropathy in pregnancy 91
see also miscarriage; perinatal mortality
fetal monitoring
hypertension in CKD 160–1
maternal dialysis and 66–7
fetal outcome, lupus nephritis 100–2

fetal wellbeing, assessment 40
in CKD 40–1
in diabetic nephropathy 119
fibroids 210
fibromyalgia 98
Flt_1 11, 12
alternative splicing 13
soluble *see* $sFlt_1$
fluid balance
acute pyelonephritis management 184
pre-eclampsia-related renal impairment 195–7
fluid loading, in pre-eclampsia 196
fluid overload, prevention 195
fluid restriction, post-delivery 196
fluid volume status, maternal
acute shifts, preterm birth in dialysis and 64
management to improve pregnancy outcome 65
follicle-stimulating hormone (FSH) 168, 172
Food and Drug Administration (FDA) 132, 133, 135
furosemide 144

ganirelix 172
general practitioners, postpartum follow-up 55
gentamicin, intravenous 185
gestational age, confirmation, in hypertension in CKD 160–1
gestational diabetes, glucocorticosteroid use and 134
glomerular capillaries
acute thrombosis 179
changes in pre-eclampsia 190, 191
glomerular capillary pressure 5
increased 112
glomerular disorders, renal tubular function assessment 37
glomerular endotheliosis 151, 190, 203
glomerular fenestrae 11
glomerular filtration rate (GFR)
antenatal care 33
cardiovascular risk and 150
in CKD 4, 33, 40, 132–3, 149
in diabetic nephropathy 112, 118
estimated (eGFR) 22, 25, 149
increase in normal pregnancy 4, 33, 71, 189, 209
reversal by nitric oxide synthase 6
increase mechanisms 3, 5–8
haemodynamics 5
vasoactive factors 5–6
measurement methods 33
in pre-eclampsia 189
renal impairment definition 96
in renal transplant recipients 71
superimposed pre-eclampsia in CKD 40
glomerular hyperfiltration 112
glomerulonephritis
crescentic, pauci-immune necrotising 96
diagnosis by renal biopsy 202, 203
primary 37
rapidly progressive 96, 97
glomerulus
in pre-eclampsia 190, 191
VEGF actions 11
glucocorticosteroids *see* corticosteroids
glucose, decreased proximal tubular reabsorption 36
glycaemic control 112, 113, 115, 122
glycosuria 36, 210
gonadotrophin-releasing hormone analogues 172
gonadotrophins
adverse effects 172–3
for assisted conception 172
secretion 168
goserelin 172
granulomatous vasculitis 104
guidelines
antenatal care in CKD 41
breastfeeding whilst on drug use 133
drug use in pregnancy 132–3
European Best Practice 76, 234

haematocrit
erythropoietin indication 238
measurement 38
haematuria 216–18
asymptomatic dipstick (ADH) 216–17
in lupus nephritis 97
macroscopic 217
in cystitis 210, 211
renal biopsy complication 202, 203
microscopic 23, 56, 216–17
renal trauma causing 217
in vasculitic nephritis 96, 97
haemodiafiltration 64, 65
haemodialysis
pregnancy outcome and 63, 170
regimen to improve pregnancy outcome 65
timing/duration 63, 65
see also dialysis

haemoglobin
decrease in CKD 142
glycosylated (HbA_{1c}) 112, 122
in normal pregnancy 237
target levels 143
renal transplant recipients 238
haemolytic anaemia
microangiopathic 180
see also HELLP syndrome
haemolytic uraemic syndrome/thrombotic thrombocytopenic purpura (HUS/TTP) 179–81
clinical features 180, 193
differential diagnosis 193
management 180–1
pre-eclampsia *vs* 180, 193
HbA_{1c} 112, 122
HELLP syndrome 13, 75, 193
differential diagnosis 193
recurrence 197
Henoch–Schönlein purpura 99, 103, 104
heparin
in nephrotic syndrome 35
see also low-molecular-weight heparin
hepatitis B 236–7
hepatitis C 235–6
herpes simplex infection 237
human chorionic gonadotrophin (hCG)
assisted conception 172
fetal wellbeing assessment 40
HUS/TTP *see* haemolytic uraemic syndrome/thrombotic thrombocytopenic purpura (HUS/TTP)
hydralazine 159, 194
in severe pre-eclampsia 195
hydrochlorothiazide 144
hydronephrosis 183, 211, 224
loin pain due to 212
management 215
'physiological' 209, 212
pre-existing, before renal transplant 224
hydrops fetalis 139, 144
hydroxychloroquine 39
lupus nephritis 100, 102
hypercalciuria 66, 214
hyperemesis gravidarum 173
hyperkalaemia, in acute renal cortical necrosis 181
hyperlipidaemia, renal transplant recipients 239
hypermagnesaemia, iatrogenic 66
hyperparathyroidism 66
primary 239
secondary/tertiary 240
hyper-reflexia 40
hypertension
adult, after ciclosporin *in utero* association 138
childhood, in vesicoureteric reflux 89
risk after pre-eclampsia 197
risk quantification in CKD by 25
hypertension (maternal)
antenatal care 32–3, 154, 160
blood pressure target 156, 158, 160, 194, 232
chronic 150, 153–4, 194
complications 153–4
pregnancy outcomes 153–4
severe 153
in CKD 149, 150
management *see below*
maternal evaluation 154
mechanisms 150, 156
superimposed pre-eclampsia 151, 153, 155–6
see also pre-eclampsia
definition 32
in diabetic nephropathy 112, 114, 117, 121
drugs exacerbating
erythropoietic-stimulating agents 143
glucocorticosteroids 134
duration of pregnancy and 155
gestational 189
laboratory assessment 154
in lupus nephritis 101, 105, 107
management 32, 39, 149, 155–8
antenatal 193–4
antepartum assessment 160
antihypertensives *see* antihypertensive therapy
complicated hypertension 157–8
diuretic cautions 144, 160
fetal evaluation 160–1
initiation, blood pressure level 156, 157, 160, 232
mild essential hypertension 156–7, 160, 161
in pre-eclampsia-related renal impairment 193–5
rationale 195
in renal transplant recipients 229, 231, 232–3
secondary hypertension 157–8
severe hypertension 158
in severe pre-eclampsia 195
'tight' *vs* 'less tight' (CHIP trial) 157, 161

postpartum 197
postpartum follow-up 55
pre-existing 150
pregnancy outcome 31, 32, 90, 153–4
lupus/vasculitic nephritis 101, 105
preterm birth associated with dialysis and 63
prevalence 149
prophylaxis 155–6
renal biopsy 203
in renal impairment, risks 26–7
in renal transplant recipients 76–7, 229, 232–3
management plan 231, 232
secondary 149, 150
management 157–8
sequelae (long-term) 197
systolic 149
uncontrolled, pregnancy outcomes 27
in vasculitic nephritis 105
see also pre-eclampsia
hypertensive encephalopathy 158
hyperventilation of pregnancy 66
hypocalcaemia 239, 240
hypocalciuria 156
hypoglycaemia 182
hypoglycaemic agents, oral 241
hypogonadism 226
hypophosphataemia, dialysis associated 66
hypotension
in acute fatty liver of pregnancy 182
dialysis-induced 64
septic shock *vs* low intravascular volume 184

ileal conduits 219
immune system
effect of *in utero* exposure to immunosuppressants 80
neonatal abnormalities, renal transplant recipients and 138
immunosuppressive drugs 39
breastfeeding risks with 49
in utero exposure, effect on children after 80, 81, 171
in lupus nephritis 105–6, 200
minimisation in renal transplant recipient 234
prepregnancy counselling advice 24–5
renal transplant patient, anaemia 238
see also corticosteroids; *individual drugs*
infertility
rates in renal transplant recipients 82
treatment for 171
see also fertility treatment; subfertility
infliximab 106
information sharing, pregnancy outcome in dialysis patients 64
informed decisions, by women
midwife's role 48
pregnancy outcome optimised in dialysis 64
see also decision making
interferon, avoidance 236
International Society for the Study of Hypertension in Pregnancy (ISSHP) 189
interstitial nephritis 91
intracytoplasmic sperm injection 83
intrapartum care, by midwives 48
intrauterine contraceptive device (IUCD)
azathioprine interference 136
renal transplant recipients 82
intrauterine growth restriction (IUGR) *see* fetal growth restriction
intravascular volume 38, 141
red blood cell volume/mass 141, 142, 237
reduced, in hypotension 184
see also plasma volume expansion
intravenous fluids 38
intravenous immunoglobulin 76
in lupus nephritis 106
intravenous urography (IVU) 213
in vitro fertilisation, renal transplant recipients 83
iron
intravenous 143
loss, in haemodialysis 66
supplements, renal transplant recipients 238
iron dextrose 238
iron sucrose 238

Joint National Committee in USA, 7th Report (JNC7) 151
J stents
double-J ureteric stents 214, 215
ureteric obstruction 224

KDR (VEGFR2) 11, 12
kidney 217
injury *see* renal trauma
rupture 183
single 182
structural abnormalities, prepregnancy counselling 23
see also entries beginning renal

labetalol 158–60, 194
contraindication 195

prepregnancy counselling advice 24
renal transplant recipients and 232
in severe pre-eclampsia 195
lactate dehydrogenase (LDH) 75, 184
lamivudine, avoidance 237
lanthanum carbonate, avoidance 239
leucopenia, azathioprine association 135
liver transaminases, abnormal 40
loin pain 211–14
acute renal obstruction 183, 224
causes 211–12
management 215
low birthweight infants
azathioprine association 135
ciclosporin association 137
dialysis association 63, 67
renal transplant recipients 79
urinary tract infections associated 234
lower urinary tract *see* urinary tract, lower
low-molecular-weight heparin (LMWH) 35
in diabetic nephropathy 115
in dialysis patients 66
lupus
cerebral 106
diagnosis 96–7
extrarenal disease 98–9
extrarenal flares 99, 101–2
renal disease *see* lupus nephritis
see also systemic lupus erythematosus (SLE)
Lupus Activity Criteria Count (LACC) 98
lupus anticoagulant 192, 241
lupus arthropathy 98
lupus nephritis 95–109, 102
active, laboratory features 97, 102
antenatal care 36, 107
autoantibodies 97, 102
creatinine levels 96, 98, 102
diagnosis 97
disease activity 98
disseminated intravascular coagulation 101, 103
epidemiology 95–6
extrarenal flares 101–2
histological classification 97
maternal/fetal outcome 100
hypertension and 101, 105, 107
immunosuppression 105–6, 139
pregnancy outcome 100, 102
management 39, 104–7, 192
cytotoxic/immunosuppressive therapy 105–6, 139
plasma exchange 107
steroids 105
summary/key factors 107
new onset, in pregnancy 101
postpartum flares 102, 103
postpartum follow-up 54–5, 55–6
pre-eclampsia in 100, 103, 192
pre-eclampsia *vs* 97–8, 100
pregnancy and 99–103, 192
contraindication to 99
effect on renal outcomes in 102–3
management 99–100
risk of renal decline 103
therapeutic termination 106
pregnancy outcome 100–2
factors influencing 99, 100–2
fetal loss 100, 192
maternal death 102, 103, 105, 107
preterm birth 102, 241
pregnancy rates 96
prepregnancy counselling 23
proteinuria 96, 97
renal flares 97, 98, 101, 102, 192
control/management 105, 192
intrapartum 103
postpartum 102, 103
postpartum follow-up 55–6
prediction 102
renal transplant recipients 231, 241
renal tubular function assessment 37
luteinizing hormone (LH) 168, 172

macroalbuminuria, diabetic nephropathy 112
magnesium, raised serum levels, dialysis and 66
magnesium sulphate 197
magnetic resonance urography (MRU), ureteric obstruction 185, 213
marital problems 169
maternal death
acute renal cortical necrosis 181
diabetic nephropathy 120
fluid management and 195
lupus nephritis 102, 103, 105, 107
vasculitic nephritis 104
maternal survival, after renal transplant pregnancy 83
Maternity Matters 45, 48
matrix metalloproteinase 2 (MMP2) 8
mean arterial blood pressure (MAP), mortality relationship, ESRD 152
men, psychosocial issues affecting carers 169
menstruation
in CKD 168
irregular, after renal/pancreas transplantation 226

6-mercaptopurine (6-MP) 131, 135
mesentery, in urinary tract reconstruction 219
metformin 241
methyldopa
  hypertension management 158, 159, 194
  prepregnancy counselling advice 24
  renal transplant recipients 232
methylprednisolone 105, 134
microalbuminuria, diabetic nephropathy 111, 112, 122
micturating cystourethrography (MCUG) 56, 91
midwife
  as advocate or arbitrator 49
  breastfeeding promotion and facilitation 49
  communication in multidisciplinary team 49
  experiences, of renal disease in pregnancy 47–8
  interpretation of medical information 49
  professional autonomy 47–8
  role 45, 46, 48–9
    case study 50
midwifery 45–52
  care, needs/expectations in high-risk women 47
  caseload 46
  challenges 46
  continuity of care 46–7
  medical model of care balance with 47
  normal *vs* high-risk pregnancy 46
  'risk' label in renal disease 45–6
minimal change disease, renal biopsy 204
miscarriage
  azathioprine association 135
  ciclosporin association 136, 137
  first-trimester
    assisted reproduction complication 173
    dialysis and 63
  GFR increase absent 4
  second-trimester, dialysis and 63
  see also fetal loss
mitochondrial fatty acid oxidation, inborn error 182
Modification of Diet in Renal Disease (MDRD) formula 22, 33
mTOR (metabolic target of rapamycin) 141
multidisciplinary team
  communication facilitation, midwife's role 49
  consensus views 249
  dialysis patients 64
  lupus/vasculitic nephritis 104
multiparity, renal transplant recipients 74–5
multiple pregnancies
  assisted reproduction complication 173
  renal transplant recipients 74–5
  risks associated 173
Multiple Risk Factor Intervention Trial (MRFIT) 150
mycophenolate mofetil (MMF) 39, 139–40
  avoidance in pregnancy 24, 140
  in breast milk 140
  in lupus nephritis 106
  management of use during pregnancy 140
mycophenolic acid, enteric-coated (MPA) 139–40
myelosuppression 135, 238

National High Blood Pressure Education Program (NHBPEP) 194
National Service Framework for Children, Young People and Maternity Services 48
National Transplantation Pregnancy Register (NTPR)
  azathioprine use complications 135–6
  ciclosporin use complications 137
  mycophenolate mofetil use complications 140
  renal/pancreas transplantation and pregnancy outcome 226
  renal transplant and pregnancy/graft outcome 71, 72–3, 74, 79, 241
  tacrolimus use complications 137
natriuretic systems 8–9, 10
neonatal death 26
  in chronic hypertension in CKD 153, 154
neonates
  MCUG screening 56
  outcome and impact of preterm birth 27
nephrin 190
nephritic flares 98
nephritis
  active, definition 97
  lupus *see* lupus nephritis
  new onset, in lupus 101
  pre-eclampsia *vs* 97–8, 100
  vasculitic *see* vasculitic nephritis

nephrolithotomy, percutaneous 215
nephropathy
  definition 112
  diabetic *see* diabetic nephropathy
  incipient, microalbuminuria 112
  reflux *see* reflux nephropathy
  risk and prevalence 112
nephrostomy, percutaneous (PCN) 214, 215, 216
nephrotic syndrome
  antenatal care 33–6
  complications/sequelae 35
  pre-eclampsia causing 35, 190
  protein/creatinine ratio (PCR) 35
  renal biopsy 204
  treatment 35
neurodevelopment
  children of diabetic nephropathy patients 122
  children of renal transplant recipients 80, 81
nifedipine 159, 160, 194
  prepregnancy counselling advice 24
  renal transplant recipients 232
nitric oxide (NO)
  increase in pregnancy 5–6
  release triggered by Flt_1 11
nitric oxide synthase (NOS) 6
  antibodies 6
  endothelial (eNOS) 6, 13
  inducible (iNOS) 6
  neuronal (nNOS) 6
  nNOS-α protein 6
  nNOS-β protein 6, 8
nitrite/nitrate, inorganic (NO_x) 5–6
nitrofurantoin 39, 185
nocturia 210
nonsteroidal anti-inflammatory drugs (NSAIDs) 182, 215
Nursing and Midwifery Council, Code of Professional Conduct 47
'nutcracker syndrome' 217
nutrition, pregnancy outcome in dialysis patients 66

obstetric complications
  multiple pregnancies 173
  previous pregnancies 28
obstructive uropathy
  congenital 182
  see also ureteric obstruction; urinary tract, obstruction
oedema 35
  pre-eclampsia 143
oligohydramnios 64, 65
oliguria 193
oncotic pressure, in diabetic nephropathy 118
oral contraception, renal transplant recipients 82
organogenesis 130
osmolality (plasma/serum) 37
  fall in normal pregnancy 8
  ovarian hyperstimulation syndrome 174
osteopenia, renal transplant recipients 239, 240
osteoporosis, renal transplant recipients 239
ototoxicity, furosemide 144
ovarian hyperstimulation syndrome (OHSS) 174, 210
  clomifene citrate associated 172
over-distension syndrome 183
ovum donation 7

pain
  loin *see* loin pain
  renal biopsy complication 201
pancreas after kidney transplantation 225
pancreas/kidney transplantation *see* renal/pancreas transplantation
pancreas transplantation 224, 225
  principles 225
parathyroidectomy 239, 240
parathyroid hormone (PTH), abnormal levels 239
parathyroid hormone-related protein (PTH-rP) 66
parity, diabetic nephropathy risk 122
patent ductus arteriosus 144
patterns of antenatal care *see* antenatal care
PCR *see* protein/creatinine ratio (PCR)
pelviureteric junction obstruction (PUJO) 212
perception of risks in pregnancy 45
percutaneous nephrolithotomy (PCNL) 215
percutaneous nephrostomy (PCN) 214, 215, 216
percutaneous renal biopsy *see* renal biopsy
perinatal mortality
  diabetic nephropathy 116, 117, 119
  renal transplant recipients 78
  see also fetal loss; neonatal death
peritoneal dialysis
  pregnancy outcome and 63, 170
  regimen to improve pregnancy outcome 65
  see also dialysis
pharmacokinetics
  in CKD 132–3
  immunosuppressive drugs 138

phosphate, total body, depletion, dialysis and 66
phosphate binders 239
phosphodiesterase 5 (PDE_5) 10
pituitary–gonadal axis, disturbances 168
placenta
 drug transfer across *see* transplacental drug passage
 length, measurement 40
placental abruption, chronic hypertension in CKD 153
plasma exchange
 HUS/TTP management 180, 181
 lupus nephritis management 107
plasma osmolality *see* osmolality (plasma/serum)
plasma volume expansion
 assessment 38
 diuretics effect on 144, 160
 mechanisms 8–10
  renal sodium excretion signals 9–10, 32
  volume perception in pregnancy 8–9
 in normal pregnancy 3, 4, 5, 32, 141, 142
podocytes
 foot processes, in pre-eclampsia 190
 VEGF secretion 11, 190
podocyturia 190
polyarteritis nodosa 98, 103, 104
polycystic kidney disease, adult (APKD) 56
polyhydramnios 63, 65
postpartum care
 consensus views 250–1
 renal transplant recipients 84
postpartum follow-up 53–7
 by GPs 55
 indications 54–6
 by nephrologist 54–5
 newly diagnosed renal disease 53, 54
  with heritable component 56
 plans 54
 pre-existing renal disease 55–6
 principles and rationale 53
post-transplant erythrocytosis (PTE) 238–9
post-transplant lymphoproliferative disorder (PTLD) 242
pravastatin 239
preconception care *see* prepregnancy care
preconception counselling *see* prepregnancy counselling
prednisolone 39, 134
 lupus nephritis 105
 metabolism 131
 pregnancy outcome and 134, 137
pre-eclampsia 39–40
 acute renal failure and 193
 clinical presentation 189
 in diabetic nephropathy 117
 diagnostic difficulties 117, 192
 differential diagnosis 192–3
  active nephritis *vs* 97–8, 100
  HUS/TTP *vs* 180, 193
  renal biopsy not advised for 204
  worsening renal disease *vs* 25
 hypocalciuria association 156
 increased protein excretion as marker 34, 40, 189–90
 indications for delivery 40
 in lupus nephritis 100, 103, 192
 management
  antihypertensives 193–5
  fluid balance 195–7
  postnatal follow-up 197
  see also antihypertensive therapy; hypertension (maternal)
 maternal/fetal effects 40
 nephrotic syndrome due to 35, 190
 oedema 143
 overdiagnosis 192
 plasma uric acid as marker 37, 100
 preterm birth associated with dialysis and 63
 prevalence 151
 prevention, aspirin 25, 39, 233
 proteinuria levels 34, 40, 189–90, 204
  persistence 54
 recurrence 197
 renal impairment in 189–99
  differential diagnosis 192–3
  management 193–7
  postnatal follow-up 197
  pre-existing renal disease *vs* 192
  risk of 26
 renal pathophysiology 189–91
 renal transplant recipients 77, 229
 risk factors 39–40
 risk quantification in CKD 25
 severe
  blood pressure control 195
  fluid balance 195–7
 superimposed on CKD 39–40, 192
  diagnostic features 40
  monitoring, in hypertension 160
  with pre-existing hypertension 151, 153, 155–6
  prevention 155–6
  recurrence 151
  renal transplant recipients 77